Contemporary Community Nursing

EDITED BY

S Burley BA, RNT, DN, RN, RM

Lecturer, Practice Nursing, University of Hull

E E Mitchell MEd, DNT, DN, RM, RN

British Red Cross Co-ordinator, Home From Hospital Service

K Melling MA, PGCEA, DNT, RNT, DN, RN

Senior Lecturer, Community Studies, Cheltenham & Gloucester College of Higher Education

M Smith MSc, DNT, RNT, DN, RN

Senior Lecturer, Health Studies, University of Wolverhampton

S Chilton MSc, PGCE, DNT, BNurse, DN, HV, RN

Lecturer/Practitioner, District Nursing, University of Central England

C Crumplin MA, RGN, DN, PGCEA, DNT

Senior Lecturer, Institute of Nursing and Midwifery, University of Brighton

A member of the Hodder Headline Group
LONDON • SYDNEY • AUCKLAND

First published in Great Britain in 1997 by
Arnold, a member of the Hodder Headline Group
338 Euston Road, London NW1 3BH

Whilst the advice and information in this book is believed to be true and accurate
at the time of going to press, neither the authors nor the publisher can accept
any legal responsibility or liability for any errors or omissions that may be made.

British Library Cataloguing in Publication Data
A catalogue record for this book is available from the British Library

Library of Congress Cataloging-in-Publication Data
A catalog record for this book is available from the Library of Congress

ISBN 0 340 677333

Composition in 10/12 Palatino by Anneset, Weston-super-Mare, Somerset
Printed and bound in Great Britain by J. W. Arrowsmith Ltd, Bristol

Contents

List of contributors

Eileen Barnes BSc (Social Policy) DNT DN RN
Senior Lecturer (District Nursing), University of Central England

Sandra Baulcomb BA (Hons) (Social and Behavioural Studies) DNT DN RM RN
Lecturer in District Nursing, University of Hull

Rita Bell MA (Health Service Studies) DNT RNT DN RN
Principal Lecturer, University of Northumberland

Marion Brew MSc (Health Education) BSc (Hons) Nursing DNT DN RN

Sandra Burley BA (Hons) Nursing Midwifery with Educational Studies RNT DN RN RM
Lecturer Practice Nursing, University of Hull

Sue Chilton MSc (Applications of Psychology) PGCE DNT B Nurs DN HV RN
Lecturer/Practitioner, District Nursing, University of Central England

Ann Clarridge MSc (Inter-professional Health and Welfare Studies) PGCEA RN DN DNT BSc (Hons) Nursing Studies
Senior Lecturer in Community Nursing, Southbank University

Diane Cuff MA (Medical Law and Ethics) PGCEA DNT DN BSc (Hons) Nursing Studies RN
Senior Lecturer, School of Health and Social Work, Suffolk College

Maggie Dickerson MPhil BA DN RN
Senior Lecturer Community Health Care Nursing, Buckinghamshire College

Derek Earl PGDip BA DNT DN RMN RN
Senior Lecturer in Health Studies, University of Plymouth

Eileen Groves MA (Health Care Ethics) RN DN DNT RNT
Senior Lecturer, Department of Health Care Studies, Manchester Metropolitan University

Barbara Johnson DN RN
Clinical Nursing Manager of Specialist Community Nursing Services, East Wiltshire Health Care Trust

Sarah Luft BSc (Hons) Nursing DNT DN RN
Senior Lecturer in Health Studies, University of Wolverhampton

Karen Melling MA (Ed Health Promotion) PGCEA DNT RNT DN RN
Senior Lecturer, Community Studies, Cheltenham and Gloucester College of
Higher Education

Elizabeth E. Mitchell MEd (Adult and Community Education) DNT DN
RM RN
Formerly Senior Lecturer, North East Wales Institute, currently British Red
Cross Coordinator, Home From Hospital Service

Jenny Newbury BEd (Hons) RN DN DPSN
Senior Lecturer in Health Studies, University of North London

Paul Parkin MSc (Medical Sociology) PGCE BSc (Hons) DNT DN RN ONC
Senior Lecturer in Health Studies, Brunel University College

Brian Pateman MA RN DNT DN
Lecturer, School of Nursing Studies, University of Manchester

Elaine Ryder MSc (Gerontology) BA (Health and Social Studies) DNT RNT
DN RN
Senior Lecturer, Community Health Care, Oxford Brookes University

Jo Skinner MA PGCEA DNT DN RN
Principal Lecturer in Health Studies, University of North London

Milly Smith MSc (Public Sector Management) DNT RNT DN RN
Senior Lecturer in Health Studies, University of Wolverhampton

Ann Sutton BEd, RDNT RNT DN RN
Formerly Course Director, Postgraduate Diploma in Community Health
Care Studies (District Nursing), Southbank University. Currently freelance
Lecturer.

Isobel M. Walker MN BSc (Hons) Nursing DNT DN RN
Formerly Principal Lecturer in Community Nursing Studies, University of
Central England

Anne Weeks MSc (Education) DNT RNT RN DN
Principal Lecturer, Buckinghamshire College

Preface

Introduction

It is intended within this book to explore current issues that are influencing community nursing practice. This has to be taken within the context of not only health care but also the wider issues of contemporary society.

Issues are addressed that are of current interest in community nursing. The topics are wide ranging and apply to all branches of community nursing. The authors have set out to examine concepts by presenting current knowledge and thinking on each subject. The intention is to raise awareness of the complexity and controversy that may surround a topic rather than provide a descriptive account. Careful examination of the texts by the reader will highlight the range of areas that come into play that confuse and complicate the issues under discussion. In this way chapters will provoke debate. The texts provide an excellent base for deeper reading and include many useful references that can be taken up for further exploration of each subject area.

The sections of the book focus on practice, leadership, management and the development of community nursing; these are in line with the United Kingdom Central Council's (UKCC) elements of specialist practice (UKCC, 1994).

To set community nursing in context, there needs to be an awareness of the main societal issues, some of which are considered in the following pages.

Community nurses work within a society which can often be extremely complex, comprising many different social groups, each having different social experiences. Society is seen as a social model of life with different customs and organizations which make up a civilized nation (Sykes, 1976). This preface provides a brief overview of the main societal issues affecting families, communities, individuals and thus community nurses. At the end of the preface, the reader is signposted to relevant reading.

The route to modern day health care, as we know it, has taken a circuitous pathway. It is not the intention of this book to dwell on the past but it is from these historical backgrounds that the emergence of society's health care needs and subsequent provision are seen. Abbot and Wallace (1990) suggest that the poor standard of health of recruits to the Boer War and later the First World War prompted a series of reforms in the early twentieth century to improve the nation's health. Linked to this was the Victorian attitude that physical decay was associated with moral decay. The family, essentially mothers, were made responsible for the health of other family members; childhood was identified as a special period for personal growth and children needed to be protected from contamination and vice. Therefore, mothers were discouraged from working and encouraged to rely on the male breadwinner.

As the twenty-first century approaches, Abbott and Wallace (1990) have put forward a set of assumptions about the family and about relationships between men and women, in support of what has become referred to as the New Right vision of the world. This concurs with Johnson's (1982) suggestion that 'the ideal society must rest upon the tripod of a strong family, a voluntary church and a liberal minimal state. Of these, the family is the most important' (p. 1). This nuclear family image of parents and dependent children is perhaps the accepted image held by most people. However in reality, this is not the case. The number of single-person households has increased, currently comprising those people who elect to be single parents and others who become single parents due to the ending of a relationship by, for example, death or divorce. This can lead to an increase in remarriage and step-parenting. Social trends (HMSO, 1993) states that 'the percentage of all families with dependent children who are lone parent families has more than doubled since 1971 – from 8% in 1971 to 18% in 1991, reflecting the rise in both divorce and births outside marriage' (p. 29). A traditional view of the family appears to exclude other relationships which are equally part of today's society. An understanding of the variability of relationship structures is therefore fundamental in developing sensitivity within approaches to care.

As a result of these changes in the family structure, it can be seen that society rather than the family will be called upon to provide care in the community. Thus nurses working within the community need to have an understanding of the social influences outlined above, which affect patient behaviour and the resources available to care for these patients. The changes have led to Central Government requiring that health and social needs be identified and met locally. One of the drawbacks of this model is that he who shouts the loudest will be heard, unless there are advocates who can speak on behalf of the silent, and often most vulnerable, members of society. Not only are community nurses hands-on practitioners but they also need to be pro-active in highlighting the needs of their patients to a wider audience.

Such changes may produce additional stress and anxiety. A further factor to consider with regard to social change is the demographic influence: people are living longer. Social trends (HMSO, 1993) state that 'By the year 2021, nearly one in five of the population will be over 65 – compared to only one in ten in 1951' (p. 15).

The role of women has become more focused. Abercrombie and Wardle (1988) suggest:

> Women have played a critically important part in the redefinition of the social division of labour in the last 20 years. For instance, there are many more married women in paid work today than there have been at any time in the last 100 years. However, the jobs women have tend to be ones which are relatively poorly paid and carry little authority. (p. 9)

The way in which men's work and women's work is segregated is a source of frustration and annoyance to many women as it highlights the differences in gender. The revival of the feminist movement as identified in writings by Greer, Millett and Oakley in the 1970s and later Blaxter (1990), Doyle (1995) and Graham (1993) have enabled more women to become aware of the oppression, sexism and male chauvinism which existed then and still continues to exist in our modern society. However, women are currently trying to improve their position and through Equal Opportunities legislation the inequalities are being slowly reduced.

An additional key factor to be considered is that of cultural stereotyping, which can often occur leading to social division between ethnic groups. Members of ethnic groups, even though they may be born in Britain, still suffer greater social and material deprivation compared with white people. There can be no doubt that black people tend to get poorer jobs than white people and suffer from racism and discrimination, mainly due to the colour of their skin or the beliefs that they follow. *Social trends* (HMSO, 1993) states that 'Unemployment rates are higher among ethnic minorities than among whites. The worst rate is in the Pakistan/Bangladeshi group – a quarter of the economically active are unemployed' (p. 63).

As recognized by Abercrombie and Wardle (1988), British society is in sociological terms a modern capitalist society. However, Sullivan (1992) suggests that the global economic situation following the oil crisis of the early to mid-1970s helped to precipitate both recession and inflation. It can be seen that contemporary Britain has experienced over the last decade the effects of international recession, leading to a decline in the British economy. Abercrombie and Wardle (1988) further comment that the British economy has declined more than that of most other nations in a comparable position in the world economic system. This has led to many British firms having lost out in competition with foreign equivalents, resulting in British firms restructuring, merging or being taken over; changes in ownership and internal re-organization. This restructuring has had serious effects upon employees; the outcomes have been redundancies leading to unemployment as well as retraining, resulting in jobs being redesigned so as to save money by making each worker more productive. Abercrombie and Wardle (1988) state that 'The British state has in the 1980's been either unwilling or incapable of improving the situation, preferring to allow the cold winds of capitalist competition to reshape the economy rather than intervening directly' (p. 8). The impact of such changes during a 10-year period on unemployment within the United Kingdom and overseas is demonstrated in Table 1.

Abercrombie and Wardle (1988) further suggest that industrial change inevitably affects class relations and class structure as occupation is a fundamental basis of class position. The number of manual workers has declined with an increase in semi-professional and professional jobs. The changing size and composition of British classes has arguably reduced the strength of the working class as a force for change. The upsurge in home ownership between 1979 and 1987 as identified by Monks and Kleinman, cited in Brown and Sparks (1990), shows an increase from 55 to 74 per cent of all households.

Table 1 Unemployment rates adjusted to show international comparison

Country	Annual averages			
	1978	1981	1985	1988
UK	5.9	9.8	11.2	8.3
France	5.2	7.4	10.2	10.1
Germany	3.5	4.4	7.2	6.1
(Fed. Republic)				
United States	6.0	7.5	7.1	5.4
Sweden	2.2	2.5	2.8	1.6

Source: Main Economic Indicators and Quarterly Labour Force Statistics. The Organization for Economic Co-operation and Development (OECD). *Social trends* (1990)

This is an increase of 19 per cent over an eight-year period, mainly brought about by the Government legislation 'right to buy' policy enabling more families in council accommodation to purchase their homes. This is shown in Table 1.2.

Table 2 Tenure of dwellings in the United Kingdom

	1981 %	1991 %
Owner occupied	57	68
Rented from local authority	31	22
Rented from private owners	11	7
Rented from housing association	2	3

Source: Department of the Environment, *Social trends* (1993)

Regional trends (HMSO, 1993) stated that 'The 1980s saw a substantial change in the tenure pattern of dwellings: rapid growth in owner-occupation and falls in the public and private rented sectors' (p. 51). However, the downside of this policy resulted in longer council waiting lists and a rapid rise in homelessness. During the last decade, the number of homeless families has doubled to more than 100 000. Whitehead and Kleinman (1986) estimate that more than 200 000 households are in 'non-tenure' accommodation on the fringe of homelessness, such as squatting, 'bed and breakfast', hostels and sleeping rough. This appears as relevant today as then.

All these issues have major implications for the role of community nurse in the need to support patients'/clients' rights and to respond to the change of climate in health care. The shift of emphasis from secondary to primary care brought about by the NHS Community Care Act (DOH, 1990) and ensuing legislation also holds continuing challenges for community nurses. The introduction of the concept of the market economy has led to such developments as skill mix, the need to be competitive and to work pro-actively. This will challenge traditional perceptions of role and service provision. It will bring about altered patterns of care, which will rely on greater collaboration between statutory, voluntary and private agencies, if the views of the consumer and the needs of the community for seamless services are to be addressed.

Thus community nursing will focus on innovative practice as shown, for example, in the development of Hospital at Home, working in partnership, collaborating in care and nurse prescribing. These and other issues are critically examined within individual chapters of this book. To guide the reader through the text, each chapter begins with a summary of areas to be discussed; key points are raised at the end of the chapter, enabling the reader to reflect and determine viable applications of the material to practice.

Contemporary community nursing is designed to inform and stimulate action and serve as a resource for the reader, in extending and developing their role.

Burley, S.
Mitchell, E. E.
Melling, K.
Smith, M.
Chilton, S.
Crumplin, C.
February 1997

References

Abbot, P. and Wallace, C. 1990: *The sociology of the caring professions*. London: Falmer Press.

Abercrombie, N. and Wardle, A. 1988: *Contemporary British society*. Oxford: Blackwell Publications.

Blaxter, M. 1990: *Health and lifestyles*. London: Tavistock Routledge.

Department of Health 1990: *The NHS and Community Care Act*. London: HMSO.

Doyle, L. 1995: *What makes women sick: gender and the political economy of health*. London: Macmillan.

Graham, H. 1993: *Hardship and health in women's lives*. Brighton: Harvester Wheatsheaf.

HMSO 1993: *Regional trends 28*. London: Government Statistical Service.

HMSO 1993: *Social trends 23*. London: Central Statistical Office.

Johnson, P. 1982: 'Family reunion', *Observer*, London, 10 October 1982.

Monks, D. and Kleinman, M. 1990: Cited in Brown, P. and Sparks, R. *Beyond Thatcherism: social policy, politics and society*. Buckingham: Open University Press, p. 87.

Sullivan, M. 1982: *The politics of social policy*. Guildford: Harvester Wheatsheaf.

Sykes, J.B. (ed.) 1976: *The concise Oxford dictionary* (6th edn). London: OUP.

UKCC 1994: *The future of professional practice – the Council's standards for education and practice following registration*. London: UKCC.

Whitehead, C.M.E. and Kleinman, M.P. 1986: *Private rented housing in the 1980s and 1990s*. Cambridge: Granta Editions.

Further reading

Blackburn, C. 1992: *Poverty and health*. OUP: Milton Keynes.

Bond, J. and Bond, S. 1994: *Sociology of health care* (2nd edn). Edinburgh: Churchill Livingstone.

Dalley, G. 1988: *Ideologies of caring*. Basingstoke: Macmillan Education.

Dallos, R. and McLaughlin, E. 1995: *Social problems and the family*. London: Sage.

Goffman, E. 1968: *Stigma*. Harmondsworth: Penguin.

Helman, C.G. 1990: *Culture, health and illness*. Oxford: Butterworth Heinemann.

Illich, I. 1976: *Limits to medicine*. London: Boyers.

James, A. 1993: *Childhood identities. Self and social relationships in the experience of the child*. Edinburgh: Edinburgh Unit.

Jeffreys, M. 1989: *Growing old in the twentieth century*. London: Routledge.

Jolley, M. and Brykczynska, G. 1993: *Nursing – its hidden agendas*. London: Edward Arnold.

Jones, L. 1994: *The social context of health and health work. Basingstoke: Macmillan*.

Taylor, S. and Field, D. 1993: *Sociology of health and health care*. Oxford: Blackwell Scientific.

Webb, R. and Tossell, D. 1991: *Social issues for carers*. London: Arnold.

Woodhead. M. 1991: *Growing up in a changing society, part 1*. London: Routledge.

Acknowledgements

A special note of thanks to Liz Mitchell from the editorial team for keeping us all on track and maintaining our enthusiasm.

PART ONE

Influences on the practice of community nursing

Issues that are topical and influence the practice of community nursing have been addressed in this part. The practice of community nursing is in the process of rapid change brought about through technological, economical and political influences. The roles of community nurses are undergoing major reappraisal. The issues that are involved in altering traditional roles are analysed in the chapters included in this part.

Work is also included that enables community nurses to revisit fundamental aspects of their role in relation to the concept of nursing.

The art and science of community nursing

Sarah Luft and Milly Smith

The purpose of this chapter is to take a look at the debate which surrounds the art and science of nursing. Recent years have stressed the importance of basing actions on fact. The value of research based practice has been confirmed (Briggs, 1972) and the profession can now confidently state that newly registered nurses acquire a sound theoretical base to inform practice. Today, nursing is in danger of becoming marginalized as the influences of changing trends in the NHS through new ideologies, the new management era, policy making and advanced technology take precedence. It could be argued that technical knowledge is available to a wide audience, that the tasks covered by nurses could be done by non-professionals, and that through time nurses will become redundant.

Influences of nursing

The influences on nursing have been discussed at length in many texts but it is useful to draw out some of the key areas which have been and still are major issues in the nursing debate. The 'gender' issue has been a focus from the time that Nightingale changed the image of nursing. Women reflected the values of the nineteenth century which means they were docile, subservient and obedient (Jolley, 1993). Nursing was considered by many as a natural extension of the female role which encompassed the lifespan, from pregnancy to bereavement.

Indeed the physical and psychological makeup of the sexes has always been a determining factor in the division of labour and even in the twentieth century true emancipation has still not been achieved. According to Leddy and Pepper (1993) Florence Nightingale referred to nursing as an 'art, and a calling practised by women under scientific heads' (Nightingale, 1894), the scientific heads being physicians and surgeons, who in the Victorian era were mainly men. The role of the nurse in the Nightingale era was focused on duty and following orders which was very much in keeping with the female role in society. Nightingale's ideas led to the popular image of the nurse as possessing saint-like qualities, selfless compassion and endless toiling to ease suffering (Leddy and Pepper, 1993). Kitson (1993) cites Reverby (1989) who suggested that this legacy has been hard to alter as it has proved difficult to make the transition from the culture of obligation to an active assault on oppressive structures and beliefs.

The dictionary definition of the word 'art' is 'the application of skill to production of beauty and works of creative imagination'. Gray and Pratt (1991) cite O'Brien (1990) who sees nursing as an art to incorporate the notion of artistry in nursing which can be equated with the ability of nurses to view patients holistically, and adapt their skill base to serve individual needs. The rhetoric of holistic practice has become commonplace, but as the business picture of health care emerges the 'task' culture is more likely to predominate. Nursing has also been concerned with advancing its professional status over the decades and it has generally been thought that the way forward here is to promote nursing's unique knowledge base. Thus emphasis has turned to the science of nursing with models and theories referring to the importance of a clearly documented, articulated rationale for practice. Somehow the art of nursing has lost ground, perhaps because it is not grounded in hard, objective, scientific evidence. Other influences are constantly altering the state of the health service provided and they must be considered in the discussion for the part that they play in the changing picture in nursing.

Policies

These have always been subject to change although conservative ideology has remained constant in that the emphasis is on an individual, as opposed to a collective responsibility. However, patterns of management style have created an environment where change itself has almost become constant. As the business of health takes shape, so the art of nursing needs to be voiced. Benner and Wrubel (1989) see nursing as intimate and particular – and suggest that there is no way to guarantee the success of caring. Caring in this context is a subjective experience. Managerial language and practices that seek to objectify, quantify and decontextualize, conflict with the nature of caring practices. Patients feel cared for when they are not treated merely as customers, consumers or resources. Yet politicians have been keen to emphasize the importance of consumer choice, and consumer views have been consistently audited although research studies still reveal that there are many gaps in consumers' knowledge (Gabbott and Hogg, 1994). In order to make choices people must possess sufficient knowledge. Ford and Walsh (1995) echo concern about the rapid pace of change and refer to 'liberating nursing', arguing that various reforms have resulted in a de-skilling, anti-professional agenda. Although these authors highlight the value of research based practice, they insist that nurses can become trapped if this is contained within a positive empirical, number crunching activity. McKay (1993) suggested that the favour shown to technology and psychomotor skills has hampered the development of nursing's knowledge base.

Technology

It is important not to underestimate the influence of the world-wide 'technological explosion'. There have been major developments in medical sciences as well as rapid spread in information technology. Both these areas serve to underline the scientific rationale where so much new knowledge emerges which can, in turn, more easily be shared with all members of the health professions. Keeping abreast of such advances creates its own challenges and offers new opportunities for practice to be research based. It is perhaps of even greater importance at this time to underline nursing as a caring practice whose science is guided by the moral art of ethics of care and responsibility.

Benner and Wrubel (1989) argue that there is a danger that the expert person is viewed as standing outside the situation, aloof and detached, in order to pronounce expert judgement. This is acknowledged in that they observe the paradoxical nature of nursing in a highly technical culture that is looking for sweeping technological breakthroughs. The idea here is to provide liberation and disburdenment. The technical culture needs to be a part of a social support system so that patients benefit not only from modern scientific theories but they also gain from a caring art. Wolfe (1986) refers to caring by the nurse that can conceivably strengthen the person's resistance to disease. It is nursing actions that enhance the person's usual social environment so that they are better cared for by family and friends and it is this art of intertwining social support that can be so crucial to health. According to Reihl and Roy (1980) Emanuel Kant in the last century argued that to practice without theory was blind, and that theory without practice was mere intellectual play. This way of thinking can be translated to support the art/science debate by proposing that the art of nursing without a strong knowledge base is blind but a strong knowledge base without the art of nursing devalues the professionalism of nursing.

Examination of the art of nursing

The art of nursing was gradually developed by the practitioners through experience and observation. The art of nursing is likely to have involved the use of tenacity, authority, and *a priori* methods (Kerlinger, 1986). Tenacity refers to beliefs held because they have been thought to be true. Authority relates to powerful people who expect instructions to be carried out without question. *A priori* knowledge relates to cause and effect and depends on the ability to reason. Over the years the use of these largely subjective skills laid down the aesthetics or art of nursing and this contributed to the understanding of the impact that nursing had on client health. The art of nursing, though generally unarticulated, was in existence a long time before the science of nursing became established. Chinn and Kramer (1991) regard the nature of nursing before the 1950s as a technical art that emphasized principles and procedures that were carried out with a spirit of unselfish devotion. This suggests that the art had become reduced to inflexible stereotyped practices but there remained a sense of caring that was evidenced through the selfless nature of nurses.

The art of nursing should not be undervalued; it was the starting point for the development of nursing knowledge and it has also provided direction for the focus and philosophy of nursing. Subsequent professional growth stemmed from those early ideas which became established and refined over time but the essence that was nursing remained at the heart of progress. A philosophical view of nursing suggests that nursing knowledge comes from several different foci (Carper, 1978). One aesthetic knowledge, the art of nursing, has already been mentioned. The other ways in which nurses become knowledgeable about their art, according to Carper, are personal knowing, ethical knowing and theoretical knowing. Personal knowing is about self-awareness and self-reflection and it is reasonable to assume that a professional who is working in the caring services, and attempting to understand people, ought to possess a high degree of self-awareness. Ethical knowing is required to enable the thinking processes that are associated with a professional's informed actions. This particular type of knowledge allows the complexity of situations to be duly considered. Theoretical knowing informs and facilitates the practice of nursing. Together the four types of knowing interrelate and provide the basis for nursing to stake its claim as a necessary therapeutic health profession. Though they are distinct areas they combine to form the whole experience (Leddy and Pepper, 1993).

Recent literature refers to the healing process of nursing (Leftwich, 1993; Lewis and Brykczynski, 1994) and relates it to the issues that are considered to be embodied in the art of nursing. The nature of this relationship is worthy of consideration as it may be a key factor in arguing the case for the value of nursing. Certainly Benner and Tanner (1987) recognize the value of expert intuition in nursing. They define it as 'understanding without rationale' and something that is practised by the expert practitioner through the benefit of experience. The healing process of nursing could well be the therapeutic art, the essence of nursing that was present at its beginning, and has gradually become defined and more clearly articulated. The nature of a therapeutic or healing process suggests that the act of nursing has beneficial outcomes that are distinct from the medical model of care.

The science of nursing

The science of nursing has undoubtedly progressed over recent years. The body of knowledge about the nature of nursing and the effectiveness of nursing interventions has steadily increased and with the changing academic status of nurses should continue its progress. It is a pleasure to observe nurses using their knowledge to make informed decisions about the practice of nursing care. The perception of care required comes from the art of nursing, involving the transformation of each individual patient's expressions of need by the nurse. Carper (1978) suggests that perception goes beyond recognition of need as it gathers together the information to create an experienced whole for the purpose of seeing what is there. Benner and Tanner (1987) consider the use of perception by expert nurses. Experts use pattern and similarity recognition from previous situations in a way that enhances their understanding of patients. This sophisticated interplay of knowledge and experience is very much the territory of expert practitioners. The nature of holistic care is that it takes into consideration a very broad perspective and requires a knowledge base from the social and natural sciences to support and develop the knowledge that is nursing. Chinn and Kramer (1991) make the point that all disciplines have value in their contribution to nursing care and that none takes priority . Each specific situation may call for one particular type of knowledge but because of the individual nature of health and nursing problems, demands are spread across the disciplines, each making a different but valuable contribution to the care that the patient receives.

Changing professional trends

One of the fundamental shifts that is occurring in contemporary nursing is the move towards increasing the technological aspects of nursing. This may involve the acquisition of highly complex knowledge and skills in specific areas of care. Such an interesting professional development naturally influences the way in which nursing is perceived by nurses, other health professionals and the general public. Over a period of time such major changes could influence the concept of nursing and move it away from its original philosophy. The aesthetic, personal, ethical and scientific knowledge described by Carper (1978) may change in balance with greater emphasis being placed on scientific knowledge. The burning question that arises from this must be 'Is this all that nurses want for nursing?' An interesting comment from Larkin cited by Leftwich (1993) is that following a myocardial infarction there was a feeling expressed that nurses and physicians were more interested in the patients' heart muscles and not them as people. Leftwich (1993) suggests that health professionals should explore the meanings of caring, curing and healing. Evidence supports the fact that patients have great concern that they are cared for by nurses (Ludwig-Beymer et al., 1993). At this time of rapid and exciting change nurses must establish a balanced view on just what it is that nursing involves.

There is a real need to retain the therapeutic art of nursing while accepting the challenges that are brought about by developments in health care. Nurses need to utilize the knowledge and skills that are at their disposal to support the value of nursing. Leftwich (1993) raises concerns that the lack of a clear healing role in nursing, or even the desire for such a role may eventually lead to nurses becoming functionally redundant.

Articulating the art of nursing through reflection

Much has been written in recent years about the 'reflective practitioner' and with increasing value placed on experiential learning the concept of reflection is now recognized as an important tool, and Palmer *et al.* (1994) stress that reflection can foster professional self-evaluation. However, they also acknowledge that the drive for efficiency, and cost effectiveness within health services often leaves little time for an individual nurse or group of nurses to reflect on their clinical practice. The ability to 'reflect' effectively incorporates a systematic approach so in this way it can be described as a scientific process. Accurate reflection also asks the nurse to examine how a situation arose and Palmer *et al.* cite Bines (1992) who writes about an integrated knowledge-in-action approach, much of which is spontaneous and tacit. This notion fits well with the Benner and Tanner (1987) concept of perceptive practice implying that there is also an art involved, but this is a personal art. Reflection asks a person to examine their cognitive/affective domains and so they become involved in the process and this very subjectiveness or subjectivity means that impersonal objectivity is impossible. On the other hand, once the thoughts and feelings have been expressed openly it then becomes easier for that reflection to take an objective stance. As the concept of artistry involves creative imagination the method of reflection must be an individual process, and this could come under the heading of personal knowledge. Fitzgerald (1994) refers to how knowledge is sought and makes the suggestion that although logical deductive reasoning is a form of reflection it could be limited by its nature. Schon (1991) argues that a positivist stance is suited to solving simple problems in contrived problems. For Schon knowledge is embedded in and demonstrated through the situations. The reality is that nurses are more likely to be faced with complex human artistry of everyday practice. He recognizes the clever things done 'on the job' and yet which are typically so difficult to describe linguistically and, to the frustration of positivistic scientists, impossible to control. Fitzgerald also cites Garrison (1991) who argues that attributes for effective reflection include an intellectual maturity to cope with autonomy, differing perspectives and shifting ideas. Exercising reflective practice gives nurses the opportunity to think through scenarios, contexts, knowledge and actions to examine the various relationships which emerge. They can focus on the current state of knowledge used (the hard facts) alongside the process/outcome, and consider how the art of nursing contributed to these. Ford and Walsh (1995) support the notion that reflection upon and during practice will liberate the nurse from the ritualistic dogma of the procedure manual. These authors highlight the value of research based practice, but insist that nurses can become trapped if this is contained within a positive, empirical, number crunching activity. The employment of more action/qualitative studies can uncover new areas of knowledge. L'Aiguille (1994) writes about how the process of reflection has developed an understanding of complex interpersonal and interprofessional situations lending further weight to the argument that the artistic nature of nursing is still alive and kicking. She refers to the fact that reflection in action has helped her to understand her inner disharmony and to recognize artistic knowledge and self-knowledge – all of which have contributed to a greater understanding of the meaning of nursing. Another example that describes the art in nursing is recorded by Connelly (1994), who highlights that reflecting on the listening processes employed in certain patient encounters enables recognition of the real nature of the presenting problem and this is not always related to the specific medical conditions that are presenting. Nurses are generally aware of the importance of communication skills: they acquire a knowledge base about how to sit, touch, observe and maintain eye contact, etc. How this is carried out requires empathy and artistry. Active listening is a complex activity and reflection on how the skill is applied may help to gain a deeper insight into the process. Connelly (1994) states that listening may seem risky, as it places one in the vulnerable position of silence and there is an art in handling silences but the opportunity to tune in with the patient and to understand the patient's story can be too valuable to avoid. These examples help to clarify the value of applying art to science; nurses need nursing knowledge and the art of reflection provides the opportunity to evaluate the contributions that nursing makes to care because care is more than just scientific knowledge.

Demonstrating the 'art' of the reflective process

The art of the reflective process can be demonstrated by the following fairly common nurse/patient encounter likely to occur in the community. The first reflective account is generally factual in that it outlines the key issues. The second account is more thoughtful and would perhaps be written by a nurse who has some experience, while the third account appears to be written by a nurse who has some insight and an awareness that the wider issues play a significant role in health welfare. This third account is 'different' in that the subjectivity is apparent as the nurse is prepared to examine her own feelings in relation to the encounter.

THE NURSE/PATIENT ENCOUNTER

The District Nurse is asked to visit Mrs P. who has a recurrence of an ulcer on her left leg. Mrs P. is well known to the district nursing team.

Account no. 1

'I visited Mrs P. She showed me her leg which required dressing and she had the prescription which she had been given by the doctor. I cleaned the wound and dressed it (according to protocol). I explained what I was doing and we discussed the importance of diet and exercise. Mrs P. seemed to accept everything I said.'

Account no. 2

'I visited Mrs P. and she was clearly very disappointed that her leg had deteriorated again. We discussed the possible reason for this and it became apparent that during the recent hot spell Mrs P. had decided not to wear her support tights. I understood her reasons for this but explained how important maintaining the pressure was for her legs. I then continued to dress the leg during which time we discussed her diet and exercise regimen.'

Account no. 3

'I visited Mrs P. and we both felt disappointed that her wound had broken down again. I found out that Mrs P.'s daughter had recently left the area and I got the impression that she was very lonely now. She doesn't feel able to cope with another varicose ulcer. She hates the smell and the pain gives her sleepless nights. I feel that if Mrs P. had had access to a local social support group over the past few months, perhaps she might have taken better care of herself and not discarded those support tights which are vital for her. Now, she is quite depressed and it will take a long time for the recovery process to get underway.'

The first account is descriptive and shallow and takes an objective stance. The second account contains more empathy which is demonstrated subjectively, and there is an understanding of how the situation came about. The third account is more revealing altogether and the art of caring is transmitted here. There is an understanding of the whole picture as well as the beginnings of the emergence of a new perspective on discharging patients whose leg ulcers have healed. This could perhaps lead to the formation of new knowledge with a research project undertaken to find out if attending support groups following discharge resulted in less breakdown of leg ulcers. Even this brief overview of how the reflective process can reflect both the science and art of nursing allows lots of issues to emerge. The 'art' is to allow for the formulation of the different perspectives to come through even if they do seem to create more difficulties initially. Reflection enables the assimilation of new knowledge which can be incorporated into further practice.

The exercise following this section is designed to instigate reflective art; details of the process are inserted in order to provide a comprehensive framework. This exercise is helpful in two ways; the first is that it encourages the assimilation of new knowledge and the second is that it helps to clarify and categorize the nursing practice implemented and determine which 'domain' of nursing knowledge was of key importance.

Application of theory to reflection

Carper's framework (1978) can be considered in relation to the above accounts in that all three accounts establish a degree of theoretical knowing;

personal knowing is clearly evident in the last two accounts as self-awareness presents. Ethical knowing is most evident in the third account because there is recognition of the complex nature of this situation and the part different interactions have played. The aesthetics of nursing is also most clearly demonstrated in the third account because the nurse uses subjective skills which are helping him/her to gain a better understanding of how a nursing intervention could benefit the health of the patient. Although this exercise compartmentalizes the knowing domains in order to establish the knowledge processes, the complexity of the nursing situation makes it hard to distinguish between the personal and aesthetic knowing and there are areas of overlap. The reader may like to try out the following exercise:

Think of an encounter in your field of specialist practice:

– identify the factors that influence the care of the patient/client

- social
- psychological
- physical
- environmental

– identify the particular traits of the patient/client involved that may influence the nursing situation
  – consider the interrelationships between the factors that influence care and
  – identify your own views and values on the situation taking into account the total set of circumstances and consider what it is that influences your perceptions of the situation and into which areas they fall.

– finally, what do you see as the balance of

- personal knowing
- ethical knowing
- scientific knowing
- aesthetic knowing

in the nursing care given. What belongs to the art of nursing?

Conclusion

It is difficult to discuss abstract concepts, and definitions of nursing care vary from culture to culture and nurse to nurse. The invisibility of the art of caring and healing makes it hard to draw out the knowledge and actions that should be identified as incorporating both the scientific and artistic nature of nursing. So often one hears the expression 'it's not so much what he/she said, but it's the way in which it was done'. This argument is so relevant for nurses – it is possible to observe someone carrying out technical procedures flawlessly and one cannot argue with this scientific knowledge. The professional nurse carries out sound technical procedures but is able to do so in such a way, and with such skill that the patient maintains privacy and dignity at all times. The patient is also able to participate if it is deemed appropriate and social interaction between nurse and patient can become firmly established as mutual trust and understanding develop. These points are of particular relevance in the patient's home where the nurse needs cooperation and help from the patient and carers in order to promote a healthy and healing environment. Using all the aspects of 'knowing' can build up expertise in nursing so that it can more easily be recognized both as a science and an art.

In the last century the well-known philanthropist William Rathbone employed a professional nurse called Mary Robinson to live in and care for his wife in her latter years. The experience was to transform the nature of home nursing, as Mr Rathbone recognized what a difference professional nursing meant, and he was inspired to initiate training programmes for 'District' nurses so that professional nursing would be available to the poor who desperately needed it. At this time the art of nursing began to be recognized as a valued commodity.

References

Benner, P. and Tanner, C. 1987: Clinical judgement. How the expert nurse uses intuition. *American Journal of Nursing*, **87**, 23–31.
Benner, P. and Wrubel, J. 1989: *The primacy of caring*. California: Addison-Wesley.
Bines, H. 1992: Issues in course design. In Bines, H, and Watson, D. (eds), *Developing professional education*. Buckingham: Society for Research into Higher Education and Open University Press.
Briggs, A. 1972: *The Briggs Report*. Report of the Committee on Nursing. London: HMSO.
Carper, B.A. 1978: Fundamental patterns of knowing in nursing. *Journal of Advanced Nursing Science*, **1**,1, 13–23.
Chinn, P.L. and Kramer, M.K. 1991: *Theory and nursing: a systematic approach*. St Louis: Mosby Year Book.
Connelly, J.E. 1994: Listening, empathy and clinical practice. In More, E.S. and Milligan, M.A. (eds), *The empathetic practitioner*. New Brunswick, New Jersey: Rutgers University Press.
Fitzgerald, M. 1994: Theories of reflection for learning. In Palmer, A., Burns, S. and Bulman, C. (eds), *Reflective practice in nursing – the growth of the professional practitioner*. Oxford, London: Blackwell Scientific.
Ford, J. and Walsh, M. 1995: *New rituals for old – nursing through the looking glass*. Oxford: Butterworth Heinemann.
Gabbott, M. and Hogg, G. 1994: Slim pickings. *Health Service Journal*, 20th January, Melbourne.
Garrison, D. 1991: Critical thinking and adult education: a conceptual model for developing critical thinking in adult learners. *International Journal of Lifelong Education*, **10**, 4, 287–303.
Gray, G. and Pratt, R. 1991: *Towards a discipline of nursing*. Melbourne: Churchill Livingstone.

Jolley, M. 1993: *Nursing its hidden agendas*. London, Melbourne, Auckland: Edward Arnold.

Kerlinger, F.N. 1986: *Foundations of behavioural research* (3rd edn). New York, London: Holt Rinehart and Winston Inc.

Kitson, A. 1993: *Nursing art and science*. London: Chapman and Hall.

L'Aiguille, Y. 1994: Pushing back the boundaries of personal experience in reflective practice in nursing – the growth of the professional practitioner. In Palmer, A., Burns, S. and Bulman, C. eds. *Reflective practice in nursing*. Oxford, London: Blackwell Scientific.

Leddy, S. and Pepper, J.M. 1993: *Conceptual bases of professional nursing* (3rd edn). Philadelphia: J.B. Lippincott Co.

Leftwich, R.E. 1993: Care and cure as healing processes in nursing. *Nursing Forum*, **28**, 3, 13–17.

Lewis, P.H. and Brykczynski, K.A. 1994: Practical knowledge and competencies of the healing role of the nurse practitioner. *Journal of the American Academy of Nurse Practitioners*, **6**, 5, 207–13.

Ludwig-Beymer, P., Ryan, C.J., Johnson, N.J. *et al.* 1993: Using patient perceptions to improve quality care. *Journal of Nursing Care Quality*. **7**, 2, 42–51.

McKay, S.A. 1993: Powering up our profession. *Canadian Nurse*, **4**, 35–7.

Nightingale, F. 1894: *Notes on nursing* (2nd edn). London: Duckworth.

O'Brien, B. 1990: Nursing: craft, science and art. In *Conference proceedings: dreams, deliberations and discoveries: nursing research in action*. Adelaide: Royal Adelaide Hospital, 306–12.

Palmer, A., Burns, S. and Bulman, C. 1994: *Reflective practice in nursing – the growth of the professional practitioner*. Oxford, London: Blackwell Scientific.

Reverby, S. 1989: A caring dilemma: womanhood and nursing in historical perspective. Cited in Kitson, A. (1993) *Nursing art and science*. London: Chapman and Hall.

Reihl, J. P. and Roy, C. (eds) 1980: *Conceptual models for nursing practice*. Norwalk, CT: Appleton-Century-Crofts.

Schon, D. 1991: *The reflective practitioner*. London: Maurice Temple Smith Ltd.

Wolfe, Z.R. 1986: The caring concept and nurse identified caring behaviours. *New Dimensions in Human Caring Theory*, **8**, 2, 84–93.

2 Contract culture

Derek Earl

Contract: *'A document setting out the terms of a formal agreement between people or groups'* (Concise Oxford Dictionary, 1982)

The publication of the Government White Paper Working for Patients *(Department of Health, 1989a) foreshadowed a drastic overhaul in the way that care was delivered to the nation. Against a background of ever-increasing expenditure on health and social security and only a finite amount of funding, the Government introduced comprehensive legislation that it claimed would 'promote efficiency' and 'enhance consumer choice' (Department of Health, 1990). Health care functions that traditionally had been within the same departments were to be separated out. Thus planning of community care, its implementation and evaluation could be undertaken by different organizations; the concepts of purchasers and providers were introduced and the contract culture emerged.*

Introduction

In the 1980s, the administration of Margaret Thatcher made it abundantly clear that it would encourage market forces to assume primacy in the delivery of a wide range of services, hitherto the prerogative of local and national government. The Local Government Planning and Land Act of 1980 required authorities to put highway and building construction and maintenance work out to tender. Progressively, throughout the 1980s, more and more local services were put out to contract and the 1988 Local Government Act extended compulsory competition tendering. By the end of 1992, almost £2 billion of work carried out by local government was subject to contract (Audit Commission, 1993).

The Thatcher administration saw no difficulty in extending contracting to work being carried out by the caring organizations such as health and social service departments. Some private and voluntary groups saw the writing on the wall, and as far back as the early 1980s had already entered into contractual agreements with health authorities to set up and manage services such as elder care day facilities.

Contracting

The Government justified its extension of contracting into the caring arena, a movement described by commentators as contract culture, on the following premises:

- The general public was said to be dissatisfied with the levels and standards of public service provision provided by local government, health and social service departments.
- The consumer should have primacy rather than the producer, as the latter will protect its position and not effect necessary change, unless it is forced to do so.
- Cost savings and improvements in quality can be achieved by market forces and competition.
- A legally binding contract is preferred to informal partnerships, as outcomes can be monitored more effectively, standards made explicit and accountability enhanced.
- Monopolistic state provision is broken, allowing a pluralistic approach to provision of care, which is said to be better able to meet consumer choice.
- Private and voluntary sector provision is deemed better than public sector provision as profit motive and voluntary ethic are seen as more powerful motivators than a commitment to public service. (NCVO, 1989)

Smee (1994) talks of four categories of 'players' in the 'market place':

- Purchasers – Two types of purchasing agencies were introduced by the legislation – health authorities and fundholding general practitioners.
- Providers – These included trusts, directly managed units (DMUs), the private health care sector, voluntary organizations, and general practitioners, whether fundholding or not.
- Regulators – Examples given were the National Health Service Management Executive (NHSME), having responsibility for rules and regulations affecting the marketing structure, and the caring organizations' professional bodies.
- Central policy makers – Government ministers whose policy decisions could influence how market forces would shape the caring services.

The government stated that the implementation of the health care contracts from 1991 would ensure improvements in quality and responsiveness to patient care. It laid down the contractual procedure as follows:

First, the prospective purchaser will issue statements relating to the type of services that it wishes to purchase. Included in this will be an indication of standards and quality.
The prospective provider(s) will respond, giving details as to how it will provide the services, and how the requirements for quality standards will be met and monitored.

The next stage will involve detailed negotiations between purchaser and provider. This will consider pricing, standards, monitoring mechanisms, and modes of delivery. A contractual agreement should be the ultimate result. It is expected that the cheapest bid would be successful, unless there were other important issues to be taken into account. Where there is to be a plurality of service providers, a primary provider may be awarded the overall contract, and then subcontract certain aspects of the work to other agencies as appropriate. The White Paper names an independent body, the Audit Commission, as having overall responsibility to monitor standards of care and quality issues.

The *Working for Patients* document (DOH, 1989) envisaged three types of contracts being negotiated:

- Block contracts – This has involved the least amount of disruption as against the previously held status quo. Facilities such as district nursing, health visiting or a certain number of beds at a local district general hospital would be purchased for a fixed period in time, at a specified price.
- Cost and volume contract – This has allowed the purchaser to be much more specific in terms of the service required, and expected outcomes. The purchaser would negotiate a fixed price for an agreed number of treatment sessions for the volume of patients which the provider will treat.
- Cost per case contracts – Here contracts have been negotiated to cover the costs of treatment for specific individuals. Because of the amount of work involved in researching and drawing up such a contract, these cases have not been numerous.

The Audit Commission (1992) spoke of contracts being on the one hand friendly agreements built on trust, and on the other hand being of a legally binding framework. It is clear that there is little scope for the former type of agreement in the face of the market forces that are prevailing in health care delivery systems. Smee (1994) argues that current information on costs and pricing is insufficient, leading many purchasers to rely on block contracts instead of embracing cost/volume or cost per case options. There is also a lack of information on outcomes, appropriateness of therapies, and overall cost effectiveness, that is only now being addressed by a number of organizations (Smee, 1994).

The National Health Service considered that the Korner data sets for purchasing purposes were inadequate, and replacement is being undertaken by Community Contracting Minimum Data Sets (CCMDSs) (Department of Health, 1990). The care workers have the responsibility of providing the necessary data to monitor and determine the effectiveness of the contracts. This would include:

- Financial data - for costs and pricing
- Statistical data - would include population profile, socio-economic details, geographic factors, skill mix of workers, etc.

- Monitoring procedures
- Clinical and non-clinical quality audit.

The Opposition political parties have been scathing in their criticism of the overall legislation, claiming in countless parliamentary debates, that it has led to an explosion in the amount of bureaucracy. As there is a legal responsibility on the part of the contractor to ensure contract specifications are adhered to, there is a requirement for professional management and efficient procedures, hence an increase particularly in the numbers of accountants and financial workers. This, the Opposition claims, is at the expense of the 'hands-on' carers, who have seen their numbers diminish and overall level of gradings fall.

There are many instances where instead of opening up caring to the market place, providers have continued with monopolistic delivery of services. Competition is limited in some rural areas, for instance, and areas of certain specialties such as accident and emergency care and ambulance services. Conversely, London was found to have overcapacity of provision of many services, operating in a highly competitive market. Contracts for health services with public and private providers must be publicly available once they are signed, as laid down by the Department of Health (NHSME, 1989). This is of course too late for public debate, as the deal has already been struck.

The health care trade unions, professional bodies, and consumer groups have united to voice their views that issues relating to quality of care might be of secondary consideration in the desire to save money and accept the cheapest option. The United Kingdom Central Council for Nursing, Midwifery and Health Visiting (UKCC, 1995) has expressed concern about the professions' standards in a contract culture. There is an overwhelming need to protect the public, and permit safe practices by nurses, midwives and health visitors in a climate of tight financial control, with resultant pressures on resources. In 1995, Council issued a document entitled 'The Council's Proposed Standards for Incorporation into Contracts for Hospital and Community Health Care Services' (UKCC, 1995). In it, the Council recommends that:

- A clause requiring compliance with the Code of Professional Conduct (UKCC, 1992) should be included in all contracts of employment;
- Registered practitioners in their employment should be able to satisfy the requirements of the Code;
- Arrangements should be made to ensure continued competence and professional development of registered practitioners, including PREP requirements;
- A policy should exist to permit legitimate concerns regarding standards of care to be expressed to employers;
- Mechanism should exist to allow monitoring of standards.

A key section of the UKCC's document looked at the role of support staff, a growth area much influenced by skill mix exercises and value for money reports (NHSME, 1992) which have gone hand-in-hand with the contract culture. Employers are asked to ensure that support workers should always work under the supervision of nurses, midwives and health visitors. Registered practitioners should be involved at all levels of the support workers' education and training, and the responsibility for assessment, planning, implementation and standards of nursing should remain with registered practitioners. Of particular concern is the NHSME (1992) value for money exercise, which on the basis of a dubious research framework made recommendations as to the need to replace expensive G and H grade community workers with lower grades who would of course be cheaper to employ.

From July 1993, there has been a European dimension added as a result of the European Council's Public Procurement Directory. At present, it only applies to local government work and affects matters such as the minimum number of tenders for a contract shortlist, and maximum length of time that the contracts may operate (Audit Commission, 1993) The time will surely come, however, when the EC legislation is widened to include those contracts that relate to member states' provision for the delivery of health care.

The contract culture is having an adverse effect on voluntary organizations. Where a voluntary group has been involved in a contract to bid for the delivery of certain services, it often now requires its members to enter into agreements to undertake those services. Whereas volunteers were happy to give of their time in informal arrangements on an ad hoc basis, many resent having formally to commit themselves to undertake service at a particular time and date, or to subordinate themselves to the provisions of an overall care plan. Voluntary group spokespersons report a growing disenchantment with contract culture, with many volunteers feeling alienated. The larger voluntary organizations have tended to involve themselves in contractual obligations but often at the cost of the principles which set up the movements in the beginning. There is a wealth of evidence from America where, in a similar climate, voluntary groups have launched themselves into the contractual market place, often with savage infighting, competing against other voluntary groups that they happily coexisted with before, and displaying an unaccustomed ruthlessness in removing volunteers and reshaping their organizations in a bid to win contracts. A strong dependence on contracts would not auger well for the organizations if they should subsequently lose a future bid.

A purchasing agency having statutory responsibility for ensuring care, available for residents in its area, will provide it by a combination of contracting with other agencies and direct provision (Brazier, 1988). Purchasers can therefore buy in services from other health authorities and trusts. In some places, this has encouraged mergers of trusts to create larger entities, to ensure that there is provision of a wider range of services. In others, purchasing consortia or Health Commissions have been formed whereby District Health Authorities (DHAs) and Family Health Service

Authorities (FHSAs) collaborate to carry out purchasing functions. The emergence of bigger purchasing agencies will bring with it potential disadvantages: purchasing decisions may well be taken that are insensitive to local needs and will fail to take into account the views of general practitioners and other significant interests (Ham, 1992). Trusts will earn the vast bulk of their income through contracts with various purchasers (HPSSME, 1991), and the ultimate long-term survival of trusts or any other purchasing unit and their ability to grow both in size and quality will depend on how successful they become in obtaining these contracts. As contracts are of fixed duration, officials will be constantly examining their contractual bids for future renewal. A trust that loses a contract might be in a dire situation, with the consequent uncertainty for its employees' job prospects.

The British Medical Association in its report on the White Paper (BMA, 1989) cautions that contracting could lead to hospitals being tempted to concentrate more of their efforts on profitable services, including private patients and patients from other districts, and less priority to the needs of its local population. A District Health Authority might decide to buy its services from another hospital, with disastrous consequences for the local hospital concerned.

Much controversy has been caused by self-governing NHS Hospital Trusts. Their income is derived from contracts with health authorities, general practitioner practices, the private sector, and other self-governing hospitals. The voluntary sector has here expressed concern that this situation will have an adverse effect on overall integration of the NHS services, and perhaps a bias towards money making specialisms that it can sell elsewhere (NCVO, 1989–2). A new breed of health care manager has emerged, the entrepreneur able to wheel and deal in the market place, selling health care just like any other commodity.

Conclusion

Contract culture by and large is not popular with the citizens of this nation. Before changes were introduced, consultation was promised with individual consumers of health care, carer organizations, community health councils, pressure groups, etc. The overwhelming response has been that decisions had already been arrived at and response consultations did nothing to influence decisions that had already been made. The media reflect the general level of concern with the state of the National Health Service, focusing on scandals, cuts in services, bed closures and continuous financial crises. Hardly a week goes by without exposures contrasting reduction in numbers of 'hands-on' service providers with overflowing administrators' car parks. The emotive plight of seriously ill young patients being shuttled around the country in search of scarce specialist beds is doing much to undermine public confidence in our ability effectively to manage delivery of health care. By opening up the provider response to competition, the government intended that market forces would reduce costs and improve quality of care. It is a matter for debate whether the latter aim is being achieved.

Points to consider

1 Contracts for delivery of care have to be freely available to the general public. How would you, as a member of the public, obtain copies of contracts in your area?

2 Have the UKCC's guidelines on Proposed Standards been incorporated into those contracts?

3 What effect have contractual obligations had on your professional practice?

4 How much 'blame' for scarcity of beds can be attached to contract culture?

References

Audit Commission 1992: *Managing the cascade of change.* London: HMSO.

Audit Commission 1993: *Realising the benefits of competition: the client role for contracted services.* London: HMSO.

Brazier, J. (ed.) 1988: *Reforming the UK health care system: Discussion Paper 47.* University of York: Centre for Health Economics, Health Economics Consortia, York.

British Medical Association 1989: *Special report on the Government's White paper, Working with patients.* London: BMA.

Department of Health 1989a: *Working for patients: White Paper on the future of the NHS. A summary of proposals and key issues for voluntary organisations.* London: HMSO.

Department of Health 1989b: *Working for patients: caring for the 1990s.* London: HMSO.

Department of Health 1990: *Working for patients: contracts for health services. Operating contracts.* London: HMSO.

Ham, C. 1992: *Locality purchasing: Discussion Paper 30.* University of Birmingham Health Services Management Centre.

Health and Personal Social Services Management Executive 1991: *Working for patients: HSS Trusts. A working guide.* Belfast: HMSO.

NCVO 1989: *Contracting in or out: contract culture – the challenge for voluntary organisations; guidance notes on contracting for voluntary groups no 2.* Birmingham.

NCVO 1989–2: *Working for patients: The White Paper on the future of the NHS. Summary of proposals and key issues for voluntary organisations.* London.

NHS Management Executive 1989: *Contracts for health services: pricing and openness EL (89) MB / 171.* London: HMSO.

NHSME 1992: *The nursing skill mix in the district nursing service. A report on the finding of the value for money unit.* London: HMSO.

Oxford University Press 1982: *Concise Oxford Dictionary.* Oxford: OUP.

Smee, C. 1994: The market in health care. In Hopkins, A. (ed.) *Regulation of the market in the NHS. Competition and the common good.* Royal College of the Physicians of London.

UKCC 1992: *Code of Professional Conduct* (3rd edn). London: UKCC.
UKCC 1995: *The Council's proposed standards for the incorporation into contracts for hospital and community health care services*. London: UKCC.

3 Issues in health promotion

Karen Melling and Ann Sutton

The purpose of this chapter is to explore and examine the developments and current trends in health promotion and health education in relation to the practice of community health care nursing.

This chapter will critically analyse the approaches and models of health promotion and health education. It will address the need for community health care nurses to work in collaboration with other health professionals in health education and health promotion activities. The chapter sets out to raise issues in relation to community health care nursing and their future role as health promoters. The aim is not to provide quick solutions but promote discussion regarding the development of innovative practice that will enhance the health status of the population. Consideration of how the challenges of promoting health initiatives may be met, together with a review and evaluation of the current problems that hamper this, may go some way towards developing effective practice for the future.

The need to respond now imaginatively and with flexibility has never been more important.

Introduction

The *Health of the Nation* (Department of Health, 1992) document has raised questions about the nature of health, health education and health promotion. It is therefore the intention of this chapter to attempt to explore these issues within the context of community health care nursing. The health needs of a diverse population present challenges to community nurses if they are to promote health. The development of effective health assessment strategies and the subsequent planning necessary for sensitive collaborative health promotion initiatives, require examination of these issues and the impact they have on people's lives. Therefore, consideration will be given to the approaches that health professionals may use, as health data become more available to assist in the assessment of health need. The current focus on promoting partnerships and interprofessional collaboration, together with providing services that are more assessable and acceptable to people, reinforces the view that the professional role needs to be examined. These developments will have implications for the education and training of community health care nurses if they are to be equipped to deal with the demands of providing effective health promotion support to user groups. It is now desirable that community nurses have the appropriate knowledge base and are able to work collaboratively with clients.

Health promotion, health education and healthy public policies will be discussed and examined in more detail at a later stage of this chapter.

Health

The current focus on the White Paper *The Health of the Nation* (Department of Health, 1992) perhaps reinforces the need to consider the issue of health. What is it? Can it be defined? If so by whom? Beliefs and values about health are diverse and can be influenced by age, gender, class, race, political views, where and how people live and their economic and social status. Aggleton (1990) maintains that defining health can be divided into two broad types: official definitions, indicating the views of doctors and health professionals, and those of the lay population. Perhaps the definition most familiar to health professionals is the World Health Organization (WHO) (1946) statement from its Constitution: 'Health is a state of complete physical, mental and social well being and not merely the absence of disease or infirmity' (cited in Downie *et al.*, 1990, p. 9). This statement has attracted criticism from many theorists and health professionals (Dubos, 1959; Downie *et al.*, 1990). Aggleton (1990) suggests this definition has been seen as too idealistic in specifying a state of health that is impossible to attain, and Seedhouse (1986) acknowledges that the definition and aims of the WHO are commendable but suggests that 'rigorous theoretical clarification' (p. 31) has not been applied. Therefore, without critical analysis, the definition becomes little more than a statement espousing well-meaning ideals. Seedhouse (1986) identifies four theories of health: 'health as an ideal state, health as physical and mental fitness to do socialised daily tasks, health as a commodity which can be bought or given, and health as a personal strength or ability either physical, metaphysical or intellectual' (p. 29). It is useful to consider these statements within the context of our own views and attitudes to health, and to examine how these views might be reflected by clients and consequently present implications for the practice of community health care nurses. Ewles and Simnett (1995), while recognizing the criticisms of the WHO statement on health, suggest that a positive view is offered and that consideration of social and mental well-being is welcome.

Health as a state where illness and disease are absent is commonly known as the biomedical view of health and as such has the attention of many of the lay community (Dines and Cribb, 1993). The problem for community health professionals is then how promoting health might be addressed for the sick but 'well,' and also the 'worried well', if this view of health is to be challenged.

Blaxter (1990) when reporting on the health and lifestyle survey 1984/85 found that lay views of health included a range of opinions. Men, especially those under 60 years, saw health as the norm, while younger people saw health as being physically fit and having energy and physical strength. Health was also seen as a 'reserve' or the ability to get over health-related problems quickly. Health is also seen as energy, vitality and leading a healthy life by not smoking , taking exercise and eating healthily. The health and lifestyle postal survey of 10 000 people in Cheshire on the Wirral during 1992 and 1993 (Dawson, 1994) found that many of those people wanted to adopt a healthy lifestyle in areas of exercise, alcohol consumption, diet and smoking. However, they experienced difficulty with a lack of willpower, cost, the influence of others and the enjoyment of unhealthy behaviours. These were seen as positive activities in that they contributed to reducing stress (Dawson, 1994; Graham, 1993). These findings have implications for all health professionals when they approach health promotion activities, the fact that people have health knowledge is no guarantee that it will be used or adopted, as identified by Prochaska and Di Clemente's (1984) processes of change. Finally, it is worth noting the more recent definition of health by the WHO (1984), 'Health is the extent to which an individual or group is able, on the one hand, to realise aspirations and satisfy needs; and, on the other hand to change or cope with the environment. Health is therefore, seen as a resource for everyday life, not an object of living; it is a positive concept emphasising social and personal resources, as well as physical capabilities' (p. 2). This statement advances the debate about health. The complexities surrounding the nature of health make it unlikely that a 'unified concept of health which includes all its meanings will be formulated' (Naidoo and Wills, 1994, p. 21).

Inequalities, and poverty issues have been shown to relate to health and illness (DHSS, 1980; Benzeval et al., 1995) and remain an issue at the present time. However, this issue received little coverage in the White Paper Health of the Nation (DOH, 1992) despite the fact that the WHO Health for all by the year 2000 (1978) wished to make this a central point of their strategy. 'For the first time in sixty years death rates for men aged 15–44 have begun to rise in the north'. This widening inequality has pushed Britain further down the life expectancy ratings from 12th to 17th in the 24 member states as suggested by the Organization of Economic Co-operative Development table (Guardian; Dying of poverty, Leader, 5.5.94).

The consideration of sound epidemiological data is essential if appropriate strategies for health promotion activities are to be developed both locally and nationally.

Health promotion and health education

Health promotion at the present time has followed an evolutionary process, from the public health sanitary revolution of the nineteenth century, through the health education movement of the twentieth century, to that of health promotion today.

The World Health Organization came into being following the Second World War as nations were horrified at human rights violations. Member states defined a world-wide strategy for health (WHO, 1946). Health education was a concept of the propaganda machine which focused on changing individuals' behaviour as a way of improving their own health (Rodmell and Watt, 1986; DHSS, 1976). Health education later widened its parameters to include social infrastructure and advocacy of social reform (Anderson, 1980; Crawford, 1977; Draper et al., 1980).

The term health promotion appeared during the early 1980s and replaced health education (Bunton and Macdonald, 1992). In Britain during the 1980s there was a wide proliferation of health education models drawing on the wider perception of health education. *Targets for Health for All* (WHO, 1985) was closely followed by the WHO discussion document on the 'Concept and Principles of Health Promotion' formulated from the Ottawa Charter (WHO, 1986). Frequently these terms are used in an interchangeable way which can cause confusion, for example, during the 1980s when some Health Education Units changed their name to Health Promotion Units. Rawson and Grigg (1988) suggest that many units did so without any identifiable role change.

Health education and health promotion: is there a difference?

The term health promotion has more recently entered the health vocabulary but has it replaced health education? During the 1984 WHO Conference in Copenhagen on 'Concepts and Principles of Health Promotion' the principles of health promotion were adopted as outlined in the discussion document (WHO, 1984) and stated as follows:

1 Health promotion involves the population as a whole in the context of their everyday life, rather than focusing on people at risk from specific diseases.

2 Health promotion is directed towards action on the detriments or causes of health.

3 Health promotion combines diverse, but complementary methods or approaches.

4 Health promotion aims particularly at effective and concrete public participation.

5 While health promotion is basically an activity in the health and social fields and not specifically in medical service, health professionals – particularly in primary health care – have an important role in nurturing and enabling health promotion. Health professionals should work towards developing their special contribution in education and health advocacy.

Additionally, the Regional Programmes in Health Education and Lifestyle (WHO, 1981) identified the key focus and strategies for action in primary care. These were that health care should be less narrowly focused on medical services; consumers should participate in the planning and implementation of care, and move towards self-help and self-care.

Health carers should promote positive health and healthy lifestyles in the community, and preventable diseases and disability should be eliminated or reduced through immunization, screening and patient/client education, this being supported in government policy with the introduction of the reports *A Vision for the Future* (DOH, 1993a) and *New World, New Opportunities* (DOH, 1993c). Tones *et al.*'s view of health promotion is that it incorporates 'all measures deliberately designed to promote health and handle disease' (1990, p. 3). More recently Bunton (1992, p. 4) argues that health promotion is 'not only a new form of health care provision but also a new form of social regulation and control'. He raises the issue that health promotion programmes have entered the lives of people in many ways and run the risk of invading privacy and civil rights.

Tones and Tilford (1994) see health education as any planned activity which promotes health or illness related learning, that is, some relatively permanent change in an individual's competence or disposition. Health education can be viewed as a way by which nurses help patients or clients by understanding their condition through open discussion, by giving information and by exploring the patients' views and feelings about a health matter together (Macleod Clark and Latter, 1990).

Successful health education is dependent on active client or patient participation at all levels of goal setting, planning and decision making (Macleod Clark and Latter, 1990). Additionally, the promotion of self-esteem, autonomy and the ability to value the beliefs and attitudes of others is fundamental (French, 1990). Health education from the outset needs to consider the issue of evaluation and the need to build into any health education programme opportunities for this to take place, at the same time fully involving patients or clients.

French (1990) warns of the dangers of simplifying complex data in order to get the message across. Many health messages are complex, therefore it is important to use methods which enable complex issues to be considered rather than adopt approaches that give simplistic advice or solutions.

Health education has been seen as helping people to change their behaviour and consequently their lifestyle, but where this is the sole aim it has been considered more recently as a form of victim blaming (Crawford,

1977; Ewles and Simnett, 1995). French (1990) reinforces this by declaring that health education is concerned with enabling people (client-centred and empowerment) to set and develop their own agendas for health. Health professionals may, by enabling the appropriate support, assist either individuals or groups to meet this end.

As stated earlier, the second part of health promotion includes public policies. The new public health movement is developing new approaches across the political spectrum, an example being *Health of the Nation* (DOH, 1992). Within this policy it is suggested that everyone has a responsibility for improving their own health, as well as improving family, home, school hospital and workplace environments, through healthy initiatives. However, the main focus of this policy is on individual behaviour change, for example, by reducing the smoking population. The government sees its main task as ensuring that individual departments work together towards common objectives by appointing a ministerial cabinet committee to monitor and assess the progress of this strategy for England, and to ensure 'proper co-ordination of UK wide issues affecting health. Community health care nurses are in a prime position to be practically involved in this development either through their role as a professional or as an individual, they may influence both community and work place settings' (Fieldgrass, 1992).

The aim of interested parties is to promote the development of healthy public policies, thereby enabling environmental changes to take place. Individuals may lend their support to community action, by making use of all aspects of recycling which are available in the community. The use of seatbelts, lead-free petrol, the demand for traffic control and park and ride schemes, all enhance active community participation in making the community a healthier and safer place.

Ashton and Seymour (1988) suggest that health professionals need to consider:

1 The need for positive indicators in place of negative ones and for qualitative and small area data, examples being the development of practice profiles.

2 The need to focus on context as well as people.

3 Doing things from where people are; the development of local initiatives to meet local needs such as carers' support groups.

4 The need for true stories to be told.

5 Assessment of the health promoting capabilities of community nurses are becoming increasingly involved in assessing local community health needs.

An example of the latter is the Participatory Rapid Appraisal Approach (Ong, 1991) where, in conjunction with members of the local community, health needs are identified along with possible resources and solutions. Having profiled the practice population, care provision can be assessed and action taken on identified needs; strategies can be revised according to the profile information provided by the primary health care team. The need to develop community profiles and case load analysis will enable the delivery of health promotion activities from a sound database and will facilitate the future planning of resource allocation (Tinson, 1995).

Deficits in health gain which cannot be met from within the practice will be highlighted and evidence made available to management, or local communities. Action then can be taken in incorporating this health need into the 'contract', such as employing a specialist health promotion officer or specialist community nurse.

The context today

Social, demographic, legislative and health care change have led to developments in the education and training of community nurses (DOH, 1993b; UKCC, 1990; UKCC, 1994) and therefore present implications for the delivery of nursing practice. This situation will cause health professionals to reflect on the health needs of the patient and client groups. How are these needs to be assessed, approached and effectively met?

In order to focus the discussion there would appear to be a need to clarify the issues and concerns that have influence on the community nurses' role as a health promoter.

The White Paper, *The Health of the Nation* (DOH, 1992) acknowledged the important contribution of the WHO *Health for all by the year 2000* (1978) in its formulation of a strategy for health in England. This document (DOH, 1992) places emphasis on the development of public policies, healthy surroundings, healthy lifestyles 'by increased knowledge and understanding of how the way people live, affects their health' (p. 14). Health services are further charged with the responsibility of identifying and meeting the health needs of the local population and achieving a balance between health promotion, disease prevention, treatment and rehabilitation. The primary health care services are seen to have a major role in using their expertise and skill to work with other professionals in developing alliances and collaborative actions to explore the potential of health promotion and develop targets to meet the national strategy (Fieldgrass, 1992). Furthermore, the National Health Service and Community Care Act (1990) highlights the responsibility of health authorities to assess the state of the health of its population, in order to purchase the provision of appropriate treatment and services which encompass the promotion of health, and the prevention of disease. This Act indicates the need for health professionals, and community health care nurses in particular, to identify clearly their role in meeting the health needs of patients and focuses attention on the importance of developing effective working relationships with other professional groups, for example social workers, if a cohesive and congruent health care programme is to be achieved (Fieldgrass, 1992).

The introduction of Project 2000 nurse education and training (UKCC, 1986), which emphasized the need for nurse education to focus on health rather than disease, further saw the need for a practitioner in the community who would take a leading role in health promotion. The need for specialist preparation to undertake the task of the promotion of health for the well population was recognized in both Project 2000 (UKCC, 1986) and in the Report of the Post Registration Education Practice Project (UKCC, 1990). The development of an effective health promoter is seen to be dependent upon the acquisition of a high level of knowledge and skills. The document *Targeting Practice* (DOH, 1993b) highlights principles of good practice for nurses, midwives and health visitors undertaking health promotion activities and draws attention to the need for innovation, evaluation and quality assurance. In order to consider these commendable aims it is worth returning to the WHO, *Targets for Health for All* (1985) report, which emphasized the need to involve those receiving care in the planning process. This appears to offer a way forward for health professionals, if they are to provide a service that promotes collaborative action and is more accessible and acceptable to the population. Linked to the idea of a partnership of care is one of empowering individuals to take responsibility for their health and to be involved in making informed choices. These ideas are implicit in *The Health of the Nation* (DOH, 1992), National Health Service and Community Care Act (1990) and the report *Neighbourhood Nursing – A Focus for Care* (DHSS, 1986).

This has implications for both the relationship between the nurse and the patient and between differing groups of nurses. Consequently, how the education and training process prepares nurses to develop their role, from one that has traditionally been prescriptive or directive, to one that allows for the empowerment of those giving care and those receiving it, needs to be considered. Empowerment emphasizes mutual goal setting and decision making, therefore this will not be successful unless both persons are committed to the process (Hokanson Hawks, 1992; Williams, 1995).

Current health concerns, such as substance abuse, HIV and AIDS (DOH, 1992) together with a 34 per cent increase of elderly in the 75–84s age range, and a 43 per cent increase in people over 85 years is expected between 1984–2001 (Smith, Jacobson and Whitehead, 1988). This also serves to focus attention on the need for community health care nurses, to have well-developed skills in preventive health care. There is a need, too, to be effective in taking a pro-active approach in the development of health promotion initiatives (Ross, 1990). Patients and clients can expect to see their own general practitioners' practices producing their own charters for the practice population (DOH, 1995).

Therefore, in consideration of the prevailing factors it would appear that there is now a requirement for community nurses to consider how to offer a service that is responsive to patient and client-identified health needs, is effective within a budgetary framework and focuses on health promotion in the provision of quality care.

Models and approaches to health promotion and their practical application

Much has been written and many models offered in the development of health promotion. Rawson (cited in Bunton and Macdonald, 1992) suggests that 'models have been imported from other disciplines' (p. 207), and cites the health belief model as an example. Rawson and Grigg (1988) identified 17 published taxonomies of collections of health education models in Britain alone. The development of models continues, those most commonly in use being Caplan and Holland (1990), Beattie (1991), French and Adams (1986), Tannahill (1985) and Tones and Tilford (1994).

There has been much debate regarding approaches versus models. It is the writers' view that the approaches to health promotion (Ewles and Simnett, 1995) are in fact the processes employed in achieving health promoting activities, and it is the models of health promotion that provide the overriding theoretical and philosophical framework.

While many community health care nurses assess a health promotional need using a model of nursing, the health need of the community at large must not be ignored. The effective use of community profiles and caseload analysis will assist in the enhancement of health promotion practice which would fall within the framework of the Health Action Model. The 'health action' model as described by Tones and Tilford (1994) identifies the many influences both internal and external which affects individuals in their enhancement of health.

It is well recognized that there are five broad approaches (Ewles and Simnett, 1995) which can be applied to health promotion activities:

- *Medical or preventive* This approach focuses on the prevention of illness and disease. Medical experts are seen to play a key role in interventions which reduce mortality and morbidity.
- *Behavioural change* Encourages individuals to adopt a healthier lifestyle which focuses on the individual's own life activities using health as a property of the individual.
- *Educational* Informs individuals by developing their knowledge base, thereby enabling them to make an informed choice. However, the choice may not be the one the health promoter prefers.
- *Client centred* This approach enables individuals to determine when and if to change their own and community lifestyle. Using a bottom-up approach, individuals are empowered to take control of their own decision making.
- *Social change/radical* Focuses on socio-economic and environmental issues. Changes in policy at local or national levels 'to make healthy choices easy choices' is often the focus of this approach.

These approaches are further described by Ewles and Simnett (1995).

A popular model as previously mentioned is the cycle of change model (Prochaska and Di Clemente, 1984; Prochaska *et al.*, 1992), which has been described as a 'revolving door model' (Tones and Tilford, 1994) and is frequently used by community health care nurses in attempting to change the health behaviour of individuals. This model is based on a cycle of five stages of change, these being precontemplation, contemplation, action, maintenance and a possible fifth stage being relapse, where the cycle may start again with precontemplation. This model accepts that there may be failure or setbacks in changing behaviour which may be due to outside influences, both social and environmental, however, it does give a framework for the community health care nurse to support the patient/client in attempting to change their health behaviour.

Health promotion is multi-faceted, and for health promotion to be enhanced within the community, nurses must be aware, and be prepared to deal with their prejudices. Role conflict, both inter and intra, may occur where the nurse sees her role simply as providing care and treatment or health checks (Clarke, 1991). This may be reinforced where other team members hold similar opinions. Therefore, it is important that a clear philosophy regarding each member's role within the primary health care team is agreed concerning each member's ideology.

Members working within the team need to be aware of the strengths of the other team members in order that they can maximize the skills they share. The use of practice profiles should enable a common health philosophy to be developed in order to meet the health needs of the practice population. Through regular auditing of the practice profile, outcomes can be measured, aims reviewed and where necessary differing approaches and models used. For example, a practice identified smoking cessation, where all community health care nurses were asked to identify carers and members of their families who would be interested in giving up smoking, to try out the effectiveness of nicorette patches. This represents a behavioural change approach to health promotion. Where health needs are identified, nurses can be more pro-active regarding health promotion activities. These activities need not be confined to one discipline only. Another example of innovative practice and an extension of the roles is health visitors and district nurses setting up and running a 'drop in' advice shop on market day in a rural town. There would appear to be more opportunities arising for nurses in terms of educational, empowerment and social change approaches to be used in the community than the traditional medical, behavioural change approaches which have been used to date.

Issues relating to the educational approach may be seen as a community nurse dilemma, as the whole culture of nurse education is one of delivering 'expert' knowledge. The 'social ritual' process which all professionals go through reinforces the belief that their knowledge is best. The caring philosophy of 'I know what is best for you, so do as I say', differs from the educational approach where information is offered and may be rejected. With this rejection comes a lack of self-worth, lack of personal value which may have a negative effect on the community health care nurse. This may then lead to the 'victim blaming' phenomenon (Ewles and Simnett, 1995).

One example is where a person suffering from heart disease is 'blamed' for their condition because they are overweight and smoke, but the reasons for being overweight and smoking are ignored.

In striving to meet *The Health of the Nation* (DOH, 1992) targets, certain individuals and groups in society are classified as being at risk of disease, an example being people who smoke or who are overweight. Individual behaviour change would be viewed as an appropriate approach. However, in the majority of incidences this change of behaviour cannot be maintained. Therefore, the emphasis must be placed on changing the underlying factors, if this change is to be permanent (Illich, 1975). It must be recognized that health professionals are unable to take sole responsibility for change. This is where collaboration with other agencies is of paramount importance.

Social change and radical approaches must be seen as a way forward for the improvement of health. As the role of the community health nurse develops, so opportunities will arise to address locally socio-economic and environmental issues. Developing a changing policy at local level 'to make healthy choices easy choices' may involve nurses in a more political arena than previously. The lobbying of local councillors, general practitioner fundholders and social services need not only be on an individual basis but can be addressed through community action groups or self-help groups.

Empowerment is very much at the forefront of current health promotion. Hokanson Hawks (1992) suggests empowerment as being the interpersonal process of providing the resources, tools and environment to develop, build and increase the ability and effectiveness of others to set and reach goals for individual and social ends. It could therefore be said that central government through changing the power base in introducing the NHS and Community Care Act (DOH, 1990) focuses on the individual need for health care. Fundamental to this concept is the role of purchaser and provider. Currently general practitioners purchase services to meet the needs of their patients, the main drawback being that fiscal resources are finite. The introduction of the *Patient's Charter* in 1993 could also be seen as a demonstration of the shift in power to the people, in principle, but in reality, are people being given a choice in the treatment they receive?

Conclusion

The future holds many opportunities and challenges to develop the nature of community health care nursing practice. The achievement will be through knowledge that is grounded in research-based practice. The identification of health need and health gain which is based on the local population's perception of health is paramount, if community health care nursing is to achieve its goal of 'Health for All'. The use of approaches and models of health promotion is to be actively sought. Working in partnership with patient and clients, using client-centred approaches, draws attention to the need for highly developed skills of communication.

The development of interprofessional alliances will allow for collaboration between different health professionals and other agencies This will enable the development of innovative practice to be responsive to health need. Only through effective evaluation of these approaches can outcomes measure a response to health need. Opportunities are now available for community nurses to lead the way in positive health promotion and health education activities.

Points to consider

1 How may the role of the community health care nurse enhance the health of the community?

2 What problems might the community health care nurse meet when fulfilling the role of a health promoter?

3 Should community health care nurses be more political in order to achieve healthy public policies?

4 What are the issues in health promotion and health education at the present time?

References

Aggleton, P. 1990: *Health*. London: Routledge.

Anderson, D. 1980: Blind alleys in health education. In Seldon, A. (eds) *The litmus papers*. London: Centre for Policy Studies.

Ashton, J. and Seymour, H. 1988: *The new public health*. Buckingham: Open University Press.

Beattie, A. 1991: Knowledge and control in health promotion: a test case for social policy and social theory. In Gabe, J., Calnan, M. and Guy, M. (eds), *The sociology of the health service*. London: Routledge.

Benzeval, M., Judge, K. and Whitehead, M. 1995: *Tackling inequalities in health: an agenda for action*. London: King's Fund.

Blaxter, M. 1990: *Health and lifestyles*. London: Tavistock.

Bowling, A. 1991: *Measuring health. A review of quality of live measurement scales*. Milton Keynes: Open University Press.

Bunton, R. and Macdonald, G. (eds) 1992: *Health promotion: discipline and diversity*. London: Routledge.

Bunton, R. 1992: More than a woolly jumper: health promotion as social regulation. *Critical Public Health*, **3**, 2, 4–11.

Caplan, R. and Holland, R. 1990: Rethinking Health Education theory. *Health Education Journal*, **49**, 1, 7 –12.

Clarke, A. 1991: Nurses as role models and health educationalist. *Journal of Advanced Nursing*, **16**, 1178–84.

Crawford, R. 1977: You are dangerous to your health: the ideology and politics of victim-blaming. *Journal of Health Services*, **7**, 663–80.

Dawson, J. 1994: Health and lifestyle surveys: beyond health status indicators. *Health Education Journal*, **53**, 3, 300–33.

Department of Health 1990: *The NHS and Community Care Act*. London: HMSO.

Department of Health 1992: *The health of the nation*. London: HMSO.

Department of Health 1993: *Nursing in primary health care. New worlds, new opportunities.* London: HMSO.

Department of Health 1993a: *A vision for the future.* London: HMSO.

Department of Health 1993b: *Targeting practice: the contribution of nurses, midwives and health visitors.* London: HMSO.

Department of Health 1995: *Patient's charter.* London: HMSO.

Department of Health and Social Security 1976: *Prevention and health: every bodies' business.* London: HMSO.

Department of Health and Social Security 1980: *Inequalities in health. The Black report.* London: HMSO.

Department of Health and Social Security 1986: *Neighbourhood nursing – a focus for care.* London: HMSO.

Dines, A. and Cribb, A. (eds) 1993: *Health promotion concepts and practice.* Oxford: Blackwell Scientific.

Downie, R.S., Fyfe, C. and Tannahill, A. 1990: *Health promotion models and values.* Oxford: Oxford University Press.

Draper, P., Griffiths, J., Dennis, J. and Popay, J. 1980: Three types of health education, *British Medical Journal*, **281**, 16 August, 493–5.

Draper, P. (ed.) 1991: *Health through public policy: the greening of public health.* London: Green Print.

Dubos, R. 1959: *The mirage of health.* New York: Harper and Row.

Ewles, L. and Simnett, I. 1995: *Promoting health: a practical guide.* London: Scutari Press.

Fieldgrass, J. 1992: *Partnerships in health promotion: collaboration between the statutory and voluntary sectors.* London: Health Education Authority.

French, J. 1990: Boundaries and horizons, the role of health education within health promotion. *Health Education Journal*, **49**, 1, 7–10.

French, J. and Adams, L. 1986: From analysis to synthesis. *Health Education Journal*, **45**, 2, 71–74.

Graham, H. 1993: *Hardship or health in women's lives.* Brighton: Harvester Wheatsheaf.

Hawe, P., Degeling, D. and Hall, J. 1990: *Evaluating health promotion. A health worker's guide.* Sydney: Maclennan and Petty.

Hokanson Hawks, J. 1992: Empowerment in nursing education: Concept analysis and application to philosophy, learning and instruction. *Journal of Advanced Nursing*, **17**, 5, 609–18.

Illich, I. 1975: *Medical nemesis.* London: Calder and Boyars.

Leader 1994: Dying of poverty. *The Guardian*, 5.5.1994.

Macleod Clark, J. and Latter, S. 1990: Working together. *Nursing Times*, **86**, 48, 28–31.

Naidoo, J. and Wills, J. 1994: *Health promotion foundation for practice.* London: Baillière Tindall.

Ong, B.N. 1991: Researching needs in district nursing. *Journal of Advanced Nursing*, **16**, 6, 638–47.

Prochaska J.O., Di Clemente, C.C., Velicier W.F. and Rossi J.S. 1992: Criticisms and concerns of the transtheoretical model in light of recent research. *British Journal of Addiction*, **87**, 825–83.

Prochaska J.O. and Di Clemente, C.C. 1984: *The transtheoretical approach: crossing traditional foundations of change.* Illinois USA: Homewood.

Rawson, D. and Grigg, C. 1988: *Purpose and practice in health education.* London: Southbank Polytechnic/HEA. Cited in Bunton, R. and Macdonald, G. (eds) (1992), *Health promotion: discipline and diversity.* London: Routledge.

Rodmell, S. and Watt, A. (eds) 1986: *The politics of health education.* London: Routledge and Kegan Paul.

Ross, F. 1990: *Key issues in district nursing.* London: District Nursing Association.

Seedhouse, D. 1986: *Health: the foundation for achievement.* Chichester: John Wiley and Sons.

Smith, A., Jacobson, B. and Whitehead, M. (eds) 1988: *The nation's health: a strategy for the 1990's.* London: King Edward's Hospital Fund for London.

Tannahill, A. 1985: What is health promotion? *Health Education Journal,* **44**: 167–8.

Tinson, S. 1995: Assessing health need: a community perspective. In Cain, P., Hyde, V. and Howkins, L. (eds), *Community nursing dimensions and dilemmas.* London: Edward Arnold.

Tones, K., Tilford, S. and Robinson, Y. 1990: *Health education: effectiveness, efficiency.* London: Chapman and Hall.

Tones, K. and Tilford, S. 1994: *Health education: effectiveness, efficiency and equity* (2nd edn). London: Chapman and Hall.

United Kingdom Central Council for Nursing, Midwifery and Health Visiting 1986: *Project 2000 – a new preparation for practice.* London: UKCC.

United Kingdom Central Council for Nursing, Midwifery and Health Visiting 1990: *The report of the post registration education and practice project.* London: UKCC.

United Kingdom Central Council for Nursing, Midwifery and Health Visiting 1994: *The future of professional practice – the Council's standards for education and practice following registration.* London: UKCC.

Williams, J. 1995: Education for empowerment: implications for professional development and training in health promotion. *Health Education Journal,* **54**, 1, 37–47.

World Health Organization 1946: *Constitution.* Geneva: WHO.

World Health Organization 1978: *Report on the primary health care conference Alma-Ata.* Geneva: WHO.

World Health Organization 1981: *Regional programmes in health promotion and lifestyle.* Copenhagen: WHO Regional Office for Europe.

World Health Organization 1984: *Health promotion: a discussion document on the concepts and principles.* Copenhagen: WHO Regional Office for Europe.

World Health Organization 1985: *Targets for health for all.* Copenhagen: WHO Regional Office for Europe.

World Health Organization 1986: Ottawa charter for health promotion. *Journal of Health Promotion,* **1**, 1–4.

4 Needs of older people

Elaine Ryder

The issue of population ageing is central in considering the current arrangements in Britain for the provision of care within the community. To achieve a healthy future for old age and promote the health of older people, knowledge and understanding of ageing and ageing processes are fundamental. Assessment of consumer needs underpins current health policy with the intention that services can be delivered more effectively.

This chapter explores the implications of such changes in relation to older people. By examining the nature of needs of older people, the complexity of assessment of needs of this group of people becomes evident. This calls into question the knowledge and skills of community nurses in the provision of effective care for older people, in the community, who currently remain a relatively powerless group within society.

Introduction

Against a background of major change in community health care delivery, community nurses are identifying areas of expertise within their role. As older people figure significantly within community nurses' caseloads, one such area of expertise is that of working with older people, to facilitate the identification of needs and appropriate interventions.

While the focus of this paper is to analyse issues in relation to the needs of older people, political influences and population trends will initially be explored to place this examination in context.

Political influences

As early as 1979, the Royal Commission on the National Health Service (HMSO, 1979) recognized that meeting the health needs of older people was one of the major challenges facing the service and that everything possible should be done to enable older people to remain independent, healthy and in their own homes. The Report recommended that all professions concerned with care of older people should receive more training in understanding their needs. Political policies have influenced approaches to the care of older people in the community. Older people have been identified as a priority group for community care initiatives (Redfern, 1991) in a number of statements (DHSS, 1976, 1977, 1981, 1987, 1988). However, the current programme of reforms that the National Health Service (NHS) is undergoing are seen by Ham (1993) as 'More fundamental than any experienced since its inception in 1948' (p. 1).

The major impact of these reforms relates to delivery of services to patients and the organization and financing of the NHS and local authority community care services. Services are envisaged (DOH, 1989a) as becoming more responsive to users' needs, with an emphasis on increased efficiency with resources. NHS contracts or service agreements will be negotiated between health authorities/general practitioner (GP) fundholders as purchasers of care, and hospitals/units (including NHS Trusts) as providers of care, and, as such, contracts will specify quality, quantity and cost of services to be provided.

These reforms with their emphasis on increased competitiveness, cost-effectiveness and consumer choice have implications for older people, in so far as changes within general practice resulting from the Review give fundholding GPs practice funds for purchasing a defined range of services for their patients. This may have the potential of increasing the vulnerability of older people because of the pressure on competitive services. This, in turn, may mean priority being given to acute treatments rather than to care for older people which is often lengthy, expensive and uncertain (Potrykus, 1991; Tombs, 1991). There is, therefore, cause for concern for protecting the rights of older people in this new health care market economy (Potrykus, 1991; Tombs, 1991).

In relation to community care services, assessment of individual care needs is seen by Ham (1993) as the cornerstone of the new arrangements, along with care management systems, to secure the most appropriate packages of care for individuals. However, the arbitrary separation between health and social care (DOH, 1989b) runs the inherent risk of older people falling through the net and may result, according to Glover (1991), in a greater burden on carers. It is the community nurse, practising at the forefront of policy implementation, who is in a key position to ensure the delivery of effective community nursing care to older people. In view of the implications of an ageing population, and changing organizational requirements and resource levels, Raynor (1990) sees the community nurse as being in a prime position to take the lead in working with older people in the community.

Having highlighted the major changes of the NHS reforms and consequential issues of concern for older people, the next stage is to clarify the meaning of 'older people' and the implications of population trends, in order to offer underpinning to the exploration of 'needs'.

Who are older people?

Chronological age, that is the standard retirement age (UK), is often used as the basis for defining age – this is still seen as a convenient age limit for defining old age, but Bond and Coleman (1992) point out that as fewer and fewer people are actually retiring at this age, such universally used definitions of old age must be used with caution. Rhetorically, old people are a national 'priority care' group but care of old people in the community is still mainly carried out by the least qualified staff and is directed more towards geriatric care which emphasizes diseases of old age rather than through gerontological enquiry, i.e. the scientific study of old age and ageing processes (Warnes, 1989). Such enquiry recognizes the complex, multi-dimensional process of ageing and the needs of older people themselves, within an intergenerational framework (Willcocks, 1992). Gerontological enquiry should help to modify some of the negative reactions to population ageing and older people that still prevail and equate ageing with problems, hardship, illness and negative experiences. Ageing is a normal biological process which cannot be prevented but much can be done to reduce disease, increase fitness and improve social consequences of growing old in society today. There is evidence, according to Phillipson and Walker (1986), of the generally disadvantaged position of old people in society and the dominance of ageism.

Ageism, as suggested by Cornwell (1989), or negative discrimination on grounds of age, can affect any age group, but in contemporary Britain is most commonly practised against old people. It is this that marks out the health care they receive as different from that offered to younger patients. Cornwell (1989) found that one of the most common complaints of older people themselves, and their carers, was their stereotyping as 'the old'. The use of blanket terms such as 'the elderly' and 'the retired' conveys, according to Victor (1991), 'an image of a homogeneous social group devoid of internal social divisions and differences. This is one of the most enduring of all stereotypes of old age' (p. 169).

Population trends

In order to reflect individual differences, it is of paramount importance that primary health care teams, by means of profiling their populations, identify the size and characteristics of their population of older people so that needs can be identified and services and expertise targeted effectively and efficiently. Antonson and Robertson (1993) suggest that arrangements for community care should take account of the views of those in need of help. In this way, health services can be based on needs of individuals, groups and communities and not just on those defined by professionals. Health needs can be met through partnerships with consumers. Their study identified that community nurses would be in a good position to identify unmet needs and, in particular, work with carers.

White (1989) suggests that, with the increase in the older population, the current emphasis on primary health care, the importance attached to preventive health and the continuing attempt to reduce hospital mean stays in a wide range of specialties, far greater knowledge and demands will be placed on community nurses in the future. Hence, their educational needs will increase rather than remain static.

The projected increase (OPCS, 1986) in the relative size of the older population in the next 20 years, is fairly slight, from 9.0 million in 1981 to 10.8 million in 2001. In Britain, there will be a large increase of smaller cohorts in extreme old age, i.e. 75–84 and 85+. Older people are the group that are seen as requiring the most social security expenditure and medical support, with the very oldest among them expected to have the greatest need. However, Perls (1995) suggests that a rethinking of this prevailing view of ageing as advancing infirmity may be needed as he was surprised to find that 'the oldest old were often the most healthy and agile of the senior people under my care' (p. 50).

Women tend to live longer than men and therefore outnumber men by 2:1 in the 75 years and over age group, and women tend to marry men older than themselves. For both these reasons, widowhood is very common (OPCS, 1989). A greater number of older people now live in their own homes (Ross, 1991) and, conversely, the proportion of older people living with relatives, other than a spouse, has fallen, although it must be emphasized that living alone does not necessarily imply lack of familial support. The implications are that extreme old age is a life stage that may feature greatest material poverty, at a time when extra expenses, for example, for heating and transport, may accrue, particularly for those in poor health. Dependency in old age can be increased or even created by reduced income, poor housing and other disadvantages, arising from the relatively low status assigned by society to older people. History has influenced the current cohort of older people, in so far as some have never married and have no children and fewer kin networks, thus limiting sources of support. The projected reduction in the relative proportion of young elderly means that fewer relatively fit people in the 65–74 age group will be able to support the increasing number of frail much older kin. The stated policy of the Department of Health and Social Security (1981) was to maintain older people at home rather than in residential care. Very little assistance, either informal or formal, is received by carers (Jones and Vetter, 1984) leading to a great deal of distress and psychological morbidity. Despite these pressures on carers, Arber et al. (1986) found that service provision appears to be provided where no family is available rather than to assist carers in their support.

With the increase in the older population, older people are a group of growing importance and they are heavy users of health and social services, which is of particular relevance to providers of health and social support.

Clarke's study (1984) showed that community nurses spend most of their time working with older patients. With the number and proportion of older people in the UK population projected to increase, demands for caring for older people will require innovation in care delivery. Such practice must be underpinned by education and research in the field of gerontology (Ryder, 1994) so that this growing section of the population are able to maintain their optimum health.

Community nurses are uniquely placed among professional groups to work with and identify the need for appropriate nursing intervention in the community, to understand the physical and emotional burden borne by carers, to note consequences of early discharge and to draw attention to some of the issues of supporting people within the community, in particular in relation to the special needs of older people at home.

Needs of older people

Two major recommendations that are reflected within the community care reforms relate to assessment of needs and individual choice in determining the meeting of such needs. Assessment of individual needs is seen as the approach to identifying special-needs of older people and, as highlighted earlier, is seen by Ham (1993) as the cornerstone of the new arrangements in moving towards a needs led service. McWalter et al. (1994) see needs assessment as central to the work of practitioners in health and social services, particularly in relation to the reforms. However, Ormond (1994) stresses that assessment of needs is important not only for the older person but also for their carer, in order to create services that are more responsive to need.

Ong (1991) recommends a more systematic approach to the assessment of needs of individuals and the translation of such needs into a care plan. Ong (1991) also recognizes the importance of the role of carers and raises four questions, seen as central to this approach: 'How do clients define their needs? How do carers define their needs? How do professionals assess needs of client and carer? What skills can each professional offer to respond to identified needs?' (p. 639).

Such questions emphasize the importance of in-depth examination from the patients' and carers' perspective, when assessing needs.

If community nurses are serious about understanding people's needs, they have to acknowledge these needs are socially constructed and closely bound up with identities and expectations, which is of particular significance for the life histories older people bring to their assessments. Ong (1991) also suggests that the way clients define themselves, the relationship between carer and client, carer's self-perception, the theoretical and practical approaches in nursing and many structural factors, play a significant role in the definition of needs.

The basis of decision making is seen as the professional assessment of patient needs which is linked closely to the relationship between the patient's health and carer well-being, including the social, psychological, economic and physical costs of caring. Needs-led assessment is seen as focusing upon identifying needs of those assessed with a view to determining how those needs might be met rather than the suitability of patients for particular services. Reassessment procedures offer excellent opportunities to ensure services change with changing needs of the patient and that inappropriate provision is minimized. For this to occur, staffing levels must be such that caseload size allows for more than a reactive response to referrals.

Need is a relative concept implying elements of both factual information and value judgements. Therefore, assessment of need must be understood in terms of the person or group making the judgement and implies there is no single definition of need. This is recognized by McWalter et al. (1994) who suggest that assessment of individual need should be considered in terms of 'normative' need, i.e. need as defined by the professional; in terms of 'perceived' need, i.e. defined as what people see to be their needs; in terms of 'expressed' need which is seen as perceived need turned into action and in terms of 'comparative' need, i.e. the comparison of need between similar populations and uptake of services. In addition to assessment of needs and identification of appropriate interventions, unmet needs must also be identified, as Dowrick (1993) points out, as the incidence of unreported health problems is very high among older people. This reflects the importance of community nurses being engaged in proactive, sensible, knowledgeable assessments of older people's health needs (McWalter et al., 1994). Taking this into consideration, Caldock (1993) suggests assumptions cannot be made about levels of knowledge and skills of practitioners and the broadening of assessment to include the knowledge and value of multidisciplinary team working would positively reflect a gerontological approach to assessment of needs.

However, multidisciplinary working requires a shared understanding of common concepts to ensure clear and accurate communication and common comprehension of practice. The nature of such interprofessional collaboration should be of a kind that is based on providing the best and most appropriate package of care rather than on misunderstood arbitrary professional boundaries.

The assessment of needs of older people, according to Ormond (1994) is dependent upon a clear explanation of the purpose of assessment and the process should involve qualitative, in-depth interviewing with individual older people and their carers. Effectiveness is seen as dependent on three key conditions: first, the acknowledgement by professionals of the need to engage in a power shift to an exchange of mutual enquiry with style being adapted to individual situations; secondly, finely tuned listening skills which rely on this power shift having taken place and thirdly, sufficient time devoted to assessment of health needs of both the individual older person and their carers. Adequate time for proper and thorough assessments (Ormond, 1994) is also supported by Barrett (1994) who points out that

' "Quick fixes" are neither possible or desirable – speedy 30 or 40 minute assessments are not acceptable in child protection work nor should they be seen as appropriate for older people. They are a manifestation of ageist practice' (p. 269).

Hence, the evidence offered reflects the complexity of undertaking a thorough needs-led assessment and therefore assumes, according to Allen *et al.* (1992), a high level of individual professional expertise to enable services derived from the reality of older people in need to be of a high standard. The fundamental principle underlying such an assessment is to offer choice to older people and their carers in relation to the community care services that are delivered. But how much say do older people and their carers actually have in the services they receive, in the decisions about how, when and where the services are delivered and in who provides them? Cornwell (1989) indicates that developing choices and flexibility for older people is an area in which considerable development is needed. So often recognition of the range of heterogeneous needs of older people is overlooked with need being seen as homogeneous. Studies such as those by Cornwell (1989) and Allen *et al.* (1992) have found little evidence of older people being able to operate as informed consumers because of the limited knowledge of availability of services both by the older person and their carers, with carers only finding out when they are at breaking point. This lack of knowledge on availability was found to reflect a lack of knowledge by community nurses with services being concentrated on those with greatest need. However, Allen *et al.* (1992) found that in reality there sometimes appeared to be a conspiracy of silence regarding availability because practitioners were concerned about a potential increase in demand and increased cost implications. Community nurses need to be aware that older people are seeking more information on what is available, what the roles are of the different personnel and how they can access services.

In order to meet the range of needs that may be identified through assessment, community care reforms indicate that complex packages of care would be available to enable older people to remain at home. However, evidence is limited regarding the actual delivery of such complex packages and generally they are seen to relate to only one or two services, with older people having little choice as to what goes into their personal care packages and that rationing was the order of the day. Waters (1995) likens this effect of dwindling resources to the game of 'pass the parcel' where:

> The parcel is the responsibility for meeting the needs of the (older) patient. The music of 'care in the community' plays in the background and the parcel is held by social services, until the money runs out; then it is passed to the health services, until resources begin to dwindle. At this point the relative is left holding the parcel. Ultimately it is the patient and his/her carer who are left in the difficult position of not being able to afford full-time care at home, yet not really wanting to relocate to a nursing home. Are we really providing choice for people? (p. 221)

Cornwell (1989) suggests that older people do want to have their health problems taken seriously and not just seen as age related. In the same study, older people expressed their wish to be consulted about visits to their home and, despite the fact that a range of people may be involved in their care, felt their problems were being 'dealt with' as opposed to feeling truly 'cared for'. The range of service providers is also highlighted by Waters (1995) who suggests that older people requiring rehabilitation can pass through the hands of many different service providers and this can often result in fragmented and poorly coordinated care packages.

The nature of choice not only relates to availability of services or agencies but also to the role of carer. Small qualitative studies (Finch, 1985; Bell *et al.*, 1987; Anonymous, 1988) reflect carers' feelings of having no freedom to choose to be a carer and is linked in their role in relation to obligation, family responsibility and duty as much as feelings of love and affection. Carers also express the fact that their role as carer often begins years before it is recognized and is one that builds up gradually. Cornwell (1989) found that this burden of caring is also reflected by older people themselves who are fearfully appreciative of how destructive being a burden can be to a close relationship, which begs the question: informed choice? Or does choice equate with availability or a response that reflects no alternative? Hence, Government statements that emphasize a needs-led service and consumer choice are at odds with the manifestation of a resource constrained supply of care, i.e. in reality a needs-led approach is operating within an organizational framework where resources govern availability and are being targeted at those most in need.

Lack of availability of resources is starting to mirror the experience in America where for most older people the situation, according to Harding (1995), is not a happy one. People who need long-term care pay for it themselves until they have exhausted their assets, a process known as 'spending down'. In Britain, many older people who thought the state would look after them in old age are having to pay large sums for their care. This has arisen from the dividing line between health care, free at the point of delivery, and social care, which is chargeable. The prospect of having to impoverish oneself in old age and then become dependent on 'welfare' is a cause of great anxiety to most older people. Approximately 75 per cent of the older population are, according to Shaw (1993), able to get about and need minimal assistance. In spite of these figures, the popular stereotype of equating older people with physical and mental deterioration persists. Focusing on disease and malfunction only serves to foster a blinkered view of the processes of ageing; assessment of needs, Wade (1993) suggests, should focus towards things a person can do and likes to do.

This comprehensive approach to need is also supported by Williamson (1981, cited in Shaw, 1993) who suggests:

Need is not confined to the relatively narrow field of therapeutics but it is expanded to include medical, psychological and social need. Nor is the determination of need confined to the individual old person but it is enlarged to include the needs of the family of which the old person is a member and, indeed, the needs of their local community in so far as the community is involved in supporting the individual old person. (p. 23)

It is important, therefore, to locate older people in an intersecting system consisting of biological, psychological and social elements. Traditionally, policies and programmes have been concerned with the pathological aspects of ageing and this has contributed to a distorted perception of old age. While the part played by disease remains an important one, a pathological model of ageing can be seen as an inadequate basis for understanding the complex problems of old people. Needs assessment should consider primary, secondary and tertiary prevention. Many old people are well and, as recommended by Victor and Higginson (1994), can benefit from programmes of care delivery which concentrate on health promotion, as many interventions are as effective in older people as those of middle age.

The provision of available, high standard assessment presents many challenges, some of which have already been alluded to and include issues such as funding, staff education, confidentiality, team relationships and interactions with a range of community agencies, general practitioners and hospitals and even such practical matters as the written form of assessment. Wade (1993) recognizes the value and influence of different perspectives within the multidisciplinary ethos required for community care. Furthermore, Kerkstra and Beemster (1994), Bull (1994) and Slack (1994) all highlight the positive contributions that such a diverse knowledge base can bring to needs assessment of older people, who have a right to highly skilled, effective nursing care.

Conclusion

This exploration of the needs of older people has identified that needs assessment of individual older people and their carers is a complex, highly skilled activity that requires knowledgeable community nurses, who are able to work in partnership with older people, who are able to devote time to elicit need and who are able to participate in the delivery of community health care through multidisciplinary team working.

This chapter has highlighted the fact that, within current health care policy, older people remain a relatively powerless group in society and, according to Luker (1988), straddle professional boundaries. Hence, it is of fundamental importance that consideration is given to the following key questions, which have direct bearing on the quality of care that is provided in order to meet the needs of older people.

Points to consider

1 Studies such as Ford (1995) demonstrate the effectiveness of care delivered by qualified practitioners. Where does the individual older person's right to such care lie within current, economically driven, community nursing grade mix reviews?

2 Community nurses are ideally situated to reaffirm their commitment to working with older people. What evidence can community nurses present to demonstrate that gerontological knowledge informs this specialist aspect of their role?

3 To what extent are the changes in the provision of continuing care services for older people consumer driven – is this more rhetoric that reality?

4 How can community nurses reconcile the apparent contradiction between the present emphasis of consumer choice and the reality of resource constrained supply of care, with access apparently controlled by 'assessment' and participation in it controlled by 'care management'?

5 To what extent do primary health care services offer support for carers? Is support for carers seen as a priority by community nurses, particularly if such additional support brings no obvious financial benefits to primary health care services?

References

Allen, I., Hogg, D. and Peace, S. 1992: *Elderly people: choice, participation and satisfaction*. London: Policy Studies Institute.

Anonymous 1988: Ethnic minority carers – the invisible carers. *Health and Race*, April/May.

Antonson, M. and Robertson, C. 1993: A study of consumer-defined need amenable to community nursing intervention. *Journal of Advanced Nursing*, **18**, 1617–25.

Arber, S., Gilbert, N. and Evandrou, M. 1986: Gender, household composition and receipt of domiciliary services by elderly disabled people. *Journal of Social Policy*, **17**, 2, 153–75.

Barrett, D. 1994: Watching your language. *Health Visitor*, **67**, 8, 269.

Bell, R., Gibbons, S. and Pinchen, I. 1987: *Patterns and processes in carers' lives: action research with informed carers of elderly people*. London: Health Education Council.

Bond, J. and Coleman, P. 1992: *Ageing in society – an introduction to social gerontology* (2nd edn). London: Sage Publications.

Bull, M. 1994: Use of formal community services by elders and their family caregivers 2 weeks following hospital discharge. *Journal of Advanced Nursing*, **19**, 503–8.

Caldock, K. 1993: A preliminary study of changes in assessment: examining the relationship between recent policy and practitioners' knowledge, opinions and practice. *Health and Social Care in the Community*, **1**, 3, 139–46.

Clarke, L. 1984: *Domiciliary services for the elderly*. Beckenham Kent: Croom Helm.

Cornwell, J. 1989: *The consumers' view: elderly people and community health services*. London: King's Fund Centre.

Department of Health 1989a: *Working for patients*. London: HMSO.

Department of Health 1989b: *Caring for people*. London: HMSO.

Department of Health and Social Security 1976: *Priorities for health and social services in England*. London: HMSO.

Department of Health and Social Security 1977: *Circular CNO (77) 8 Nursing in primary health care.* London: DHSS.

Department of Health and Social Security 1981: *Growing older.* London: HMSO.

Department of Health and Social Security 1987: *Promoting better health.* London: HMSO.

Department of Health and Social Security 1988: *Community care: agenda for action (Griffiths report).* London: HMSO.

Dowrick, C. 1993: Self-assessment by elderly people – a means of identifying unmet need in primary care. *Health and Social Care in the Community,* **1**, 5, Sept. 289–96.

Finch, H. 1985: *Health and older people: attitudes towards health in older age and caring for older people.* London: Social and Community Planning Research.

Ford, P. 1995: What older people value in nursing. *Nursing Standard,* February, **9**, 20, 25–8.

Glover, R. 1991: Evolution or extinction? *Journal of District Nursing,* **9**, 12, 18–19.

Ham, C. 1993: *The new National Health Service.* Oxford: Radcliffe Medical Press.

Harding, T. 1995: Into the wilderness. *Community Care,* 27 April, 3 May, 20–1.

HMSO 1979: *Royal commission on the national service report.* London: HMSO.

Jones, D. and Vetter, N. 1984: A survey of those who care for the elderly at home: their problems and their needs. *Journal of Social Science and Medicine,* **19**, 5, 511–14.

Kerkstra, A. and Beemster, F. 1994: The quality of assessment visits in community nursing. *Journal of Advanced Nursing,* **19**, 1205–11.

Luker, K. 1988: The nurse's role in health promotion and preventive health care of the elderly. In Wells, C. and Freer, N. (eds), *Ageing population – burden or challenge?* pp. 155–61. New York: M. Stockton Press.

McWalter, G., Toner, H., Corser, A., Eastwood, J., Marshall, M. and Turvey, T. 1994: Needs and needs assessment: their components and definitions with reference to dementia. *Health and Social Care in the Community,* **2**, 4, 213–19.

Ong, B. 1991: Researching needs in district nursing. *Journal of Advanced Nursing,* **16**, 638–47.

OPCS 1986: *Mid 1985 population estimates for England and Wales.* OPCS Monitor PP1 86/1. London: OPCS.

OPCS 1989: *General household survey.* London: OPCS.

Ormond, K. 1994: Wise words. *Health Service Journal,* August, p. 28.

Perls, T.T. 1995: The oldest old. *Scientific American,* January, 50–5.

Phillipson, C. and Walker, A. 1986: *Ageing and social policy.* Aldershot: Gower.

Potrykus, C. 1991: The numbers game. *Health Visitor,* **64**, 6, 180–1.

Raynor, M. 1990: The changing role of the district nurse. *District Nursing Association Newsletter,* **III**, 2, 6–7.

Redfern, S (ed.) 1991: *Nursing elderly people* (2nd edn). Edinburgh: Churchill Livingstone.

Ross, F. 1991: Nursing old people in the community. In Redfern, S. (ed.), *Nursing elderly people* (2nd edn) pp. 465–84. Edinburgh: Churchill Livingstone.

Ryder, E. 1994: Gerontology within district nurse education. *Journal of Advanced Nursing,* **20**, 430–6.

Shaw, M. 1993: *The challenge of ageing* (2nd edn). Edinburgh: Churchill Livingstone.

Slack, J. 1994: Rationing resources. *Elderly Care,* **6**, 5, 37.

Tombs, A. 1991: Doubts about elderly care. *Health Visitor,* **64**, 6, 181.

Victor C, 1991: *Health and healthcare in later life.* Milton Keynes: Open University Press.

Victor, C. and Higginson, I. 1994: Effectiveness of care for older people. *Quality in Health Care,* **3**, 210–16.

Wade, B. 1993: *The changing face of community care for older people: year 1, setting the scene.* London: RCN, Daphne Heald Research Unit.

Warnes, A. 1989: *Human ageing and later life – multidisciplinary perspectives.* London: Edward Arnold.

Waters, K.R. 1995: Pass the parcel: care of the elderly in the community. *British Journal of Therapy and Rehabilitation,* May **2**, 5, 221–2.

White, R. 1989: Caring for and caring about the elderly – defining dynamics. *Senior Nurse*, **9**, 6, 22–4.

Willcocks, D. 1992: Gerontology. Only another 'ology'? *Generations Review*, **2**, 2, June, 2–5.

Williamson, J. 1981: Practical assessment of the geriatric patients. Besançon. In Shaw, M. 1993: *The challenge of ageing* (2nd edn). Edinburgh: Churchill Livingstone.

5 A right to health care?

Eileen Groves

The language of rights has become an integral part of our socialization process, the notion of rights being applied to many aspects of living. People frequently talk of their rights both legal and moral, in relation to a wide variety of issues. For example, rights to freedom of speech; to free choice; rights to particular benefits, entitlements or welfare services.

Rights, if indeed they exist, inevitably bring with them corresponding duties or obligations from others. That is, having rights to act in a particular way or rights to certain services has implications that 'someone' has a duty or obligation to enable those rights to be realized.

Conflicts and dilemmas arise when the number of people claiming a particular right exceeds the resources available to meet those claims and those duties and obligations become untenable.

In recent years health care professionals and the general public have become increasingly embroiled in the language of rights in relation to health care services and to expectations of certain standards of care and treatment. This has been reinforced by the publication of The Patient's Charter *(DOH, 1995) which sets out rights of entitlement and the standard of service one might expect to receive from the National Health Service (NHS).*

But to what extent can we continue to exercise a right to health care, legally or morally, in today's climate of free market ideology within the National Health Service, and given the ever increasing difficulties of dealing with scarce resources? If it were agreed that despite such difficulties there still remains such a right, is there also then a duty to provide whatever that health care need might be even if it is for unusual, very expensive or prolonged care and treatment?

As provision becomes more problematic and the chasm between the rhetoric of patients' rights to NHS health care and the reality of providing such care widens, there will be implications for all health care professionals. Nurses cannot remain indifferent to such issues. Working at the coal-face of health care provision there is on the one hand an expectation that they will meet the rights and needs of patients and clients, yet on the other there is the need to work within tightly controlled budgets which may make this an impossible task.

This chapter seeks to explore the nature of rights and the extent to which we might expect to have health care needs met given the current resource allocation issues.

A right to health care?

'The National Health Service is a service for everybody. For many people and their families it is the most important public service in their lives' (Bottomley, 1995). *The Patient's Charter* (DOH, 1995) on Rights and Standards throughout the National Health Service (NHS) lists many rights and expectations which individuals should receive, and on the issue of access to services states that 'You have the right to receive health care on the basis of your clinical need, not on your ability to pay, your lifestyle or any other factor' (p. 5).

The question of entitlement to health care was acknowledged as long ago as 1948 in the United Nations Universal Declaration of Human Rights which states that 'Everyone has the right to a standard of living adequate for the health and well-being of himself and his family, including food, clothing, housing and medical care and necessary social services, and the right to security in the event of unemployment, sickness, disability, widowhood, old age or other lack of livelihood in circumstances beyond his control' (Article 25).

This statement recognizes the concept of health care in its widest holistic context and is clearly not confined simply to the right to medical care. Health care is now recognized as a 'public good' rather than a 'private good' that one is expected to buy for oneself (Charlesworth, 1993). The World Health Organization reaffirmed in its declaration of Alma Ata of 1978 that 'health . . . is a fundamental human right and that attainment of the highest possible level of health is a most important world-wide social goal, without distinction of race, religion, political belief, economic or social condition' (WHO, 1978 p. 2). In order to attain a high standard of health it may be necessary at some time in one's life to access health care. But can people in today's market led health care environment, with the difficulties of scarce resources, still work with the ideology of 'a right to health care'?

This paper seeks to explore the nature of rights, how they apply to today's NHS, and just how absolute such rights are, if indeed, they exist at all.

Introduction

The language of rights is extremely complex and the nature of rights to which an individual may lay claim are many and varied and may encompass a whole range of legal and institutional rights as well as moral rights. It is the intention within this paper to select those aspects of rights which may be usefully and practically applied to the question 'Do individuals have a right to health care'?

Any discussion on rights of entitlement to a service or commodity brings with it equally compelling debate on issues such as:

• Do we each have equal rights, or do some have more rights than others?

- How can we ensure that individuals with rights are treated equally, fairly and justly?
- If there is a right to health care, are there ever situations in which an individual might forfeit those rights?

It is anticipated that an exploration of the question of rights to health care will likely raise more questions than it offers answers and also raise further issues for discussion. Before exploring the nature of rights and whether we have been granted a right to health care, it is perhaps worth taking time to look at what is meant by care and in particular health care.

Health care

A dictionary definition of the word 'care' offers a multiplicity of concepts, all of which merit definition in their own right. The Oxford Minidictionary (1988) offers the following definition: 'serious attention and thought, caution to avoid damage or loss, protection, supervision, worry and anxiety, to feel concern, interest or liking, and that to "take care of", is to take charge of the safety and well-being of, or to deal with'.

Such definitions of care could be applied to the care of inanimate objects which one covets or of animals. Ye· · arly here are all of the elements one would hope to find in the care of t. e who are ill or vulnerable in any way. It can come in the form of practical assistance to ensure their protection, safety and well-being and/or in showing concern and interest in that person.

These notions of 'care' for one another are a part of living with and providing for one another which gives meaning and value to our existence. We all at some time or other in our lives are the providers or recipients of care.

The subject of care and caring is diverse in itself (Brown, Kitson and McKnight, 1992) and some elements defined as care may conflict or be difficult to harmonize, for example, the practical aspects of care and the emotional/attitudinal aspects of care (Griffin, 1983). However, the concern of this paper is to explore whether people have a right to professional health care.

Care may be said to become professional when an individual through illness, acute or long-term, experiences a loss of autonomy such that he or she becomes unable to care for all their basic needs or is unable to function at an acceptable level. Those who would care for them in a lay capacity may experience difficulty in providing that acceptable level and require professional intervention which may be medical or care, in its more holistic concept. Is there at such times a 'health care right'?

Rights

Rights may be legal, civil or institutional. This includes rights that are granted to people by means of legislation or rights that are conferred on individuals or groups as a result of their belonging to a particular organization which gives them certain entitlements. Fromer (1981) suggests that we have two categories of rights. The first is option rights, which are essentially concerned with personal freedom, although clearly not total freedom (freedom within set boundaries, that is not infringing on other people's rights). The second is welfare rights, which are primarily concerned with benefits and legal entitlements, for example the right to free education. Another group of rights is said to be moral rights or natural rights: rights which. for moral reasons, ought to be protected.

The importance of establishing rights and the influence of rights in our lives is reflected by Professor Dworkin (1981) who suggests that 'Individual rights are political trumps held by individuals' and further that 'they are crucial in representing the majority's promise to the minorities that their dignity and equality will be respected' (p. 205).

John Locke, an influential seventeenth-century philosopher and proponent of the concept of natural law, defended the rights to 'life, liberty and estate' as being God-given moral rights which man had a right to defend if necessary by force (Gillon, 1992). It is such sentiments which have formed the basis of various national and international declarations of human rights, such as the United Nations Declaration of Human Rights (1948).

Yet, not all human rights as listed in such declarations are natural rights. The right to education, to health care, to legal representation are human rights brought about through legislation but are not natural rights. Some rights require positive action by another action, to ensure an individual's rights are fulfilled. The rights to goods or services is an example; others require negative action, for example, a right not to be harmed. As Gillon (1992) suggests rights are justified claims that require action or restraint from others while Fromer (1981) contends that the granting of rights automatically implies corresponding duties and responsibilities; one cannot exist without the other.

Therefore, if there is a right to health care, using the justified claims approach, then by implication someone has a duty or responsibility to enable that right to be exercised. Such rights are referred to as claim rights. However, it needs to be recognized that a right is not necessarily something to which we have to make a claim but something to which we have claim. But can the duty to provide for a claim be absolute if that claim right is to a commodity which is in short supply, as are some forms of specialized health care? Downie and Calman (1994) suggest that for there to be a right to receive, the right should be 'practicable'. This appeal to practicability can be seen as being implicit and, to some extent, explicit in the Mission Statements of many of the newly formed NHS Trusts, many of which indicate that their particular range of health services will be provided within available resources. What remains unclear is the concept of a right to health care. Perhaps the question should be, is there a moral right to health care? Philosophers involved in the study of bioethics have conflicting views on whether health care should be or can be considered as a right. Some put forward strong argument that all health care is something everyone should receive regardless of the cost (Brody, 1986), others argue that the best that can be claimed is a decent minimum of health care (Fried, 1992; Buchanan, 1978). Still others argue that there is no such thing as a right to health care and that such an expression is nothing more than a dangerous slogan (Fried, 1982).

Beauchamp and Childress (1989) put forward two premises for believing that there is a moral right to health care. The first suggests that there are similarities between health care and other needs which have conventionally been protected by governments, for example, provision of adequate resources for protection from the threats presented by crime, fire and pollution. Health care they claim has parallels. The main difference is that such protection of external threats constitutes a general social good as opposed to the predominantly individual good afforded by health care. There are however aspects of health care, such as health promotion, health education and screening which might be said to be for the greater social good. It could be argued that individual health should be afforded that same parallel of protection by means of adequate resources to provide for individual health care needs.

The second argument Beauchamp and Childress (1989) offer to support a moral right to health care is that ill-health is largely a matter of unpredictable bad luck or misfortune over which the individual has little control. Unlike the costs of the basic necessities of life, it is difficult to predict the cost of health care thus those who are unfortunate enough to be disadvantaged by ill health over which they have little control ought, in the interests of justice, be able to access such health care; this should enhance their opportunity to regain functional capacity or prevent possible further deterioration. Johnstone (1989) makes an interesting and equally compelling argument in defence of a moral right to health care. She observes that as health care has the power to promote life and well-being, both of which are moral ends, and enhances potential for other moral interests such as autonomy, it would be morally wrong to deny the right to such care.

It is questionable whether the two types of rights, claim rights (through legislation) and moral rights can be compared in this way as both may be seen to be equally valuable concepts within their own sphere. However Thompson et al. (1988) would suggest that legal rights have the stronger persuasion and are paramount as they state 'moral rights have only the strength which existing social consensus and convention give them, and impose only moral obligations on others, whereas legal rights may be enforceable through the courts' (pp. 109–10). Just how far the law might be expected to intervene, when the claim right to health care is not met in accordance with the National Health Service Act (DHSS, 1977) or Patient's Charter Standards (1992, 1995), will be addressed later.

If it is agreed that there is a legal and/or moral right to care, it is important to recognize that individuals have the right not to exercise that right, that is not to use the health care services offered to them. This can of course create dilemmas for some health care workers, who may have difficulty in accepting such a choice and choose then to take a paternalistic approach to care, i.e. giving care on the basis of acting in another's best interests. In many cases the choice to opt out of health care will only affect the patient concerned; indeed in law, to continue care or treatment in such circumstances would constitute the crime of battery or trespass against the person. However the dilemmas may be compounded when such a choice may affect the health of others, as in cases of infectious disease.

In the main however, health care workers are concerned with acting as advocates to patients and clients in ensuring that their rights and entitlements to health care are met. One of the great difficulties for health care professionals working in today's health care environment is the dilemma created by on the one hand taking on that role of advocate, and on the other working within tightly controlled budgets and management structures. All health care workers through education and training and through professional Codes of Conduct have placed upon them rights, duties, responsibilities and principles which are encompassed within a deontological (duty based) ethical framework; do as you would be done by and treating people as individuals and not as a means to an end (Kant, 1785). They are increasingly working within policies and management structures which could be classed as utilitarian, that is principles which demand that one strives to achieve the greatest good to the greatest number of people. In practice, this means that all activities are determined by the goal of maximizing good and utilizing resources to obtain the best cost-effective benefits. This will mean that some will lose out. Health care workers are finding that increasingly they are caught in the middle, being aware of the wants, needs and rights of patients and clients, being mindful of their advocacy role, but feeling powerless to reach a solution.

The introduction of the purchaser provider system within the NHS has meant that health authorities have moved towards entering into contracts to purchase packages of care. These have to be achieved within tightly controlled budgets, and based on perceived health needs of the locality rather than, as in the past, perceived medical needs. The result is that the right to health care may in theory still be claimed. However the care required may not necessarily be there on the doorstep, in which case the principles of equality of entitlement and equality of access to health care, as stated in the NHS Act (1977), might well be questioned.

Entitlement to health care

One of the fundamental principles in the founding of the National Health Service (1948) was from each according to his means, to each according to his needs. This in practice meant that each individual should contribute financially through taxation and National Insurance contributions and that, regardless of the amount of contribution made, each should receive what he or she needs (Rumbold, 1993). Such contributions were considered to give everyone the right to claim health care when needed.

Leading on from that underlying philosophy, two of the key objectives of the National Health Service at its inception were:

• to provide equality of entitlement to health services;
• to provide equality of access to those services.

These objectives have continued to be central tenets in subsequent health service reviews. The National Health Services Act (1977) states in section 1 that it is the Secretary of State's duty to continue the promotion in England and Wales of a comprehensive health service designed to secure improvement in the physical and mental health of people in those countries and in the prevention, diagnosis and treatment of illness and for that purpose to provide or secure effective provision of services in accordance with the Act. It further suggests in Section 3 that the Minister has a duty to provide a whole range of services and health care provision to meet all reasonable requirements, the significant part of the statement being 'to meet all reasonable requirements'. This duty is in turn delegated to health authorities. Therefore any failure to perform such a duty under Section 3 of the Act would be the responsibility of the health authority concerned.

Meeting all reasonable requirements: it might be argued whether a heart/lung transplant or being sustained indefinitely on a life support machine and all the associated care that such intervention entails, could be considered a reasonable requirement, or access to reproductive technology for infertile couples. Who is to decide on what is a reasonable requirement? More importantly who has the right to make those decisions at either a macro or micro level?

It is easy with hindsight to be critical of the naivety of the NHS creators in 1948, who expected that in providing a right of individuals to free spectacles, free dentures, free surgical procedures and medical care when necessary, that all would have their health care needs met. Modern medical technology has advanced far beyond the bounds of anyone's expectations. Even within the last decade, few would have envisaged that kidney or heart/lung transplants, for example, would be an everyday occurrence and make the logistics of medicine and the delivery of health care an ongoing problem. Unfortunately, as has been witnessed over the years following the inception of the NHS, demand is not self-limiting as was once thought, but is very much relative to supply and demand. As soon as new treatments or procedures are developed there will be a waiting list for that service. It would also be easy at this point to enter into debate about what might be classed as ordinary or extraordinary treatment or means of sustaining life and how far rights to such care can be claimed, but that is an issue which merits its own discussion.

Mason and McCall Smith (1994), begin their debate on health resources and dilemmas in treatment with this statement:

> Even if a basic material is widely available, the cost of harvesting, treating or assembling it put some restraint on its use; moreover, the manpower required for distribution and exploitation of the finished product is always going to be limited. Applying this to medicine, it is clear that it is impossible to provide every form of therapy to everyone – some form of selective distribution is inevitable. (p. 248)

The very nature of selective distribution implies that not all will have their health care needs met and their right to health care is made subject to competition with others who may claim to have equal rights to the same commodity. Much of the sophisticated care available, plus increasing life expectancy, means that people require health care for longer periods of time and the question of rationing and prioritizing becomes a part of the scenario.

A further dimension to the problem lies in the fact that many people, through general education, health education and the media, are now much more aware of their rights in many aspects of life, including the right to health care. The *Patient's Charter* (1992, 1995) highlights the various choices available to people and their rights to obtain health care treatment and services. The subject of distributive justice within the health care setting has been the centre of much debate over recent years and many attempts have been made to provide ethically acceptable solutions based on various theories of justice. These have included a range of selection systems based on such criteria as age, medical need, personal criteria, individual merit or even a lottery system has been proposed as the fairest way of distributing health care resources. Others have produced complicated formulae in an effort to quantify in terms of cost and expected health gain outcomes for a particular individual undergoing a particular health care procedure. The best known of these is the system of quality adjusted life years (QALYs). According to Williams (1985) the essence of a QALY is that it takes a year of healthy life expectancy (following health care intervention) to be worth 1, but regards a year of unhealthy life expectancy to be worth less than 1. In essence, the general idea is that a beneficial health care activity is one which generates a positive amount of QALYs and an efficient health care activity is one where the cost per QALY is as low as possible. A high priority health care activity would therefore be seen to be one where the cost per QALY is low, and a low priority activity is one where the cost per QALY is high. Clearly the whole arena of distributive justice in the context of a right to health care is vast and in all these forms of selection or the QALY approach there are ethical implications which demand further study.

Limits to health care entitlement

Are there ever situations when it might be claimed that an individual has forfeited a right to health care, for example, in the case of so-called self-inflicted illness: the smoker who develops lung disease, the alcoholic who develops liver failure? Harris (1992) suggests that there seems to be something unjust about the possibility of rescuing someone who has deliberately put themselves in danger, rather than someone who for no fault of their own has become in need of help.

One of the difficulties in subscribing to such views in relation to health is that there are so many less obvious ways in which health might be put at risk, for example, through what is eaten, work done, social or sporting activities, all of which might have an equally detrimental effect on health status. Is there any way in which one's age should affect one's right to health care?, for example, the premature neonate or the elderly. One might be seen to have had a 'fair innings', the other requiring very intense and expensive support until mature enough to be independently viable. This also applies to new technology which allows for treatment of the foetus *in utero*. Do those who are mentally ill or those with learning disabilities have the same rights as others? There is clearly another moral debate running through such questions: at what stage in life's continuum and in what situations are we afforded or denied rights? Answers to such questions will depend largely on how people are valued and indeed on how we determine the nature of personhood (Harris, 1992). This is a vitally important area for discussion. The views of people in positions of securing health care provision are determining the purchasing of local health services. The result may be that some individuals are unable to have their right to a particular health care need met.

The legal position

To date the law has offered conflicting views on how it sees the right to health care as being enforceable through the courts. It may be that now the *Patient's Charter* (1992, 1995) is firmly established and local trusts are publishing their service contracts, that more cases may be coming through the courts and thus case law may become established. Much of the case law available is concerned with a right to medical care rather than health care in its more holistic context.

In 1980, four people from the same health authority took legal action claiming that due to shortage of facilities they had waited an unreasonable length of time for orthopaedic surgery. They claimed the Secretary of State and the health authority were in breach of their duty to provide care and as such were denying their right to health care. The court decided it could not intervene and the case went to the Appeal Court. As expected, the reasonable requirement argument was used and Lord Denning considered that claim of a failure of duty could not stand as the actions taken were not totally unreasonable (Kennedy and Grubb, 1994).

In 1987, the case of 'Walker', a baby whose surgery had been postponed five times because of a shortage of skilled nursing staff in paediatric intensive care, did not receive much support either from the trial judge. He suggested that the court was not the place for such decisions to be taken and should not be asked to intervene (Kennedy and Grubb, 1994). More recently the case of 'Child B', a case involving a child requiring treatment for leukaemia and being refused by the trust on the grounds of expense and poor overall prognosis for the child, has brought about a mixed response. The High Court ruled that treatment should be given whilst the Court of Appeal on the same day overruled that decision and supported the trust's action. Kennedy and Grubb (1994) suggest that it is likely the law will develop in three different ways:

firstly – cases relating to complaints about inadequacies in the delivery of care, that is, breach of duty on the part of the health authority in providing a service which falls short of the required standard as a result of reduction of resources;
secondly – cases relating to non-provision where it is said the service should be provided;
thirdly – cases relating to curtailed provision due to reduced resources which adversely affects the patients care.

Conclusion

The author has attempted to use a legal and ethical perspective and draw together some of the very pertinent and current issues relating to the right to health care in today's market-led health service.

In this time of great change within the health care arena, new treatments, new health care initiatives and services are being introduced daily and one thing can be certain, as soon as new treatments and approaches to care are made available there will be a queue of people who would benefit from such care. The balance between an individual's right to health care, whatever their health needs may be, and the issue of scarce resources would seem to be a delicate one and, in today's climate of free market ideology, an insoluble one.

The importance of determining whether there is a moral right to health care is of great significance as clearly legal and civil rights can be given or taken away by those in decision-making positions, whereas rights based on widespread moral intuition and grounded in moral values are much more endurable and powerful (Gillon, 1992). If we have a moral right to health care then such care should be readily available and accessible whenever and wherever the need arises and not be dependent on the political persuasions of the day.

References

Bottomley, V. 1995: *The Patient's Charter and you*. London: Department of Health.

Beauchamp, T. and Childress, J. 1989: *Principles of biomedical ethics*. Oxford: New York.

Brody, B. 1986: Equality and rights in medical care. Cited in Johnstone, M.J. (1989) *Bio-ethics*. London: Bailliére Tindall.

Brown, J., Kitson, L. and McKnight, T. 1992: *Challenges in caring*. London: Chapman and Hall.

Buchanan, A. 1978: Medical paternalism. *Philosophy and Public Affairs*, 370–90.

Johnstone, M.J. 1984: The right to a decent minimum of health care. In Johnstone, M.J. (1989) *Bio-ethics*. London: Baillière Tindall.

Charlesworth, M. 1993: *Bioethics in a liberal society*. Cambridge: Cambridge University Press.

DHSS, 1977: *The National Health Service Act*. London: HMSO.

DOH 1995: *The Patient's Charter and you*. London: DOH.

Downie, R.S. and Calman, K.C. 1994: *Healthy respect– ethics in health care*. Oxford: Oxford Medical.

Dworkin, R. 1981: *Taking rights seriously* (3rd edn). Cambridge: Duckworth.

Fromer, M.J. 1981: *Ethical issues in health care*. St Louis: CV Mosby.

Fried, C. 1982: Equality and rights in medical care. In Johnstone, M.J. (1989) *Bio-ethics*. London: Baillière Tindall.

Gillon, R. 1992: *Philosophical medical ethics*. Winchester: Wiley & Sons.

Griffin, A.P. 1983: A philosophical analysis of caring in nursing. *Journal of Advanced Nursing* **8**, 289–95.

Harris, J. 1992: *The value of life*. London: Routledge.

Johnstone, M.J. 1989: *Bio-ethics: a nursing perspective*. London: Baillière Tindall.

Kant, I. 1785: *Groundwork of the metaphysics of morals*. (Trans.). Cited in Acton, H.B. (1970) *Kant's moral philosophy*. London: Macmillan.

Kennedy, I. and Grubb, A. 1994: *Medical law* (2nd edn). London: Butterworths.

Locke, J. 1690: *Second treatise on government* (Translation) (1966). Oxford: Blackwell.

Mason, J.K. and McCall Smith, R.A. 1994: *Law and medical ethics*. Edinburgh: Butterworths.

Oxford Minidictionary 1988: (2nd edn). Oxford: Oxford University Press.

Rumbold, G. 1993: *Ethics in nursing practice*. London: Baillière Tindall.

Thompson, I.E., Melia, K.M. and Boyd, K.M. 1988: *Nursing ethics*. Edinburgh: Churchill Livingstone.

United Nations 1948: *The universal declaration of human rights*. New York: United Nations.

WHO 1978: *Alma Ata primary health care*. London: HMSO.

Williams, A. 1985: The value of QALYs. *Health and Social Services Journal*, (July), 8, 3–5. Cited in Seedhouse, D. (1988) *Ethics: the heart of health care*. Chichester: J. Wiley and Sons.

Advocacy: possibility or ploy?

Elizabeth E. Mitchell

In this chapter, the origins of the concept of advocacy are examined, together with one interpretation of the present position of advocacy within community nursing. There are legal and ethical considerations to take into account. The reader is urged to reflect on the implications of initiating advocacy within their field of practice. It seems to be assumed that part of a nurse's responsibility is to act as an advocate for patients and carers. If this is to be done, it is necessary to understand the concept and realize the responsibilities that may follow. Many philosophical and practical issues require consideration and some of these are drawn into the discussion within this chapter. There appears to be a strong case for considering a moratorium on advocacy by nurses, pending legal interpretation, while continuing (legally) to speak out on behalf of people they seek to serve.

Introduction

The primary intention of this paper is to explore current concepts of advocacy and to set in context the origins of its inclusion within nursing practice, as well as some of the legal and ethical considerations.

It seems that the word 'advocacy' has been introduced to nursing with apparent ease; from general discussion, it appears to be thought of as a 'good thing' and something that nurses do anyway. But is this not what was, and maybe in some quarters still is, said about the process of nursing? However, just as empirical examination found this is not to be so (NERU, 1986), it is pertinent to look more closely at the implementation of advocacy.

One of the difficulties in researching 'advocacy' from a community perspective, is that much of the information has come from hospital sources, mainly in mental health and psychiatric fields, with little community nursing material available, although the use of advocacy by nurses in other countries is to be found, for example America and Australia.

Origins of the concept

Involvement of nurses in issues wider than immediate 'nursing' were being extolled as early as 1908, with words that seem strangely contemporary. Dock (1908) states 'I am ardently convinced that our national (nursing) association will fail of its higher opportunities . . . if it restricts itself to the narrow path of purely professional questions and withholds its interest and sympathy and its moral support from the great, urgent, throbbing social claims of the day' (p. 895).

Although Meredith (1987) contends that there were many dissenters to this view of the nursing role, that wider vision has persisted. Rogers (1970) states 'A profession exists for social means. Its direct responsibility is to the people it purports to serve' (p. 15).

Advocacy is not new within a legal framework; in Scotland, it is used at the Bar, as someone who professionally pleads the case for another. In addition, throughout the UK, lawyers and other legally trained individuals may assist persons to exercise or defend their rights (Gathercole, 1986). The International Council of Nurses (1973) states that the nurse acts as patient's advocate, protecting and promoting the rights and welfare of the patient. The advocacy role within hospital nursing in the United States of America in the 1970s and 1980s is well documented (Annas and Healey, 1974; Abrams, 1978; Donahue, 1978; Jenny, 1979; Gilligan, 1982; Kohnke, 1982; Zussman, 1982; Nelson, 1988) and worthy of study. However, the evidence appears to be of wide and varying interpretations of the concept. The current usage within nursing seems to have been prompted by the WHO 1st Health Promotion Conference Charter, in which advocacy for health was highlighted as part of health promotion activities. The WHO (1986) reiterated this two years later as 'the challenge for a move towards the new public health by reaffirming social justice and equity as the prerequisites for health, and advocacy and mediation, as the processes of their achievement' (p. 26). WHO Nursing (1986) speaks of the 'obligation of nurses to act as patient advocates' and the 'universal imperatives' to give care that allows clients to make choices for themselves and contributes most to client functioning. The United Kingdom Central Council for Nursing Midwifery and Health Visiting (UKCC, 1989) also highlights the value of the role of patient or client advocacy, seeing it as an integral and essential aspect of good professional practice. Although the meaning is not made clear, nurses are warned that it is not to be seen as an adversarial activity. But the consequences for a nurse undertaking a role of advocate, even when they feel that the activity is in the best interest of the patient, seems hazardous, if in the judgement of an employer, that activity is ill-advised and therefore indefensible.

However, Pyne (1992) maintains that it is a mandatory requirement that each nurse safeguards and promotes the interests of patients and clients, while the UKCC (1992) requires that each nurse, midwife and health visitor report such things that could jeopardize standards of practice, care and safety to 'persons in authority'. But is that advocacy – and does the reporting free the nurse from any further responsibility?

There is currently no basis in law for the role of advocacy if the adult recipient is incompetent to give consent (Dimond, 1989). And if they are competent? Tingle (1988) suggests that there is no absolute, right answer to the issue of advocacy as a nursing role, although it must be seen as combining both ethical and legal complexities. If this is so, then there is a need for nursing to show an awareness of those uncertainties, thus hopefully safeguarding not only the nurse but also the society they seek to serve.

Legal issues

There are legal issues. Although a patient may have a legal and moral choice to treatment, it may not follow that the nurse has a responsibility, either legally, or morally, to act as patient's advocate (Wicker, 1991). Moreover, Wicker (1991) seems to imply that the nurse is working under obligation to the law to prevent future litigation, rather than act pro-actively as advocate for the patient concerned. Following the Mental Health Act (1983) Section 114, by which approved social workers have specific duties to choose the least restrictive option for the patients, social workers are placed in the role of advocate for the person concerned (MacFadyen, 1989). However, three myths exist: that professional expertise and testimony is beyond reproach; that advocacy services are widely available; and thirdly that the legal process is traumatic for the ill person, and that therefore proceeding to claim rights may not be perceived to be in their best interest (Perlin, 1982). And if in practice, the choice of least restrictive options is limited, does that limit the role of advocacy? It may also be that informing someone of their rights is of little value, if they are unable to act upon that information; a role which stops at this stage seems very restrictive in the wider sense of advocacy as empowerment. Furthermore, an independent advocacy service may be hard to achieve, with funding often dictating an apparent allegiance between purchaser and provider.

Strong arguments are advanced for an advocate who works independently (Sang and O'Brien, 1984; Gostin, 1984), whether they are consumer, volunteer or professional. Is that possible for nurses – and do they see the need for that independence?

Although advocates are recognized in law and have right of access to information in the USA, there is no such provision in the UK. This means that the balance of power is still within the hands of the professionals, on whom the citizen advocate depends for cooperation and goodwill (Renshaw and Metcalf, 1987). Perhaps, as Rathwell (1990) suggests, there is a role for the Community Health Councils as advocates.

Healthy public policy requires strong advocates who put health high on the agenda of policy makers 'fostering the work of advocacy groups' (WHO,

1988). In the USA, this role has been taken over by the community nurse specialist (Kuehnert, 1991). They not only act as advocate for an individual or family but also work in partnership with the community and encourage self-help. Part of their role as advocate is in working to enable and empower the community to access and use mechanisms to change policies affecting health. However, the Liverpool Declaration on the Right to Health (Healthy Cities, 1988) warns that meaningful public participation also necessitates acknowledging the freedom of people to make choices and hold views (on health) with which we disagree.

One interpretation of the concept of advocacy

Although Mitchell's (1994) literature review has limitations in its collecting mechanisms, of 154 articles found, only three were of research. Without the availability of research, there cannot (yet) be research based practice in relation to advocacy. The increasing interest in the concept, with its inclusion in the trusts' mission statements, appear at times to be in response to a wish for its inclusion, rather than as an understanding of the possible implications of that inclusion.

From the literature, 19 different categories for the concept of advocacy emerge (Table 6.1). Interestingly, six of these are not identified by the district nurse teachers' survey: autonomy, policy making, consult, intercede, assist and encourage, even though two of these (assist and intercede) appear to be of significance within the literature studied. Furthermore, four categories (acting for, representing, empowerment and awareness) are seen in Mitchell's (1994) study as of greater significance to district nurse teachers than within the examined literature. Other anomalies seem to occur. The district nurses interviewed categorize advocacy as mainly concerned with supporting, representing, informing, empowering, regaining and retaining rights and partnership. Where then is the professional common ground?

Clients seem to see advocacy as supporting, empowering, informing, retaining rights, regaining rights and partnership, in line, to a varying degree, with all the other sources of information. 'Interceding' is considered only by the literature and clients, not by those who practise. However, the small numbers interviewed make this of value as a possible indicator, rather than of significance.

Four major groups of concern were identified by district nurse teachers (Table 6.2): dangers, dilemmas, needs and shifts in practice. These would need to be considered by any community nurse wishing to be advocate: a not insignificant list, on top of all other current working pressures.

Mitchell's (1994) study identifies five themes (Table 6.3 and Figure 6.1). While it needs to be remembered that these are trends found and further research may render even trends invalid, they do offer an initial framework for practitioners to use to explore their thoughts on the concept, before deciding the relevance or possibility of its inclusion in practice. The research is within a district nursing framework. However, discussions across community nursing suggest that all practitioners tend to raise similar views and concerns. What may be at variance within the range of community nursing practice is the client's interpretation of the role.

Table 6.1 Understanding of advocacy: emerging categories

	Category	Used by			
		Literature review	Distric nurset teachers	District nurses	Others
1.	Retaining Rights	X	X	X	X
2.	Regaining Rights	X	X	X	X
3.	Empowering	X	X	X	X
4.	Policy-making	X			
5.	Autonomy	X			
6.	Supporting	X	X	X	X
7.	Consult	X			
8.	Acting for	X	X		
9.	Partnership	X	X	X	X
10.	Encourage	X			
11.	Assist	X			
12.	Intercede	X			X
13.	Recommend	X	X		
14.	Promote	X	X		
15.	Defending	X	X		
16.	Representing	X	X	X	
17.	Inform	X	X	X	X
18.	Plead for	X	X		
19.	Awareness	X	X		

Source: Mitchell, E.E. Examination of the Role of Advocacy in District Nursing Practice, MEd Thesis, University of Liverpool, p. 36, figure 3.2, adapted with permission

Ethical considerations

Cookfair (1991) says that the client, if competent, should be the primary decision maker. Mitchell's research (1994) suggests that one of the reasons that advocacy needs to be discussed and explored is that it is used unknowingly as a justification to act paternalistically. Nurses do not always acknowledge rights: one district nurse felt that she had to some extent the right to tell patients what to do: 'it's for their own good'. Is this not maternalism/paternalism?

Howe (1989) sees a growing obligation for nurses to act as advocates for patients, 'allowing us to claim the six principles (five of moral philosophy and a sixth – a duty of care) on their behalf' (p. 159). However, patients may not wish it thus, seeing that 'you have to be careful of moral issues as they're essentially subjective things' (Mitchell, 1994). Do community nurses have the time and space, as well as the will, to look at patients' subjective needs?

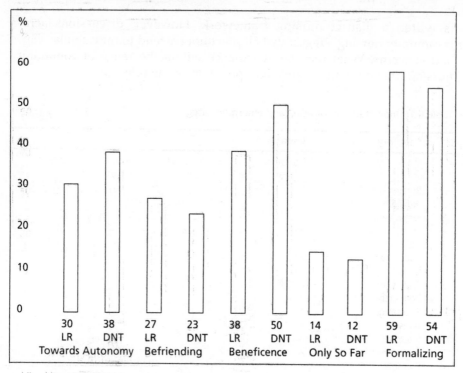

LR = Literature Review
DNT = District Nurse Teachers' Survey

Figure 6.1 Comparison of literature review and district nurse teachers' survey using the emerging themes. *Source* Mitchell, E.E. (1994)

Dyer and Bloch (1982) offer a principle of health care partnership as an alternative to an impersonal respect for autonomy as the appropriate substitute for paternalism within care; this would enable joint decision making, relationships of trust, equality and negotiation to occur and the patient's view to be seen as valid. Certainly, problems may arise from autonomy being seen as a prime ethic: the excessive weight given to impartiality and detachment might cause difficulties within the development of relationships (Harbison, 1992). If advocacy is interpreted paternalistically, patients will continue to be exposed to dominance, by nursing rather than by medical intervention. It may also be that some patients' expectations are for paternalism.

Current state of advocacy

The International League of Societies for Persons with Mental Handicap identify three types of advocacy: self-advocacy, lay or citizen advocacy and legal advocacy. In some countries, there is a fourth – crisis advocacy, taken on because often what is needed is an immediate reactive stance, as an

Table 6.2 Aspects of advocacy and district nursing practice which need to be addressed. Question 13, district nurse teachers' survey

Dangers	• district nurses whose voice is not welcome: boat rockers and Graham Pink encourages dependency • not achievable: can't be all things to all people • legally risky • conflict • paternalistical.
Dilemmas and constraints	• fear of loss of position in the new regime • resourcing for provision of quality care is severely restricted • advocacy without power • what are the parameters? • working within constrained resources, resulting in conflict • limits: need for comparison between UKCC and legal requirements.
Needs	• UKCC Code of Conduct must be strengthened • resourcing must be addressed • set advocacy in context • requires emphasis on notion of working in partnership • district nurses need to be more pro-active in advocacy • emphasis on empowerment • understanding that it is for another's needs, not self • freedom of expression • working with other professionals; enabling informed choices to be made • heightened awareness of concept • research on advocacy and empowerment, especially informed choice • research on advocacy and empowerment badly needed • protection and support for district nurses in the management system; coping strategies; ability to question • understanding of implications • unless specifically timetabled, may not be fully addressed.
Shifts in practice	• context of working with others • wider political advocacy for policy changes • advocacy could be made more avert; much more emphasis in practice • can we be advocates and providers? better advocacy moves to independence from nursing – or changes to UKCC Code of conduct.

Source: Mitchell, E.E. (1994) Examination of the Role of Advocacy in District Nursing Practice, MEd Thesis, University of Liverpool, p. 44, Table 3.2

interim arrangement, until one of the other types of advocacy can be instigated.

One influence on the concept of advocacy may be that consumers no longer see professionals as having all the answers (Breen, 1990). Mitchell (1994) found this when interviewing patients: difficulty in walking is not seen as a result of a stroke nor is improvement expected: 'I'm ninety, ninety three this birthday. Yes I am. That's what's making me feeble and losing me speech' (p. 28).

Rose and Black's (1985) definition of advocacy is as a series of problem-focused activities, to overcome situations which cannot be successfully

Table 6.3 Themes emerging from the literature review on advocacy

Theme I	Towards autonomy:
	retaining, regaining rights; empowering policy-making; autonomy
Theme II	Befriending:
	supporting; consult
Theme III	Beneficence/non-maleficence:
	acting for; partnership; encourage; assist; intercede
Theme IV	Only so far:
	recommend; promote
Theme V	Formalizing:
	defending; representing; inform; plead for; awareness

negotiated through direct service provision. This empowerment is seen as an on-going process of direct interactions, covering all contacts with all clients. People may be seen as objects (known and acted upon) or subjects (knowing and acting) (Freire, 1968, 1973). Thus, advocacy/empowerment work is directed towards two main goals: the transformation of people who have been turned into objects and the transformation of the conditions which reproduce their objectivity. The first without the second will allow the treadmill of disadvantage to continue.

Perhaps as Benner (1990) suggests, it may not be the legalistic form of advocacy that nurses need to consider but a form that arises from belonging in the same community, being a full member and participating together, in an attempt to fight off the tendency to 'discount the person' (p. 82).

Some nurses (Brown, 1986; Allmark, 1992) disagree that the role of advocacy has a place. If patients need advocates, they are being firmly relegated to the place of the dumb, weak and oppressed; they are being forced into a position of dependence on nurses, whose role should be empowerment. Others contend that many nurses have never heard of ethical issues, yet feel that they are fulfilling their role as patient advocate (Morrison, 1991).

The recent changes in the NHS (National Health Service and Community Care Act, 1990 (HM Government, 1990)) gives prominence to consumerism and patients' rights. But as Nocon (1992) points out, consumers usually have money, choice and power; without money, is it merely window dressing? Instructions from a patient to 'do what you think best' is not always the result of choice and handing over control to the health care provider – there may never have been control. A treatment box, full of prescribed items, is not seen to belong to the patient: 'That's their box in the corner; I don't touch it' (Mitchell, 1994).

So where next?

After literature overload, reflection from a weary nurse manager: 'Wonderful papers, wonderful systems, loads of language but in terms of what we have done for the patient, we haven't done a lot more. We are coercing them to accept less because there is less around' (Mitchell, 1994, p. 84).

Do we know what we are doing? Nineteen categories have been found but with no regular pattern of use apparent (Mitchell, 1994), although six are common:

- supporting
- informing
- empowering
- retaining rights
- regaining rights
- partnership.

A small patient sample shows that the above are indeed seen as part of a nursing role, but not seen as advocacy. Sang (1985) warns of the dangers of advocates taking a paternalistic role. This may be even more complex if the advocate sees in the use of Parson's (1952) formulation of the sick role, the patient's legitimate exemption from normal social responsibilities and thus the nurse's role to take over the responsibility and encourage dependency. Nurse managers are aware that the formal theoretical education may not survive the transition to the 'real world'. Perhaps in order to conform to the system, knowledge (of ethics in particular) is set aside from practice and the task is imposed on the patient, providing short-term gain.

There is the danger also that advocacy is seen to have 'always been there' and presumed to be done. It is further complicated if it is seen as a 'silent world of advocacy' (Mitchell, 1994), undertaken without patient/client involvement. This would seem to offer no independent check nor safeguard for the patient and to give no guarantee of becoming independent of the community nursing system. Thus Robinson's (1985) role of advocacy as 'smoother' could all too quickly become 'smotherer', justified as in the patient's best interest.

It could be that in response to changes taking place both within and outside nursing, community nursing behaviour is at times based on what Cherry et al. (1990) describe as 'habitual patterns from the past'. These habitual reactive roles are described as a 'Drama Triangle' (Karpman, 1968); when feeling defensive, people often move into one of three reactive positions: persecutor, victim or rescuer. In the role of rescuer, there is collusion with another's unwillingness to take responsibility, encouraging dependency. It is also possible that the more one rescues, the less opportunity there is for the victim to get out of that position. The danger seems to be that the triangle is static; it controls others by confining and determining their response. Unless community nurses are able to examine the role they are playing and that they are offering to other people, whom they seek to help, it would appear that a tradition of rescuing might prevent initiatives to act other than paternalistically, negating the ability to advocate. With the advent of trusts and the ethos of a market economy within the NHS, another danger is seen in the conflict between the needs of the individual and the demands of management. Wolfenberger (1991) explores the manufacturing of devalued people, which appears pertinent to the present changes in the NHS. He suggests that in searching for our own identity, we draw up boundaries of what we are and what we are not. There is an attempt to explain everything (vis, in trusts, the readily available annual report, the spate of open days); anything or anyone seen as uncontrollable becomes a scapegoat ('the boat rockers and Graham Pink', see Table 6.1). Wolfenberg goes on to describe the acquisition of power and status within the group, as well as economic advantage. This leads to devalued people (those outside being seen as less than those inside) and negative views towards them. Those associating with the devalued become devalued and there is at times outright persecution for helping the devalued. The climate for community nurses taking on a new role seems at best inclement. Although there seems to be consensus regarding the need for advocacy, there appears to be very little information of where it would fit in for people. It seems to be undertaken on an ad hoc basis – is it safe to leave it thus?

Another danger is that of someone who is not independent being called an advocate. There is likely to come a point when there is conflict and the patient is left, in Sacks' (1982) words, 'double thinged'. Having been led to believe they were being rescued, they may then be let down again, this time by the helper.

Is advocacy without power possible? Although it is much talked about in trusts' philosophies, there seem to be no formulae set out on methods to achieve this. If it is for the community nurse to recognize the need and pass that need on to managers for action, there must be an outcome. However, freedom of expression within a constrained and tightened management structure may not be possible; it could be argued that the nurse has real difficulties in speaking out in controversial areas, as employment becomes more and more valued. There is a recurring dilemma of the level of intervention: do you put your career on the line or go only so far (Table 6.3)? Those working in a multidisciplinary team need to resolve another problem: others in that team may find the role of advocates frightening or threatening to their retention of power or status. These could be doctors, nurses or friends and relatives of the person for whom the nurse is advocating. It may also make the actual or potential role of nurse advocate impossible if, for example, the GP becomes their employer.

Yet another area of potential problem is that of attempting to advocate for more than one person, when there are competing needs. When, for example, there is only one night sitter, can you equally advocate for two patients, representing their individual needs? The same could occur when supporting a patient's needs clashes with the also great needs of the informal carer. Unless there is independent advocacy, there is the risk of serving the one and ignoring the other. In the community, the informal carer is likely to be offering the greater input of care and, without them, the patient may not be able to remain where they wish. The community nurse often has to compromise in order to offer viability of a situation: have they then acted as advocate? O'Brien (1984) stresses the need to check out when compromise is possible – but also the need to check when compromise means a sell-out of a person's rights and dignity. Citizen advocacy is normally one of long-term involvement; with the current increase of people requiring intensive nursing care in the community, this does not seem feasible for nurses.

Sang (1985) stresses that both self and citizen advocacy are about offering considerable opportunities to redress the balance of power, to enable people who have had their power removed or never given to them to possess that power to influence the decisions which affect their lives. Jordan's (1975) question is to a Social Worker's Annual Conference but is applicable to all community workers. He asks 'Do we make decisions about our clients' lives as if they were full and equal citizens, on par with ourselves, as if to uphold their civil and social rights were to uphold our own; or do we make decisions about them, as if their citizenship was of a different, more limited kind?'

Empowering by having access to education and knowledge and the freedom to use that knowledge to the best of one's own ability may be seen as a form of advocacy (Kohnke, 1982). Even that may be fraught with difficulties: Freire (1969) argues that there is no such thing as a neutral education process. Thus, unless possible bias is openly acknowledged by those within the system, it may prove difficult to help those devalued by it. Furthermore, if the system employs the community nurses, they are likely to be seen by those outside the system to have taken on its values. There is an additional aspect; unless the consumer is asked what they wish of the community nursing intervention, it may be that nurses are so caught up in doing and saving lives that they fail to allow people 'the dignity of risk' (Perske, 1972), to ask the 'wrong' question, to make the 'wrong' decision. If so, then nurses run the risk of seeing them as 'objects: known and acted upon' (Freire, 1969, p. 80).

Copp (1986) queries whether we will make the climate right for others if not for ourselves. Community nurses may prevent others from advocating or receiving that service if they lack acceptance of people's equal rights. If a person labelled 'senile' disagrees with what the community nurse offers, it might be presumed that it is because of their mental state, rather than accepted that it is not what they want. Conversely, if community nurses accept without question the client's 'no' to help, they may disadvantage people, unless the possible outcomes of their preferred option have been openly explored.

Citizen advocacy (CA) schemes are now established in an increasing number of towns and cities. Mitchell (1994) found that either few district nurses know of their existence or, if they do, do not see a link between CA and a possible role of advocacy in nursing. Without awareness, it is difficult to direct people towards citizen advocacy. If community nurses choose not to advocate, there remains a necessity to listen to people and their articulation of their need. Is community nursing ready for the changes that it is likely to bring? As Mitchell (1994) states 'empowered they will actually say, not "this is what we would like to happen here" but "this is what you will do" ' (p. 103).

There is seen to be a place for protection and support by managers for community nurses who take on the role. In one trust, the word advocacy is in as an item, a skill. However, the database does not appear to record it. It is thus difficult to know if it is being undertaken. And the solution seems to be always within the same system. There is a need to acknowledge the present reality but also need to work towards change. Otherwise the community may become an enclosing force, just as restrictive as any official institute, from which many community nurses would choose to distance themselves.

O'Brien (1984) explains that the Georgia Advocacy Office programme is based on three main aims:

- developing an agency that can grow slowly to get the groundwork done thoroughly;
- respond to the reality in the community in order to shape the best possible response to people with needs;
- bear in mind the realities of the existing service systems.

These aims are well able to be seen within a community nursing context, with or without advocacy. One difficulty could be that part of what community nurses currently describe as advocacy seems to equate to 'only so far'. There is a risk if it is presumed that there is no route beyond.

Conclusion

As maybe always happens, more and more unrolls ahead of you as you travel. Thus we and the profession may develop. The 'themes of advocacy' and 'concepts of advocacy categories' are offered as tools to explore a wider range of literature and role interpretation by those practising advocacy.

There is a need to include the study of citizen advocacy, self-advocacy and legal advocacy in community nursing courses, exploring how the community nurse might act as pointer to the service provision by others. Meanwhile, it would seem prudent to call for a moratorium on advocacy by nurses, while continuing (legally) to speak out on behalf of people they seek to serve.

Colliere (1980) states that primary health care means giving back to people a place, their rightful place, in the study of their health problems and making the decisions that need to be made. Perhaps community nurses can work towards the stage when they do not need to give back because it will not have been taken away in the first place. Freire's (1968) 'praxis' involves the transformation of objects into subjects by workers being open to listening and being educated by the oppressed. The way to achieve this is through dialogue, 'not afraid to confront, to listen, to see the world unveiled' (Freire, 1968, p. 24), turning consumers into providers, an apt simile in the current NHS changes. It is unlikely to be easy; to use Sartre's (1959) 'subject I, object you' metaphor, it would entail movement of the power tradition, subject nurse, object patient to subject nurse person, and subject patient person, acceptance of others as having equal rights, not just rights.

Many nurses appear to be working towards autonomy of practice. If the profession believes it for itself, then it would seem at least a moral obligation to believe it for others. As an interim, people need advocates because others do not have to listen. Nurses need to be involved in the dialogue but not necessarily as advocates. With legal safeguards and independence from the system they are seeking to challenge, then maybe advocacy for nurses is possible. On the other hand, it could be a ploy to speak 'wonderful words', without offering the reality in which to implement the concept.

The reader is challenged to examine their own perceptions, using these concepts, themes and practice, then decide whether the current status is that the developing role of advocacy is a possibility – or part of a ploy, which lulls us into believing that it is already being practised, courtesy of paternalism/materialism!

Points to consider

1   Are the people you seek to help subjects or objects?

2   Do they have rights equal to yours – or rights?

3   Concomitants to advocacy are risk, heat and prevention (Copp, 1986). Do you agree?

4   Who should define the concept and role of advocacy, within the context of community nursing?

References

Abrams, N. 1978: A contrary view of the nurse as patient advocate. *Nursing Forum*, **XVII**, 3, 258–67.

Allmark, P. 1992: The case against nurse advocacy. *British Journal of Nursing*, **2**, 1, 33–6.

Annas, G.J. and Healey, J. 1974: The patient rights advocate. *Journal of Nursing Administration*, May/June, **4**, 25–31.

Benner, P. 1990: Commentary: the many faces of advocacy. *American Journal of Nursing*, **90**, 1, 82.

Breen, H. 1990: The psychiatric nurse–patient advocate? *Canadian Journal of Psychiatric Nursing*, **31**, 4, 9–11.

Brown, P. 1986: Who needs an advocate? *Nursing Times*, **82**, 72.

Cherry, C., Robertson, M. and Meadows, F. 1990: *Personal and professional development for group leaders: a training course*. Edinburgh: Scottish Health Education Group.

Colliere, M.F. 1980: Development of primary health care. *International Nursing Review*, **27**, 170.

Cookfair, J.W. (ed.) 1991: *Nursing processes and practice in the community*. St Louis: Mosby Year Book Inc.

Copp, L.A. 1986: The nurse as advocate for vulnerable people. *Journal of Advanced Nursing*, **11**, 255–63.

Dimond, B. 1989: Exercising accountability in the legal context. *Nursing Standard*, **50**, 3, 38–9.

Dock, L.L. (1987): Some urgent social claims. *American Journal of Nursing*, **7** (July 1908), p. 895. In Meredith, S. 1987: Lavinia L. Dock: calling nurses to support women's rights, 1907–1923. *Journal of Nursing History*, November, **3**, 1, 70–8.

Donahue, M.P. 1978: The nurse: a patient advocate? *Nursing Forum*, **17**, 2, 143–51.

Dyer, A.R. and Bloch, S. 1982: Informed consent and the psychiatric patient. *Journal of Medical Ethics*, **9**, 69–75.

Freire, P. 1969: *Pedagogy of the oppressed*. New York: The Seabury Press.

Freire, P. 1973: *Education for critical consciousness*. New York: The Seabury Press

Gathercole, C. 1986: Citizens first: north west. In Butler K, Carr, S. and Sullivan. F (eds), *Citizen advocacy: a powerful partnership*. London: National Citizen Advocacy.

Gilligan, C. 1982: *In a different voice*. Cambridge, MA: Harvard University Press.

Gostin, L. 1984: Foreword to Sang, B. and O'Brien, J. *Advocacy: The UK and American experience*. London: King's Fund.

Harbison, J. 1992: Gilligan: a voice for nursing? *Journal of Medical Ethics*, **18**, 202–5.

Healthy Cities Inter-Sectorial Committee 1988: *The Liverpool Declaration*. WHO Healthy Cities Project.

HM Government 1990: *National Health Service and Community Care Act*. London: HMSO.

Howe, J. 1989: Aids – the right approach? *The Professional Nurse*, **5**, 3, 156–9.

International Council of Nurses (1973) *Code for nurses. Ethical concepts, applied to nursing*. Geneva: ICN.

Jenny, J. 1979: Patient advocacy – another role for nursing? *International Nursing Review*, **26**, 6, 176–81.

Jordan, J. 1975: Speech given at *British Association of Social Workers Annual Conference*.

Karpman, S. 1968: Fairy tales and script drama analysis. *Transactional Analysis Bulletin*, **7**, 26, 39–43.

Kohnke, M.F. 1982: *Advocacy: risk and reality*. St Louis: CV Mosby Company.

Kuehnert, P.L. 1991: The public health policy advocate: fostering the health of communities. *Clinical Nurse Specialist*, **5**, 1, 5–10.

MacFadyen, J.A. 1989: Who will speak up for me? *Nursing Times*, **85**, 6, 4–5.

Meredith, S. 1987: Lavinia L. Dock: calling nurses to support women's rights, 1907–1923. *Journal of Nursing History*, **3**, 1, 70–8.

Mitchell, E.E. 1994: *Examination of the role of advocacy in district nursing practice*. MEd Thesis, University of Liverpool.

Morrison, A. 1991: The nurse's role in relation to advocacy. *Nursing Standard*, **5**, 41, 37–41.

Nelson, M.L. 1988: Advocacy in nursing. *Nursing Outlook*, May/June **38**, 3, 136–41.

Nocon, A. 1992: Punters sold down the river. *Nursing Standard*, **5**, 6, 46, 50.

Nursing Education Research Unit (NERU) 1986: *Report of the Nursing Process Evaluation Working Group, NERU Report 5*. Chaired by Friend. London: Kings College.

O'Brien, J. In Sang, B. and O'Brien, J. 1984: *Advocacy: The UK and American experiences*. London: King's Fund Publishing.

Parson, T. 1952: *The social system*. London: Tavistock.

Perlin, M.L. 1982: Mental patient advocacy by a patient advocate. *Psychiatric Quarterly*, **54**, 3, 169–79.

Perske, R. 1972: The dignity of risk and the mentally retarded. Mental retardation. In Sellin, D.F. (1979), *Mental retardation*. Boston: Allyn & Bacon Inc.

Pyne, R. 1992: Accountability in principle and practice. *British Journal of Nursing*, **1**, 6, 301–5.

Rathwell, T. 1990: Stand up for patients' rights. *The Health Service Journal*, 88–9.

Renshaw, J. and Metcalf, M. 1987: *A friend in need: citizen advocacy in Britain.* Discussion Paper No. 517/1. Canterbury: PSSRU, University of Kent.

Robinson, M.B. 1985: Patient advocacy and the nurse: is there a conflict of interest? *Nursing Forum,* **22**, 2, 58–63.

Rogers, M. 1970: Yesterday a nurse, today a manager, what now? *Journal of New York State Nurses' Association,* **1**, 2, 15–21.

Rose, S.M. and Black, B.L. 1985: *Advocacy and empowerment: mental health care in the community.* London: Routledge and Kegan Paul Plc.

Sacks, O. 1982: *Awakenings* (2nd edn). London: Picador.

Sang, B. 1985: A question of power. *Openmind,* **17**, 12.

Sang, B. and O'Brien, J. 1984: *Advocacy: the UK and American experiences* (King's Fund Project Paper Number 51). London: King's Fund Publishing Office.

Sartre, J.P. (1959): *Being and nothingness.* (Trans. Barnes, H.E.). Bristol: Methuen.

Tingle, J.H. 1988: Nursing ethics and the law. *Senior Nurse,* **8**, 2.

United Kingdom Central Council for Nursing, Health Visiting and Midwifery (UKCC) 1989: *Exercising accountability: an advisory document.* London: UKCC.

UKCC 1992: *Code of professional conduct for the nurse, midwife and health visitor.* London: UKCC.

Wicker, C.P. 1991: Legal responsibilities of the nurse. *Surgical Nurse,* **4**, 1, 16–17.

World Health Organization (WHO) International Conference on Health Promotion 1986: *Charter for action to achieve health for all by the year 2000.* Ottawa: WHO.

WHO, Nursing Division, Europe 1986: *Nursing targets for Europe.* NURS/EURO, 86.3. Copenhagen: WHO.

WHO 1988: *Report on the 2nd international conference in health promotion,* Adelaide, 5–9 April 1988: Priorities for Public Health Policy. Copenhagen: WHO.

Wolfenberger, W. 1991: *On promoting social advocacy.* Conference tapes: Newcastle-upon-Tyne, July 1991.

Zussman, J. 1982: Think twice about becoming a patent's advocate. *Nursing Life,* **6**, 46–50.

PART TWO

Managerial and leadership strategies in community nursing

The chapters included in this part address some of the areas of the community nurse's role that have become enhanced with the implementation of specialist practice. The PREP document (UKCC, 1994) uses the terms 'leadership in community nursing' and 'management in community nursing' to illustrate two of the areas of practice that are fundamental to specialist practitioners. Neither of these roles are new but the nature of specialist practice places a greater emphasis on them.

This part of the book assumes a basic management knowledge and makes no attempt to teach management skills. There are many valuable management tests that will provide the knowledge that underpins the skills required by community nurses.

7 Collaboration for care

Jenny Newbury, Ann Clarridge and Jo Skinner

This chapter is about working together for effective care in the community. Throughout the chapter there are activities to help you relate the issues to your own practice. Community nurses' roles in interdisciplinary, interprofessional and interagency collaboration are analysed and it is recognized in this chapter that there are different modes and levels of collaboration. These are discussed in relation to community nursing practice, as well as some of the factors that influence the effectiveness of working together, such as the level of organizational support and commitment for joint working and physical proximity of the parties involved. Some of the barriers to collaboration are explored, such as the competitive environment of the contract culture, incompatible philosophies, language sets and socialization of different professions and confusion over roles and responsibilities. Ways of overcoming these barriers are also identified and the characteristics of effective and ineffective collaboration are listed. Finally, the importance of collaborative working for community nursing is stressed in relation to current policy frameworks and good practice.

Introduction

In 1985, in response to the Select Committee on Community Care, the Government confirmed its commitment to the concept of collaboration. It bestowed responsibilities on local authorities and health authorities to form alliances, to promote joint planning and joint working in preparation for the implementation of the 1990 NHS and Community Care Act (DOH, 1990).

Since the introduction of the Act, changes to health and social care delivery rely on effective collaboration between workers, to ensure that clients and patients receive appropriate care from the right agency at the right time. This has special significance for community nurses. For instance, the Standing Nursing and Midwifery Advisory Committee (SNMAC, 1995) state that 'public health in nursing, midwifery and health visiting practice is about commissioning health services and providing professional care through organised collaboration in the NHS and society, to protect and promote health and well-being, prolong life and prevent ill-health in local communities, groups and populations' (p. 5).

There are clear benefits to collaboration. In particular, these include positive health outcomes for patients and families, the effective use of resources (Henneman *et al.*, 1995), increased job satisfaction for practitioners and further collaboration. Observations made by the Audit Commission show that there are some small-scale successful examples of collaboration between agencies (Wistow and Hardy, 1991).

Community nurses do not practise in isolation. They work closely with a wide variety of health and social care workers at individual practitioner level. In particular, they work in partnership with patients, clients and carers. Although community nurses may work a great deal on their own, they do work in skill mixed teams which have been growing larger. Collaboration therefore is an essential element of community nursing practice. It is often presented as 'a way forward' for health care especially in the community. However, it is not always easy, particularly when boundaries are shifting and a variety of disparate professionals is involved. Indeed, collaboration is often seen as a remedy where there is conflict (Henneman *et al.*, 1995).

ACTIVITY 7.1

1 Think about an episode of good practice in collaboration. This can be from your current or past experience. What was it about this episode that was good?

Definitions and explanations of collaboration

The dictionary definition of collaboration is 'to work in association' (Chambers, 1961) and the thesaurus offers 'partnership', 'alliance' and 'teamwork' as words which may be used as alternatives with like meaning (Collins, 1986). All these terms relate closely to community nursing practice, since community nurses collaborate in varying ways during the course of their work, for instance corporate caseloads in health visiting require sophisticated teamwork. Community nurses have to collaborate with each other to achieve certain goals that would be physically impossible or unsafe on one's own, for example, lifting patients, rehabilitation, night visits (Baly, 1981). They cover each other's work during sickness and annual leave. Hence, teamwork is essential.

The broad range of expertise required to fulfil the generalist functions of district nursing or practice nursing means that these nurses call upon and share care with other specialist practitioners, such as the stoma therapist and the continence advisor. Partnership is the key to successful interdisciplinary working of this kind.

Community nurses also form alliances with other members of the primary health care team. Interprofessional collaboration is a major responsibility within the preventative, caring and managerial aspects of community nursing practice. The UKCC (1992) Code of Professional Conduct makes it clear that nurses need to work in a collaborative and cooperative manner with health care professionals and others in providing care, and recognize and respect their contributions within the care team.

In the delivery of community care the community nurse has to relate to and work with disparate groups, including social services and voluntary organizations. Interagency collaboration is therefore another aspect to be taken on board. Thus, it can be seen that community nurses need to collaborate at interdisciplinary, interprofessional and interagency levels. In addition, of course, they must collaborate with families, patients and carers as required by the UKCC Code of Professional Conduct to work in a collaborative and cooperative manner with patients, clients and their families (UKCC, 1992).

Furthermore, community nurses are at the interface between primary and secondary health care. Foster (1991) advocated 'integration between authorities providing primary and secondary care and with social-care agencies' (p. 8–9) as the key to overcoming gaps in provision. This requires both individual good practice and an effective primary care strategy for gathering and disseminating information about health needs and integrating quality services. Hughes (1989) suggests that such collaboration is cheaper.

Table 7.1 Types and examples of collaboration in community nursing

Interdisciplinary	Interprofessional	Interagency/sector
Teamwork	Shared care	Care management
General/specialist	Primary health care team	Child protection
partnerships	Liaison/referral	Public health initiatives
Corporate caseload	Education	Education
Cover for leave	Research	Research
Education	Audit	Audit
Research		
Audit		

Modes of collaboration

In general, collaborative working emerges through the establishment of teams and networks. In this instance, networks refer to different professionals who occasionally meet but who hold common interests, whereas teams are comprised of different professionals in the same place, working towards a common goal. Collaboration means improving communication between team members, when and where to contact other members and an identified time for individual members to have face-to-face contact (Haggard, 1992).

Armitage (1983) and Bond *et al.* (1985) advance the notion that the concept of collaboration includes two interrelating ideas: that of joint working and that of a relationship which promotes creativity amongst the collaborators. This notion builds upon the suggestion made by Bruce (1980) that physical and social proximity and positive motivation are crucial factors in potential collaboration. Physical proximity certainly aids collaboration. More collaborative work may be achieved during a meeting in the corridor than in a formal setting. However, sharing a building does not necessarily mean collaboration. The socialization of different disciplines and professions can create barriers that require considerable positive motivation to overcome.

There are also two levels of collaboration. Coleman (1982) makes distinctions between high-level and low-level collaborative activities. The high levels refer to situations where there is a great commitment by the individuals reflected by their willingness to share resources, knowledge and skills for a common goal. The low level is identified when individuals accomplish their own task while merely recognizing that others are accomplishing theirs simultaneously and noting only when the two might be integrated. Most community nurses will come across high and low levels of collaboration. It is interesting to consider the extent to which physical proximity affects the level of collaboration and whether high levels can be achieved when the individual workers do not share the same work base. For instance, outreach nurses with a hospital base may find it more difficult to integrate and collaborate with community nurses based in the health centre. However, community nurses sharing the same health centre do not necessarily collaborate, especially where they do not share a common philosophy or goal.

Barriers to collaboration

Although collaboration is generally recognized as productive and useful in the provision of health and social care, there remain conflicts and obstacles to joint working. Long-standing criticisms of primary health care teams have focused on poor collaboration and lack of understanding about roles (and the potential) of team members (Poulton, 1991). Bond et al. (1985), in a major study considering collaboration in primary health care teams, identify more than 30 studies researching attitudes towards collaboration and structure and organization of teams, but they do not provide any evidence that interprofessional collaboration is happening.

Wistow and Hardy (1991), looking from a management perspective, identify five categories of barriers to effective joint working. These five categories are: structural, procedural, financial, professional and status and legitimacy. These categories encompass most of the problems which the literature on collaboration and teamwork has highlighted. Of significance is the need for organizational support. The core of any collaborative scheme is its intrinsic weakness and vulnerability in the face of organizational pressures which undermine and threaten its continuing development. According to Wistow and Hardy (1991), successful management of collaborative care is dependent upon clarity of purpose, commitment and shared ownership.

However, the political agenda with its emphasis upon competition in health and social care can militate against collaboration (Horder, 1995): Where professionals are competing for resources and contracts the idea of sharing information becomes unthinkable. This competitive environment also permeates education with institutions unwilling to divulge curriculum developments, even successful interprofessional initiatives, to their rivals in the contract war.

Care management, at the centre of community care policy, is a prime example of the need for collaboration at all levels. The district nurse or community psychiatric nurse is often the key worker and therefore responsible for assessing for community care and liaising with all other services but the dividing line between health and social care is an ephemeral one. Indeed, community nurses are at the bridgehead of health and social care. In their everyday experience these concepts appear inseparable when working in homes within a given neighbourhood (Evers, 1991). This ambiguity between health and social care is nowhere more apparent than in community care for people with learning difficulties. Community mental handicap nurses, district nurses and other community nurses develop criteria for determining the boundaries between health and social care, making arrangements to ensure that the appropriate agencies are involved and acting as an advocate for the patient or family between the various personnel (Hughes, 1989; Winn, 1990). However, Horder (1995) stresses that transfer of care to the community makes collaboration between professionals more difficult because of the scattered context in which they work. For instance, a care package may involve community nurses, who could be working in a community trust clinic or a fundholding practice, social worker or care manager who will probably be based in a social services sub-office, voluntary organizations which may be based outside the area, private care agencies, as well as other professionals from different sites. A commonality of experience may confer similar attitudes and reactions on disparate groups of professionals which can enhance cooperation and collaboration. Shared goals, especially amongst 'front-line' workers albeit from different disciplines, may also enhance cooperation. However, incompatible professional ideologies and organizational cultures between groups of health and social workers militate against successful interprofessional working and learning (Dalley, 1993). Although Dalley found most incompatibility between GPs and social workers, she found the district nurse felt very frustrated as a buffer between them.

Distinct but complementary roles have always existed within community nursing. Outside the family of community nursing, this distinctness has not always been understood. Many assumed that these roles were interchangeable, for example, the specific role of the Macmillan nurse may not have been distinguished from the district nurse; the health promotion roles of the health visitor and the practice nurse can be confused and there is no commonly accepted definition of the role of the nurse practitioner (Bryar, 1994). Such confusion does nothing to assist interprofessional and interagency collaboration. Also, there have been periods of tension and 'territoriality' in community work, often due to the lack of strategic planning and uncoordinated management changes as well as discreet areas of expertise. These differences were often tribal in nature (David, 1991; Dalley, 1993). This was evidenced following the wide-scale introduction of practice nurses and the fear felt by other community nurses of erosion of their roles (Hancock, 1991).

Ironically, many of the clashes have occurred because of differing philosophical ideas about nursing care in the community; these have had as much influence as roles, responsibilities and competences. For instance, the nature of district nursing has shifted from a paternalistic, medically orientated service, to one which is health orientated and seeks to empower patients and carers. The holistic (nursing) approach to care has been found to be appropriate in identifying needs and minimizes dependence, as opposed to a 'narrow diagnosis' (Ong, 1991). However, this shift may not be understood by GPs, other professionals and patients and carers.

As has been seen, a major issue for community nurses is the variety and different ways they need to relate to disparate groups. Child protection presents an example of the way in which community nurses must work with a wide range of individuals and groups. Health visitors and school nurses find themselves relating to social workers, the police and judiciary, nursery or school staff, community psychiatric nurses, general practitioners and paediatricians as well as the family. There is ambiguity in the power relations between all these groups related to status and employment as much as knowledge and expertise. Changes in policy and the shifting of control over resources will inevitably lead to individuals and groups of professionals feeling vulnerable and will sharpen their perception of their roles and status. The implementation of GP fundholders commissioning community nursing services in 1993 had this effect, with district nurses and health visitors feeling uncertain about their professional positions and status.

Problems occur when there is role overlap and differing perceptions about status within teams. Role overlap can lead to rivalry between professionals, as seen with the mixed reaction of doctors to nurse practitioners. It also occurs between professions in terms of defining social and health care boundaries (Huntingdon, 1981). It can also occur between the statutory and voluntary sectors.

How individuals perceive themselves in terms of their occupation and status affects their interaction with other professionals. The ideology and status attached to the occupation is acquired through education and training and is reinforced while working alongside others in the same occupation. The differences in academic levels of education and mandatory practice have pervaded the professionals' attitudes towards each other for a long time.

Pietroni (1992) discovered that, over and above professional rivalries and ideological differences, difficulties arise as a result of lack of knowledge of each other's language. Any information system within the management structure which is intended to facilitate the storage and exchange of information requires the information to be accurate, relevant and readily understood by all who seek to use it to improve patient care. One example of a language sub-set not necessarily understood universally is the introduction of marketing terminology, or budget-speak, to health and social care. It is essential to successful collaborative working that information provided by one professional will be understood by another in some other place within the organization. There is a need for a common language (Swayne, 1993).

However, as Pietroni (1992) found, there is a variety of language by which individuals' experiences as recipients of care is communicated and construed between professionals involved in the delivery of care. Even the language used to describe the recipient of care varies; patient, client, user, customer and other terms are used depending on the professional group involved. If there is such a wide variety of terminology used, the question raised is whether it is practical or even expedient to develop a common language.

Another potential barrier is the issue of accountability. For successful collaboration, there is a need to set standards of performance of all professional participants, and a need to make individuals accountable for the outcomes and audit of care. However, Engel (1994) points out that professional emphasis is normally on personal accountability, but collaboration and teamwork means accepting corporate responsibility for outcomes; it may not be easy for an interprofessional group to agree on a common goal, related objectives or appropriate distribution of tasks.

- Common goal/s
- Individual and organizational commitment
- Management support
- Respect and trust
- Common language
- Shared learning
- Reflective practice
- Includes users and carers
- Adaptability to change.

Overcoming the barriers

Whatever the obstacles may be, recent central government policy has placed considerable emphasis upon collaboration and teamwork across professional and disciplinary boundaries. But questions arise when putting policy into practice regarding the acquisition of knowledge and skills that are required for effective collaboration and teamwork. In seeking out knowledge for collaboration, it may be helpful to look at Ovretviet's (1993) three models. The first is the bureaucratic model where collaboration is imposed by a higher authority. Despite the 'top-down' approach, this form of collaboration can yield useful results by bringing professionals who would not otherwise integrate into contact with one another and offering an opportunity to learn each other's aims and methods of working (Nocon, 1994). To a certain extent, the NHS and Community Care Act (1990) and care management have imposed a bureaucratic model of collaboration in the mixed economy of care.

Ovretviet's (1993) second model comes into play when organizations establish relations based on contracts, payments for services and penalties in the event of non-compliance. This is the market model. The explosion of interprofessional collaboration between GPs and practice nurses as a result of the 1990 GP contract is an example of this model, where GPs employ practice nurses to meet the health promotion targets and run the clinics set out in the contract. Fundholding has further developed the GP's need for collaboration with community nursing staff, whose services they commission; and there is some evidence of better understanding of professional roles as a result (Jackson, 1993; Rowe, 1993).

The third model is based on association and the belief by organizations or individual professionals that collaboration has the potential to solve problems of mutual concern. This approach needs to be more flexible and exploratory than the bureaucratic model (Nocon, 1994) and is particularly useful where there is no clear solution to an issue. Work in the fields of dementia, homelessness and HIV, among others, have demonstrated the association model, with creative partnerships between the voluntary sector, outreach health and social workers and mainstream services. This form of collaboration tends to occur more naturally than others, but still requires knowledge and skills to be effective.

- Role confusion and overlap
- Tribalism
- Professional rivalries and power/status conflicts
- Competition for resources
- Disparate organization
- Incompatible ideologies and cultures
- Poor communication systems including use of language
- Emphasis on individual rather than corporate accountability.

What knowledge and skills are needed for collaboration? Key areas appear to be an ability to tolerate individual differences between people (Areskog, 1994) and understanding of the roles and views of other professionals (Horder, 1995). Awareness of the opportunities and constraints experienced by other professions and enhanced communication skills, which enable the disposal of stereotypes and generate trust between professionals, also form the basis for collaboration (Barr, 1994). Menzies (1988), however, argues that teaching people to be sensitive to each other's position is money for old rope, since most people want that anyway. However, they go back to their old situation, which does not allow them to deploy sensitivity and they slip back or become frustrated and discontented. Commitment to collaboration at policy and management levels of the organization are therefore essential prerequisites.

Engel (1994) highlights some more specific competences for collaboration particularly in teams, such as those of primary health care. An ability to adapt to and participate in change are the two most fundamental attributes. The change from acting independently to joint decision making requires a deliberate act of adapting to new circumstances, a new way of working. The most basic requirement to be able to adapt to change is the individual's own professional competence. As Engel points out, unless professionals feel confident in their own expertise and have the respect of their peers, they are unlikely to feel sufficiently secure to be willing to negotiate the distribution of tasks, within an interprofessional setting. Community nurses need to feel confident about the important role they play because of their first-hand knowledge of both localities and individuals.

Along with adapting to change, the ability to feel comfortable with ambiguity and uncertainty is needed, since the prospect of decision making and collaborating presents much uncertainty. Similarly, professionals must be able to reason critically in order to analyse favourable and unfavourable aspects of change and make decisions about discarding past beliefs and adopting new strategies. Engel (1994) likens the process to bereavement, in which there may be denial and anger before letting go something familiar. Barr (1994) found such reactions among pessimistic educators faced with introducing shared learning and fearing that values and philosophies which they held dear were being put in jeopardy.

The methods of instilling new knowledge and skills for collaborative practice have been widely debated. Shared learning between professionals is generally seen as a step in the right direction but the achievement of successful interprofessional education can be problematic. However, despite the obstacles, Barr (1994) found numerous trends either prompting or shaping initiatives in shared learning. Repeatedly suggestions have been made that social workers, nurses and other health workers should have a shared generic foundation course, to eliminate some of the cultural idiosyncrasies peculiar to different professional groups and enable more effective teamwork (Dalley, 1990; Hancock, 1991). There has been a trend for some time within higher education for shared learning in core areas between disciplines within community nursing and with social workers. But placing people in a classroom together does not necessarily lead to a better understanding of each other's roles. There is obvious cynicism regarding the effectiveness of achieving collaboration by putting different groups of professionals together in a didactic learning situation. Therefore, appropriate interactive teaching and learning methods are essential, value being added to shared learning when participants not only learn alongside each other, but also from and about each other (Barr, 1994). In addition the immense value of learning together in daily practice should not be ignored (Horder, 1995). Hutchinson and Gordon (1992) agree that over and above recognition of role is the significance of working relationships between people, built upon acceptance, mutual understanding and respect.

The contribution of reflective practice towards enhancing this learning in practice cannot be underestimated (Barr, 1994; Glennie and Cosier, 1994). By standing back and looking at one's own professional practice, the contribution of other professionals in meeting the needs of users can become clearer. As seen earlier in this chapter, Pietroni (1992) emphasizes the effect of different language sub-sets between professional groups. Not only do they use separate languages but also different modes of thought. He suggests that reflection which occurs within one language sub-set runs the danger of repeating the same mistakes over and over again. For instance, a very narrow view of a problem will be achieved with the GP reviewing the situation using a medical sub-set only focusing on terms like signs, symptoms, diagnosis, treatment, or a therapist using only a psychoanalytical sub-set with terms like projection, splitting, transference and the unconscious. Similarly a nurse using a health promotion sub-set employing only concepts such as lifestyle, risk assessment, empowerment could offer an equally narrow view and there would be little chance of successful collaboration between these professionals. For the reflective process to be really creative, leading to new solutions to old problems, there must be as much diversity as possible, with integration of language sub-sets. Pietroni advocates this integration as the way forward in collaborative work; he does however admit that to encourage a wide-range reflective process amongst professionals is not an easy task.

ACTIVITY 7.2

1 Describe an episode from your own practice which involved interprofessional and/or interagency collaboration.

2 In your opinion how effective/ineffective was the collaboration? How was this characterized? For example, levels, proximity, positive motivation, shared goals, language, status of individuals.

ACTIVITY 7.3

1 Which of Ovretviet's three models applies to your own organization?

2 Which model would you choose for your practice, and why?

Conclusion

In this chapter collaboration has been identified as a vital aspect of community nursing practice. Collaborative working will remain a high priority in the foreseeable future within current policy frameworks for health and social care. By identifying a unified specialism of community health care nursing, the UKCC has created a climate for interdisciplinary practice and education. The new standards for specialist education and practice in the community also demand pro-active, innovative work with other professionals and agencies (UKCC, 1994).

The development of GP fundholding into total purchasing means that community nurses are and will be, in certain areas, working more closely with all providers of community care commissioned by the fundholders. This includes multiprofessional evaluation and audit of services (Morris, 1993).

The mergers of health authorities and family health services authorities into health commissioning agencies also require community nurses to be involved with a wider variety of agencies and to influence purchasing across a broad range of services. Indeed, the *Vision for the Future* (NHSME, 1993a) strategy stresses the valuable input that nurses, midwives and health visitors can make to the purchasing and commissioning cycle, by working alongside other professionals to assess health needs and the impact of health interventions.

The *New World, New Opportunities* document (NHSME, 1993b) also places much emphasis upon teamwork, multidisciplinary training, collaborative research, partnerships in care and shared care as keys to progress in primary health care nursing.

Within these policy frameworks, collaboration occurs at a number of levels and requires a range of knowledge and skills to be accomplished effectively in the advancement of health care. However, there are many barriers and obstacles faced by professionals when attempting to work collaboratively. Shared learning both in educational institutions and in the workplace are seen as fundamental to overcoming some of the barriers. Organizational support for collaboration is also essential. Community nurses are in the forefront of many collaborative ventures both at the level of individual health care and at the planning and policy level. They need to use their skills to their full potential to provide integrated and comprehensive health care for users and their carers in order to guarantee responsive, creative and flexible services that are compatible with local needs (Cameron *et al.*, 1989; MacLellan, 1990) and to improve health outcomes. Community nurses are not solely responsible for enabling clients and patients to achieve health but need to coordinate their efforts with others.

ACTIVITY 7.4

1 What are your own individual strengths and weaknesses in collaborating with others?

2 Reflecting on your strengths and weaknesses, plan how you might develop your collaborative skills for your future practice.

References

Areskog, N.H. 1994: Multidisciplinary education at undergraduate level – the Linkoping model. *Journal of Interprofessional Care*, **8**, 3, 279–82.

Armitage, P. 1983: Joint working in primary health care. *Nursing Times Occasional Papers*, **79**, 75–8.

Baly, M. (ed.) 1981: *A new approach to district nursing*. London: Heinemann.

Barr, H. 1994: *Perspectives on shared learning*. Nottingham: Centre for the Advancement of Interprofessional Education.

Bond, J., Cartlidge, A.M., Gregson, B.A., Philips, P.R., Bolam, F. and Gill, K.M. 1985: *A study of interprofessional collaboration in primary health care organizations*. Crown Copyright.

Bruce, N. 1980: Cited in Bond, J., Cartlidge, A.M., Gregson, B.A., Philips, P.R., Bolam, F. and Gill, K.M. (1985), *A study of interprofessional collaboration in primary health care organizations*. Crown Copyright.

Bruce, N., Gilmore, M. and Hunt, M. 1974: *Work of the nursing team*. London, CETHV.

Bryar, R. 1994: An examination of the need for new nursing roles in primary health care. *Journal of Interprofessional Care*, **8**, 1, 73–84.

Cameron, E., Badger, F. and Evers, H. 1989: District nursing, the disabled and the elderly: who are the black patients? *Journal of Advanced Nursing*, **14**, 346–82.

Chambers 1961: *Chambers dictionary* (4th edn). Glasgow: The Villafield Press.

Coleman, P. 1982: Collaboration between services for the elderly infirm. In Ball, C., Coleman, P. and Wright, J. (eds) *Delivery of services, main report*, Vol. 1. University of Southampton, Department of Social Work Studies.

Collins 1986: *The Collins thesaurus*. London: W. Collins Sons and Co.

Dalley, G. 1990: The impact of new community management structures: an overview. In Hughes, J. (ed.) *Enhancing the quality of nursing in the community*. London: King's Fund.

Dalley, G. 1993: Professional ideology or organizational tribalism? the health service–social work divide. In Walmsley, J., Reynolds, J., Shakespeare, P. and Woolfe, R. *Health, welfare and practice: reflecting on roles and relationships*. London: Sage with Open University Press.

David, A. 1991: Survival strategies. *Nursing Times*, **87**, 13, 45–7.

DOH 1990: *NHS and Community Care Act*. London: HMSO.

Engel, C. 1994: A functional anatomy of teamwork. In Leathard, A. *Going professional: working together for health and welfare*. London: Routledge.

Evers, H. 1991: Taking extra care. *Health Service Journal*, 4th July, 27.

Foster, A. 1991: Of primary importance. *Primary Health Care*, **1**, 8, 8–9.

Glennie, S. and Cosier, J. 1994: Collaborative inquiry: developing multidisciplinary learning and action. *Journal of Interprofessional Care*, **8**, 3, 255–64.

Haggard, L. 1992: Making the team work. *Health Service Journal*, 1st April.

Hancock, C. 1991: Moving centre stage. *Primary Health Care*, **1**, 4, 11–13.

Henneman, E.A., Lee, J.L. and Cohen, J.I. 1995: Collaboration: a concept analysis. *Journal of Advanced Nursing*, **21**, 103–9.

Horder, J. 1995: Interprofessional education for primary health and community care: present state and future needs. In Soothill, K., Mackay, L. and Webb, C. (eds), *Interprofessional relations in health care*. London: Edward Arnold.

Hughes, J. (ed.) 1989: *The future of community health services*. London: King's Fund.

Huntingdon, J. 1981: *Social work and general medical practice: collaboration or conflict?* London: Allen and Unwin.

Hutchinson, A. and Gordon, S. 1992: Teamwork in primary care: how much do we know about it? *Journal of Interprofessional Care*, **6**, 1, 25–9.

Jackson, C. 1993: A tale of two teams. *Health Visitor*, **66**, 2, 41.

MacLellan, M. 1990: Not a happy picture. *Journal of District Nursing*. March, 19–20.

Menzies, I. 1988: *Containing anxiety in institutions*. Selected Essays Vol. 1. London: Free Association Books.

Morris, R. 1993: Community care and the fundholder. *British Medical Journal*, **306**, 635–7.

National Health Service Management Executive 1993a: *A vision for the future: the nursing, midwifery and health visiting contribution to health and health care*. London: Department of Health.

National Health Service Management Executive 1993b: *New world, new opportunities*. London: Department of Health.

Nocon, A. 1994: *Collaboration in community care in the 1990's*. Sunderland: Business Education Publishers.

Ong, B. 1991: Researching the needs of district nursing. *Journal of Advanced Nursing*, **16**, 638–47.

Ovretviet, J. 1993: *Co-ordinating community care: multidisciplinary teams and care management*. Buckingham: Open University Press.

Pietroni, P.C. 1992: Towards reflective practice – the languages of health and social care. *Journal of Interprofessional Care*, **6**, 1, 7–16.

Poulton, B. 1991: Does your team really work? *Primary Health Care*, **11**, 2, 11–12, 14.

Rowe, J. 1993: Isolation fears. *Health Visitor*, **66**, 2, 42.

Swayne, P. 1993: A common language of care? *Journal of Interprofessional Care*, **7**, 1, 29–35.

Standing Nursing and Midwifery Advisory Committee 1995: *Making it happen: public health – the contribution, role and development of nurses, midwives and health visitors*. London: Department of Health.

United Kingdom Central Council for Nursing, Midwifery and Health Visiting 1992: *Code of Professional Conduct*. London: UKCC.

United Kingdom Central Council for Nursing, Midwifery and Health Visiting 1994: *The future of professional practice – the Council's standards for education and practice following registration*. London: UKCC.

Winn, L. (ed.) 1990: *Power to the people*. London: King's Fund.

Wistow, G. and Hardy, B. 1991: Joint management in community care. *Journal of Management in Medicine*, **5**, 4, 40–8.

8 Sharing in partnership

Diane Cuff

This chapter will explore the manifestations and challenges of 'sharing' in the community health care nurse–patient relationship, with particular reference to older patients. In the first section the concept of partnership is examined, as portrayed by various authors. From the existing definitions the theme of sharing emerges as an essential requisite for 'true' partnership, one in which both partners have equal contributions to make to the caring process. Key opportunities for sharing are then explored separately drawing on relevant literature.

The value of forming partnerships between professional and patient or client is well established in health care literature from across both sides of the Atlantic and has been largely unchallenged by those of us working in nursing. Urging a more collegiate relationship between care providers and receivers has grown out of the ideology of consumerism. In the health care setting consumerism has been translated as implying that the customer, namely the patient, has by right a voice in determining the nature of care to be provided and how it should be delivered so that it meets their needs and expectations. By increasing customer involvement in these areas, the relationship between health professionals and patients has needed to change. Such changes are perhaps best represented in the position statement drafted by the Royal College of Nursing (1987) which states that 'each patient has a right to be a partner in his own care planning and receive relevant information, support and encouragement from the nurse which will permit him to make informed choices and become involved in his own care' (p. 16).

Having a right to be a partner in care has not surprisingly been a reoccurring theme in much of the subsequent professional literature and health policy, though the term partner is not always explicitly used. However, few papers have looked critically at the ideal of partnership nor examined its meaning. In the first instance this paper will attempt to remedy this absence by exploring the concept and derive from this suitable definitions and meanings. Following this an in-depth examination of the nursing behaviours which contribute to partnership formation will be undertaken. While this text is intended for community health care nurses (CHCNs), illustrative examples are drawn mainly from the wider forum of nursing.

What do health care professionals mean by 'partnership'?

Before embarking on the main discussion concerning the characteristics or attributes of nurse–patient partnerships, it would be helpful to know more about what this concept means within both nursing and especially community health care nursing. The quest for a definition proved to be more difficult than expected, for while partnership is often referred to in texts and policy documents, few have taken the trouble to explain what they meant by it. Only one entire text was found devoted to the topic of partnership in nursing, and in its review of definitions it offers a simple view of partnership as 'an alliance between two or more people involved in a shared venture' (Christensen, 1990, p. ix). In this instance the two people concerned are the nurse, or the community health care nurse (CHCN), and the patient. The use of this latter term has caused some controversy regarding its associations with passivity and submissiveness. Despite these concerns this title is still commonly used within nursing texts and one to which many nurses can readily relate.

Nursing is not alone in developing partnerships, as evidenced by the writings of authors such as Pugh and De'ath (1989) and Bastiani (1993) on the type of relationship between schools, teachers and parents. The definitions they have provided offer greater insight into this topic and might be easily translated across the professional boundaries. Pugh and De'ath (1989) for instance describe working partnerships between school and parents as being 'characterised by a shared sense of purpose, mutual respect and willingness to negotiate. This implies a sharing of information, responsibility, skills, decision making and accountability' (p. 68). In a similar vein Bastiani (1993) supports Pugh's description while adding to it the features of sharing aims and goals, power and ownership.

The verb that is common to all three of these definitions is 'to share', implying partnership is essentially an interactional process. 'Sharing' conjures up images of two or more people participating in joint or collaborative experiences. To share, according to the Oxford English Dictionary (1993) is 'to take part in an action or experience' which when applied to the nursing context would perhaps translate as taking part in the caring experience. None of these definitions of sharing really encapsulates what it means to share in a partnership, or the costs and benefits of such sharing. Further clarification may arise in future discussions of the nature of 'sharing' as a prerequisite for creating partnerships between both community health care nurses and their patients. Pugh's and Bastiani's definitions provide a useful framework to structure these discussions:

- sharing of – information
- sharing of – planning and decision making
- sharing of – responsibility
- sharing of – control and power.

Sharing of information

Nurses have a key role as information brokers yet they do not always respond adequately to this demand. Ford (1990), a freelance journalist, gives an example of this failure in recalling the frustration felt as a patient when staff repulsed his request for information about himself and the hospital routines. He states, 'When I asked for information about my health, I was met with, at best, surprise and, at worst resentment. On one occasion after my weight had been recorded and I inquired what it was, a nurse asked me incredibly: "Why do you want to know?" ' (p. 59).

This short extract speaks volumes about the lack of empathy and sensitivity shown by some nurses when dealing with patient requests for information. Neither is this an isolated incidence as both research and health ombudsman complaints often reveal patients to be ill-informed (Wilson-Barnett, 1989). Why then do nurses appear to devalue the importance of such communication or respond to this obvious need?

Information sharing should form a central part of the normal dialogue between nurse and patient for two key reasons. Several researchers have shown that when nurse and patient exchange personal information this enables them both to build up a better understanding of each others' values, assumptions, experiences and needs. Sharing this type of information therefore symbolizes a sense of trust between both parties and puts them at ease (Sheppard, 1993; Fosbinder, 1994). Self-disclosure has been found in differing contexts to act as a springboard to psychological closeness thereby allowing patients to see the nurse as a human being. This closeness then opens the doors to sharing mutual respect, trust and openness. By contrast, maintaining strict professional boundaries is more likely to restrict exchanges of information and limit sharing.

There is also evidence to support mutual sharing of information as being instrumental in increasing positive care outcomes (King, 1981; Jewell, 1994). Trojan and Younge's (1993) study of home care nursing found that where patient and nurse spent time together getting to know each other the knowledge gained enabled a growing commitment towards achieving the patient's health goals. Where this sharing was found to be limited or absent, there appeared to be a far greater tendency for patients to re-enter the health care system, particularly where it was an elderly patient (Trojan and Younge, 1993). Similar concerns about re-admission have been echoed in recent reviews of discharge policies (Tierney et al., 1993). Failures to communicate are often at the root of poor discharge outcomes especially where the elderly patient is concerned. These findings indicate that sharing information can be fundamental to identifying the true needs and problems of patients and developing more effective strategies for resolving them.

Information sharing between nurse and patient may often be inhibited by the confusing effects of technical language and jargon used. Ashworth et al. (1992) warns against the use of 'impenetrable and unexplained professional and technical terminology' (p. 1433) on the grounds that it can generate feelings of inadequacy and embarrassment, for fear of appearing 'ignorant'. While proliferation of professional jargon and technical terms may be seen as an unavoidable consequence of the growing complexity of health care, this exclusivity of language and its side-effects should not be ignored. Nurses often are not immune to this problem and seek to compensate for it by rephrasing or rewording the information in 'layman's' terms. Unfortunately, this helpful response can be interpreted as further emphasizing the patient's lack of membership, reinforcing that they are indeed outsiders (Ashworth *et al.*, 1992).

Apart from the content of language and its exclusivity, a failure to recognize and value the patient's agenda can be another barrier to effective information sharing (Hewison, 1995). Where this happens the patient's real needs often go unrecognized and the patient's right to access pertinent information concerning their health status is restricted or denied. This has consequences beyond being ill-informed as it affects their decision making. When the withholding of health information from the patient is intentional then strong ethical objections can be raised. All too frequently in the past both doctors and nurses have decided if, and when, certain information can 'safely' be given. While such decisions may be well intentioned and aimed at promoting the best interests of the patient, it is always dangerous to assume anyone other than the patient knows what is 'best' for them. Such behaviour fundamentally stems from a lack of respect for a person's autonomy. Ashworth *et al.* (1992) concluded, from her study of patient participation, that were nurses truly to believe and accept patients as unique and worthy of treatment as individuals, then they could not fail to recognize them as a knowledgeable expert on how illness, treatment and operations affect them personally. Who else could intimately know about the impact a health problem had on self-concept, role and relationships with significant others, other than the patient? Sadly this is often not reflected in the sources of information and knowledge often used to profile patients' needs. Few have as yet sought the consumers' perspective on many health concerns.

Given that there is much to recommend sharing information, community health care nurses may need to question existing practices. This would entail developing and maintaining self-awareness and self-knowledge as important processes for recognizing internal barriers to sharing information (Chavasse, 1992). Changing individual practices may equally depend on whether the organizational climate is open in its communications with its employees as well as patients. Nurses, as employees, may themselves need to feel they too have access to important information concerning themselves and their work before they can then reciprocate by sharing information with their patients.

Sharing planning and decision making

Much of what has just been discussed around sharing information and knowledge might equally apply to this next dimension. Again several authors, on both sides of the Atlantic, have strongly supported patient involvement in planning and decision making (King, 1981; Macleod Clark and Latter, 1990; Wright, 1990; Orem, 1991). The premise of such recommendations are that patients, as active participants in care, are seen to be exercising their personal autonomy. There are, however, considerable differences between the importance given to autonomy in the USA in comparison to the UK. In the States the right to autonomy and participation has been legally recognized by the Patient Self-Determination Act 1991 which requires all hospitals, nursing homes and health agencies to advise patients of their rights to accept or refuse medical care.

Recently within the UK, there has been some movement towards giving legal recognition of patients' rights in this area, most notably with regard to advanced directives (BMA, 1994; Robertson, 1995). Furthermore, the right to refuse treatment has even been acknowledged by the courts on several occasions (Kennedy and Grubb, 1994). However, such court rulings are not always a true reflection of actual health care practices. Documentary evidence presented by the media, giving personal accounts of patients' or carers' experiences, suggest that patients' stated treatment preferences, or refusal, of further life saving intervention have on occasions been overridden or ignored by nursing or medical staff (BBC2, 1994). What is so often disturbing about these practices is that the views or preferences of others (such as doctors or colleagues) are placed above those of the patient thereby contravening the nurses' professional code of conduct (UKCC, 1994).

At the very beginning of this chapter it was pointed out that nursing has a mandate to involve patients in planning and decision making. This is not new to the health arena; in the late 1970s the World Health Organization (1978) recognized people had both 'a right and duty to participate individually (and collectively) in planning and implementation of their health care'. Several more recent reviews, policy statements and Acts of Parliament have placed a duty on health care providers to seek ways of increasing their involvement of service users at both the individual and organizational levels (NHS and Community Care Act, 1990; *Strategy for Nursing*, DOH, 1989; *Working in Partnership*, Mental Health Review Team, DOH, 1994; *Patient's Charter*, DOH, 1991). In the context of this paper, sharing and decision making at the individual level will concern itself with the opportunities for the shared planning of care, agreement of individual goals and aims, and the selection of appropriate interventions afforded by community health care nurses. Whether these directives are successful in encouraging practitioners to involve patients more in decision making and planning remains to be seen, though often such top-down approaches fail because of the lack of any sense of ownership. It may further help the cause if community health care nurses were to recognize the mutual rewards to be gained from adopting this approach. Perhaps the most beneficial outcomes from sharing planning and decision making are empowerment and positive patient care outcomes. There are many on the caseloads of community health care nurses who represent the vulnerable in our society, the frail elderly, chronically ill, those with learning disabilities, all of whom could benefit from being enabled to share in the process of reaching health care decisions and determining interventions. Achieving more positive care outcomes is equally affected by the mutual investment that sharing in this activity entails. Patients are more likely to play their part in the care process if they have been actively involved in setting the goals.

Despite these incentives there are factors which can equally restrain the sharing of planning and decision making. Again, a major influence is the organizational climate itself. Where controlling and non-participative management styles are commonly practised, the staff often feel disempowered and consequently ill-equipped then to empower others (Foster and Mayall, 1990; Stevenson and Parsloe, 1993). Much importance needs to be attached by the organization to fostering a climate of reciprocity and trust so that contributions from staff and their active involvement in planning and decision making is valued.

In today's NHS cost effectiveness and cost savings seem to be valued above democratic decision making processes and the involvement of subordinate staff or patients. These demands can influence the priorities and lead practitioners or their managers to favour only the clinically proven interventions. While this might to some extent improve clinical outcomes, this is at the expense of consumer choice and involvement. By denying choice, the exercise of autonomy is again restrictive and patients are expected (sometimes reluctantly) to conform to the nurse's wishes rather than their own. In a social care context, Raymond (1989) encountered service users who talked about feeling 'pressurized', having to 'knuckle under' and 'bite their tongue' when interacting with the professional, while in health care Waterworth and Luker (1990) made similar observations of what they coined 'reluctant collaborators'. Responses of this kind are often reactions to existing power differentials. Vulnerable service users, including patients, can be made to feel unable to assert their preferences and choices for fear that in doing so they might prejudice their chances of receiving services. It is possible that past encounters with domineering professionals have affected the way in which certain patient groups, in particular older patients, respond to professionals. Community health care nurses, as the gatekeepers to services, need to be sensitive to the considerable power they exert over others, especially that which comes from the ability to provide or deny access to caring services. This might explain why it is that some older patients and their carers tend to adopt acquiescing and conforming behaviours. Perhaps this is simply a defence mechanism used to avoid upsetting the professional and ensuring they receive some form of service, even if it is not the one that they most want or need.

Age has also been shown to influence involvement in decision making.

Biley (1992) found in a small study of acute surgical patients that those least likely to want to participate in this activity were the older patients. She was unable to show what produced this reluctance, highlighting a need for further research in this area. Explanation might be that the effort needed for adjusting to the idea of sharing planning and decision making is too difficult or complex to make. This may be especially so when people are ill. It seems entirely plausible to suggest that older and frailer patients are going to need whatever reserves of energy they have for just coping with the impact of their illness and achieving recovery or rehabilitation. Even so, community health care nurses need to be careful of simply accepting the patient's wishes and thus taking over the responsibility for all decision making. When the patient then wants to reassert their authority with regard to making choices about care, it can be all too easy for these overtures to be ignored and paternalism intervene. To avoid this scenario community practitioners can again turn to Biley's findings for potential solutions.

According to Biley, patients, including those who were elderly, can feel out of their depth and unqualified to make judgements and decisions about their care. She found some were comfortable with making certain types of decisions but felt there were some types better left to the nurse. Biley categorized these groups of decisions into those where 'the nurse knows best' and those where 'the patient knows best'. In the former, recognition was given to the extensive range of technological and theoretical knowledge and expertise nurses use to inform decisions concerning nursing interventions, whereas in the second category the important deciding factor was the personal and intimate knowledge that a patient possessed about things of importance to them. Shared planning and decision making in this format recognizes that both partners have an equal, but different, role to play. Working together and sharing decision making using this model requires both partners to negotiate those areas to be entrusted to the nurse's judgement alone and those where the patient's own views would be paramount. There are, however, several pragmatic limitations to this way of working which could affect its widespread use in practice. Finding the time to negotiate these parameters of decision-making may deter many hospital-based nurses from bothering, though in the community setting the relationship can develop over longer periods. Some practitioners may also be put off by arguing the difficulty of ensuring that the identified parameters are sufficiently comprehensive for both current and even future planning and decision-making needs. This in itself is difficult to predict in some complex changing care situations; however, not having an entirely airtight agreement is no justification for not trying to ensure the patient has some voice in respect of their care. Clearly any such agreements ought to be formalized within normal care plans, otherwise those involved in the care delivery would not be privy to what has been agreed and act accordingly, though any agreement of this kind, as with all advanced directives, cannot be considered as binding and unchangeable. Community health care nurses need to be sensitive to any changes that might influence what has hitherto been discussed, for instance growing confidence and willingness to join in decision making on the part of the patient signals the need for review, as would any deterioration in their condition. This emphasizes the need for vigilance in monitoring and reviewing opportunities afforded for sharing in the planning and decision-making process. Finally, even if these issues are dealt with there is then the question of whether both parties involved possess the necessary skills for the bargaining and negotiation that Biley's divisions of decision making would entail. In addition, the existing power imbalances, can, according to Trnobranski (1994), interfere negatively with the process of negotiation. Despite these barriers, the practitioner should not be put off finding and trying out new challenging ways of promoting greater involvement of patients, of all ages, in the area of decision making and planning. Otherwise the importance of sharing such activities as an empowering strategy may continue to be largely overlooked and devalued.

Sharing of responsibility

Having advocated that patients are allowed to be involved in decision making and planning, it seems logical to assume that with this comes a share of the responsibility and accountability for the outcomes of care. This, however, has implications on the legal standing given to the part played by the patient in their care. How the employer might view the accountability of their employee in these informal partnership arrangements must also receive consideration. Indeed, given these possibilities, it seems surprising that so little in the literature on participation or partnership discusses this issue. Responsibility can give an immense sense of self-worth and value to the patient. The trust that is implied by working together, to achieve shared goals, is a measure of how much the nurse recognizes and values the patient's contributions.

While these are the possible rewards, the other side of the coin may not be so appealing and attractive to patients. Outside of health care, any partnership would mean that both partners would equally share in the responsibility if things went wrong and so incur any penalties. On these terms, responsibility and accountability within a partnership is a two-way process in that both parties are held liable for the costs of failures, as well as reaping any rewards. However, in health care the situation is somewhat different in that a patient does not choose to go into hospital or be visited by a community nurse. Any agreements they make therefore cannot be viewed in the same way. Even so, to consider that a patient has a duty to be involved in planning and decision making implies some sense of obligation being owed. This could imply that penalties might be incurred if a patient did not dutifully participate in their care.

In the caring context patients who do not conform to nursing expectations or refuse care are often penalized in a variety of ways. Both in the hospital and community the difficult and demanding patients are avoided, passed from nurse to nurse and their needs largely ignored (Stockwell, 1972; Hewison, 1995). Nurses thus make the rules and mete out the punishment to those who break them. Apart from this informal system of judging acceptable behaviour, there are the more formal standards of the law. It is in this setting that the question of whether patients can ever be held legally responsible for their part in the caring process and thus accountable for the consequences presents an interesting challenge. As yet no case of this kind has appeared before the English courts, the only guiding precedents come from the North American courts. The term used for this type of complaint is 'contributory negligence' which means that the actions of the patient are shown to have contributed to the consequences of any negligent action by their doctor. A small number of cases heard in the North American courts in the 1980s led Picard to offer the following interesting observations (Kennedy and Grubb, 1994). First, it was held by the courts that any contributions made to care, by either patient or doctor, could not be viewed as equal, given the disparity of knowledge and the fact that the 'patient may be ill, submissive, or incapable of acting in their own best interests' (p. 492). The second observation was that any contributory negligence would have to be dependent on whether the patient met the standard of care expected of the 'reasonable patient'. What the courts might deem as 'reasonable' was linked to the knowledge the patient, as lay person, possessed about the relevant medical matters. From this, Picard forecast future changes to the court's present positions on the basis that while, up to the mid 1980s, Canadian and American courts had placed a somewhat low expectation of this knowledge, this was likely to change. Her prediction was that as the patient's knowledge and participation in health care becomes the norm, then the courts might thereby place greater expectations on the patient to contribute to their own health care and assume a proportional responsibility for outcomes directly affected by their contributions.

The case of Schliesman v Fisher (1979) illustrates Picard's principles well. Schliesman was a diabetic patient who suffered a below knee amputation; he alleged this was caused by his doctor's withdrawal of prescribed diabetic medication. In his defence, the doctor contended that this particular patient's history of non-compliance had led him to consider the patient unsafe to use the drug. On hearing this case, the presiding judge expressed concerns about the respondent's failure actively to control his illness, given that it was deemed to be within his power to do so. He noted that while the loss of leg could be attributed in part to the withdrawal of treatment, some of the blame lay with the patient. It was deemed of some significance that the respondent could have played a substantial part in bringing his diabetes under control, in line with his doctor's advice, but he had failed to take any action. This suggests that patients might potentially be held accountable by the courts for the part they play in their care. As a consequence, any failure on their part to meet agreed outcomes could be taken into account when apportioning legal liability. On the surface this judgement sounds just, however, unfortunately proving contributory negligence is not all that easy given previous experiences in the North American courts (Martineau *v* Nelson, 1976; Schliesman *v* Fisher, 1979).

Any such existing legal or moral duty to share responsibility and accountability would still only apply to those patients who are autonomous and so able voluntarily to consent to their part in the planning of care. It thus follows that in wanting to enable patients to take some responsibility for health, nurses must ensure that any non-compliance and unwillingness to share responsibility is not simply judged as a symptom of limited mental capacity and incompetence. Mental competence in this sense is simply being judged on the basis of what professionals perceive as rational decision making. In the past, and even present, paternalistic health professionals have tended to override the wishes of patients who are old, with failing mental health, or learning disabilities, deeming their expressed choices to be either 'irresponsible' or 'irrational'. Judgements are often based somewhat erroneously on what the professional themselves would have chosen to do, mental incapacity therefore appears to depend on whether the patient agrees, rather than disagrees, with what the professional considers is best (Kennedy and Grubb, 1994).

This particular version of 'nurse knows best' is disempowering, it assumes that the patient does not have the capacity to cope with such responsibilities. This pattern of behaviour can also be noticeable in nursing leadership styles. Working patterns in the community have fostered a high degree of autonomy in community health care nurses, often involving little questioning of the authority of these professionals over staff or patients. In some instances the power and control this independence fosters has produced management styles which do not permit staff or patient participation. Past studies in nursing have repeatedly shown that patients, as well as workers, reject such autocratic and authoritarian approaches (McIntosh, 1986; Foster and Mayall, 1990). Despite this knowledge the continuing traditional hierarchies within management of community nursing services only serve to reinforce leader dominance and the controlling of subordinates, namely other grades of staff or patients.

Failing to share responsibility can also be attributed to inadequacies within professional education. Meyer (1993) experienced a reluctance amongst staff to involve family and relatives in care provision in a hospital ward. A number of nurses felt ill-prepared for providing patient or carer education and support. Sharing responsibility therefore requires an ability to judge what can be safely shared with others. Otherwise patients may find themselves in the position of receiving too little responsibility or too much. Too much responsibility can also occur as a result of other deficiencies in the service where the resources are limited or inadequate; consequently the patient is left to cope with perhaps only minimal support. Sharing therefore presents challenges to conventional management structures which recognize only individual responsibility and accountability.

Sharing control and power

This final section draws together many of the threads from earlier discussions to consider whether the sharing of power and control with patients is ever achievable? From the consumers' perspective some have argued that while sharing goals and decision making are possibilities, the hope of acquiring a more equal share of the power is unlikely (Family Rights Group, 1991). The presence of power differentials between patients and health professionals has long been debated (Friedson, 1975; Miles, 1991). Therefore it should come as no surprise to community health care nurses that as the authority figure and professional expert they will often be perceived by their patients, in particular elderly patients, as very powerful individuals. The existence of such power has enabled community practitioners to exert considerable influence over patients' behaviours and health.

The nature of power is that those who possess it have the potential ability to influence another person or group (Moorhead and Griffin, 1992). Power defined thus is capable of manipulating people to achieve desired responses, indicating the potential for misuse and abuse of power especially where vulnerable individuals are concerned. To prevent this patients and the public at large need some form of internal or external regulation to protect them from the whims of powerful professionals. It would be naive to suggest that practitioners' own moral code of conduct offers sufficient protection given the pluralistic nature of health care, therefore the UKCC, as the professional regulatory body, has disciplinary functions aimed at protecting the public. They also provide nurses with a code of conduct which currently suggests that any influence exerted by nurses on patient's behaviours would always need to be in the patient's best interest. The danger is that the patient's interests can be manipulated or misinterpreted to represent the nurse's interests or the interest of others.

Power when used in this way often creates dependency and removes autonomous control from the patient, whereas a more legitimate use of power would be to enable and empower patients to reassert control over their own health and well-being. These contrasting uses of power are similarly reflected in Hokanson Hawks' (1991) analysis of power within nursing. From her review of the literature two distinctive categories of power emerged which were defined as the 'power over' and the 'power to'. 'Power over' is allied to the power bases identified by French and Raven (cited in Moorhead and Griffin, 1992) as being legitimate, reward, coercive, expert and referent. Power of this kind seeks to dominate, it relies on professional authority and expert knowledge as the source of legitimacy and justification for some of its oppressive nature. Patients were often exposed to this form of power given the 'paternalistic philosophy that previously dominated health care' (Trnobranski, 1994). In the past subjection to 'rigid ward routines and unquestioning hospital rules and regulations' (Morgan, 1984) often resulted in patients losing their identity, self-esteem and independence.

Disempowered by this process the patients responded by adopting passive and submissive behaviours. Repeated exposure to these patterns develops an expectation on the part of the patient that nurses, or any other health professional, will always assume control. The consequences of these established patterns are still evident amongst older patients today (Hewison, 1995), and other equally vulnerable groups. A study by Rees and Wallace (cited in Evans and Kearney, 1996) into consumer participation within social care found that it was economically and educationally disadvantaged individuals who exhibited submissiveness and deference to expertise and authority. Many older patients also fit into this category by virtue of their lack of educational opportunities and limited financial resources. By contrast the well educated, economically secure service users were more confident with officialdom and were the ones who actively wanted to share decision making (Evans and Kearney, 1996).

An unfortunate consequence of accepting the submissive responses of patients is that it can lead nurses into believing they have the right to give directions, orders and make the rules (Hewison, 1995). Kendall's (1993) small study of health visitors clearly indicated that controlling behaviours were still a feature of practitioner and client interactions, in particular in contacts with families from the lower social classes. Partnership as a form of professional–client relationship was reserved largely for those deemed 'worthy', such individuals tended to belong to the middle classes. Similar observations were made in the district nurse–patient relationship back in the late 1970s. McIntosh (1979) found that district nurses interacted differently to those in 'poor homes' as opposed to those from the middle classes. In the former setting nurses tended to adopt a more dominant role, 'good naturedly issuing orders to any members of the household they could enlist' (p. viii). While this study was undertaken some 15 years ago, Kendall's more recent findings suggest it would be erroneous to assume that patients are no longer subjected to such discrimination and paternalistic practices.

It would appear that the mere presence of 'power over' seems to create structures which either intentionally or unintentionally encourage such controlling practices. The influence of other health professionals who thrive on their power and status and cling to their trappings of power with a limpet-like tenacity (Kennedy, 1988; Baistow, 1994) may in part be responsible for such nursing behaviours. Macleod Clark and Latter (1990) recognized that these behaviours needed challenging and thus urged all nurses, including those working in the community, to confront their control over power. They pointed out that nurses needed to recognize that partnership really means handing back power to the patient. Therefore the proposed solution was for 'nurses to divest themselves of the power, status and authority which they associate with being a professional' (p. 31). To many community health care nurses this might seem a somewhat drastic step and entail an unacceptable loss of power and control thereby damaging their professional standing alongside other professional groups. However, on closer inspection, their advice is not advocating that nurses become 'power neutral' or 'powerless', but recommending the divestment of 'power over'. By retaining and developing the scope for 'power to' the gateway to further sharing and partnership remains firmly open.

'Power to', according to Hokanson Hawks (1991), is a wholly different form of influence aimed at enabling and empowering rather than dominating. Its primary purpose is gate-opening as opposed to gate-keeping. According to Rogers (1983), for power to be an enabling and empowering process, knowledge, information and decision making must be shared. Mutual goal setting and working together are likewise associated with 'power to' (Hokanson Hawks, 1991). One source of 'power to' available to experienced community health care nurses is their possession of valuable information and specialist knowledge that may be of help with meeting the needs of a patient. It is through the channelling of professional expertise and knowledge, and the sharing of it with patients, that effective care can be instigated and agreed goals met.

Power which enables people is sensitive to the organizational climate and requires a very different attitude and approach by those in authority, especially those managing the services. Authoritarian styles of management and hierarchical decision making stifle the opportunities for sharing and partnership. What is needed are changes similar to those adopted in primary nursing. A decentralization of management structures has been shown to facilitate greater nurse autonomy and the sharing of power between nurses (McMahon, 1991; Wright, 1991). This has subsequently encouraged greater sharing of control and power with the patient, illustrating the impact that empowering one group of individuals can have in other relationships.

Empowerment is thus a potentially powerful tool, which Raymond (1989) claims can offer nurses a new source of role legitimacy and *raison d'être* (Baistow, 1994). He contends that instead of allying itself to medicine to acquire or maintain power, nurses would be better off seeking power and authority through their interactions with patients. By adopting this strategy community health care nurses, in collaboration with colleagues working in other settings, could realign the boundaries of professional power and control; diverting power away from professionals, or any other powerful group, to those who have been traditionally disempowered within health care.

Conclusions

The diverse nature of community health care nurses' practice suggests that the opportunities to develop sharing relationships and partnership will differ. Finding out what comfortably fits into a particular setting and planning considered strategies is in itself a useful sharing exercise, one in which all interested parties, nurses and patients, might wish to participate.

While this may seem simple, sharing in the professional context needs to be consciously nurtured and integrated into the practitioner's repertoire of skills. Some community health care nurses may have lost the skill or never fully experienced this way of working. What is most needed to facilitate this process is for practitioners to feel empowered to bring about such changes in their practice. For this to happen sharing and partnership must become accepted and established into the educational processes. This is starting to happen with the increasing emphasis on shared learning within the new specialist practitioner programmes (UKCC, 1994). In this context, novice or experienced practitioners can begin to share with other disciplines and appreciate their contributions to primary health care. By facilitating collaborative working in the classroom new insights can be gained into existing roles and existing power differentials safely challenged. These learning opportunities might then pave the way for more meaningful sharing and partnership with patients and clients.

Points to consider

1 Identify any driving or restraining forces currently operating in your work setting that might be influencing the extent to which you and others are able to share information and decision making with patients.

2 Explore the feasibility of community health care nurses adopting Hokanson Hawk's notion of 'power to' as an alternative to the more traditional model of professional power and control.

3 Reflect on how open you are, as a practitioner, to sharing in its many forms. Consider what factors have influenced you in the past that have empowered or disempowered you for working in partnership.

4 Discuss the opportunities that you as a student community health care nurse have had either within the classroom or out in the practice setting to work in partnership with your teachers. Consider to what extent these educational experiences directly influence the relationship you might develop with patients.

References

Ashworth, P., Longmate, M. and Morrison, P. 1992: Patient participation: its meaning and significance in the context of caring. *Journal of Advanced Nursing*, **17**, 1430–9.

Baistow, K. 1994: Liberation and regulation? Some paradoxes of empowerment. *Critical Social Policy*, **42**, 34–47.

Bastiani, J. 1993: *Your home school links*. New Publication Educational.

BBC2 1994: *Taking liberties: not for 222*. 12th May.

Biley, F. 1992: Some determinants that affect patient participation in decision making about nursing care. *Journal of Advanced Nursing*, **17**, 414–21.

British Medical Association 1994: *Statement on advanced directives* (revised version). London: BMA.

Browne, A. 1993: A conceptual clarification of respect. *Journal of Advanced Nursing,* **18**, 211–17.

Chavasse, J.M. 1992: New dimensions of empowerment in nursing – and challenges. *Journal of Advanced Nursing,* **17**, 1–2.

Christensen, J. 1990: *Nursing partnership: a model for nursing practice.* London: Churchill Livingstone.

DOH 1989: *Strategy for nursing.* London: HMSO.

DOH 1990: *NHS and Community Care Act.* London: HMSO.

DOH 1991: *Patient's charter.* London: HMSO.

DOH 1994: *Working in partnership: a collaborative approach to care.* Mental Health Review Team. London: HMSO.

Evans, D. and Kearney, J. 1996: *Working in social care: a systemic approach.* Aldershot: Arena.

Family Rights Group 1991: *The Children Act (resource pack).* London: FRG Publications.

Ford, A. 1990: Patients are worms. *Nursing Times,* **86**, 15, 59.

Fosbinder, D. 1994: Patient perceptions of nursing care: an emerging theory of interpersonal competence. *Journal of Advanced Nursing,* **20**, 1085–93.

Foster, M.C. and Mayall, B. 1990: Health visitors as educators. *Journal of Advanced Nursing,* **15**, 286–92.

Friedson, E. 1975: Dilemmas in the doctor/patient relationship. In Cox, C. and Mead, A. *A sociology of medical practice.* London: Collier Macmillan.

Hokanson Hawks, J. 1991: Power: a conceptual analysis. *Journal of Advanced Nursing,* **16**, 754–62.

Hewison, A. 1995: Nurses' power in interactions with patients. *Journal of Advanced Nursing,* **21**, 1, 75–82.

Jewell, S.E. 1994: Patient participation: what does it mean to nurses? *Journal of Advanced Nursing,* **19**, 433–8.

Kendall, S. 1993: Client participation in health promotion encounters with health visitors. In Wilson Barnett, J. and Macleod Clark, J. (eds), *Research in health promotion.* London: Macmillan Press.

Kennedy, J. 1988: *Treat me right: essays in medical law and ethics.* Oxford: Oxford University Press.

Kennedy, J. and Grubb, I. 1994: *Medical law: texts and materials.* London: Butterworth.

King, I. 1981: *A theory for nursing: systems, concepts, processes.* New York: John Wiley.

Macleod Clark, J. and Latter, S. 1990: Working together. *Nursing Times,* **86**, 48, 28–31.

Martineau *v* Nelson 1976: 246 NW 2d 409 (Sup Ct Minn).

McIntosh, J.B. 1979: The nurse–patient relationship. *Nursing Mirror Supplement,* January 25, i–xi.

McIntosh, J.B. 1986: *A consumer perspective on the health visiting service.* Social and Paediatric Research Unit, University of Glasgow.

McMahon, R. 1991: Power and communication issues in primary nursing. In Ersser, S. and Tutton, E. (eds), *Primary nursing in perspective.* London: Scutari Press.

Meyer, J. 1993: Lay participation in care: threat to the status quo. In Wilson Barnett, J. and Macleod Clark, J. (eds), *Research in health promotion.* London: Macmillan Press.

Miles, A. 1991: *Women, health and medicine.* Milton Keynes: Open University Press.

Moorhead and Griffin 1992: *Organisational behaviour* (3rd edn). Boston: Houghton and Mifflin Co.

Morgan, A. 1984: Learning to interact. *Journal of District Nursing,* April, 20/22/24.

Orem, D.E. 1991: *Nursing concepts of practice* (4th edn). St Louis: Mosby Year Book.

Oxford English Dictionary, 1993.

Pugh, G and De'ath, E. 1989: *Working towards partnership in the early years.* London: National Children's Bureau.

Raymond, Y. 1989: Empowerment in practice. *Practice,* **1**, 5–23.

Rogers, C. 1983: *Freedom to learn in the 80s.* Columbus: Charles E Merrill; New York: Mcgraw-Hill.

Robertson, G.S. 1995: Making an advanced directive. *British Medical Journal*, **310**, 6974, 236–8.

Royal College of Nursing 1987: *In pursuit of excellence: a position statement on nursing*. London: RCN.

Schliesman *v* Fisher 1979: 158 Cal Rptr 527 (Cal CA).

Sheppard, M. 1993: Client satisfaction, extended intervention and interpersonal skills in community mental health. *Journal of Advanced Nursing*, **18**, 246–60.

Stevenson, O. and Parsloe, P. 1993: *Community care and empowerment*. York: Joshua Rowntree Foundation.

Stockwell, F. 1972: *The unpopular patient*. London: Royal College of Nursing.

Tierney, A.J., Jose Closs, S., Hunter, H.C. and Macmillan, M.S. 1993: Experiences of elderly patients concerning discharge from hospital. *Journal of Clinical Nursing*, **2**, 179–83.

Trnobranski, P.H. 1994: Nurse–patient negotiation: assumption or reality? *Journal of Advanced Nursing*, **19**, 733–7.

Trojan, L. and Younge, O. 1993: Developing trusting, caring relationships: home care nurses and elderly patients. *Journal of Advanced Nursing*, **18**, 1903–10.

UKCC 1994: *Professional code of conduct* (3rd edn). London: UKCC publications.

Waterworth, S. and Luker, K.A. 1990: Reluctant collaborators: do patients want to be involved in decisions concerning care? *Journal of Advanced Nursing*, **15**, 971–6.

Wilson-Barnett, J. 1989: Limited autonomy and partnership: professional relationships in health care. *Journal of Medical Ethics*, **15**, 12–16.

World Health Organization and United Nations Children's Fund 1978: *Primary health care: international conference on primary health care*. Alma Ata, USSR.

Wright, S. 1990: *My patient, my nurse*. London: Scutari Press.

Wright, S. 1991: Facilitating therapeutic nursing and independent practice. In McMahon, R. and Pearson, A. (eds), *Nursing as therapy*. London: Chapman and Hall.

9 Teamwork and skill mix

Sandra Baulcomb and Sandra Burley

Teamwork is suggested to be the most effective way to deliver services to a variety of individuals or groups (DHSS, 1986), yet it still remains problematic in reality (Audit Commission, 1992). It is the purpose of this chapter to examine the concept of teamwork, trace its development and examine the type, purpose and functioning of the client's team, network association teams and formal teams (Ovretveit, 1993), within which community nurses work in the primary health care setting. The chapter will explore the advancement of teamwork through shared educational provision and team building workshops and examine the main developments of the skill mix debate using the primary health care team as a vehicle to promote discussion and elucidate salient and relevant issues.

Throughout the chapter, the reader is encouraged to examine their individual team contribution as preparation for discussion with other team members in order to expose areas of commonality, highlight and acknowledge unique aspects of their role and identify areas for team growth and development.

Introduction

Specialist community practitioners should channel their activity toward the provision of care and services for identified communities or population groups as well as individuals living in the community (UKCC, 1994).

The range of services available have to meet an ever expanding demand for provision based upon the assessment and identification of the communities' health needs. Work focuses on targeted health promotion activity, intervention and care provision for the acute, chronic and terminally ill (WHO, 1974), offered within a framework that promotes independence and choice for clients (DOH, 1991, 1995), while being mindful of the constraints of finite resources.

In the late 1980s, 50 per cent of the NHS workforce were employed as nurses, midwives and health visitors (Central Statistical Office, 1992), resulting in a cost of £7 billion out of a total NHS expenditure for 1992–1993 of £27.4 billion (HM Treasury, 1992). These escalating costs caused increasing concern for community nurses in fulfilling the governments edict for cost containment against the balance for the provision and delivery of a quality, appropriate and needs led service (DOH, 1990).

As well as offering an appropriate range of care and services, community nurses are required to develop services that are signposted through the *Patient's Charter* (DOH, 1991, 1995) which are accessible, acceptable, equitable, person centred, health promoting and multisectorial; that is, involving assessment of other aspects affecting individuals such as the environment and social and personal aspects which influence the health status of the target population (WHO, 1978).

Brief consideration needs to be given to the current factors influencing team working, these being primarily government health policy, i.e. the inception of GP fundholding, community trusts (DOH, 1989a), the effects of clinical grading (Beardshaw and Robinson, 1990), the recent developments in community nurse education (UKCC, 1994), alongside the nursing profession's call for increased autonomy of its practitioners.

Teamwork has become increasingly relevant to primary health care provision with the emphasis on the move toward a primary care-led NHS (DOH, 1994), with continuing support for the development of community services in line with the government White Papers such as *Caring for People* (DOH, 1989b), *Working for Patients* (DOH, 1989a) and the subsequent implementation of the NHS and Community Care Act (DOH, 1990) and the push toward a more pro-active and preventive approach to service provision (DOH, 1992).

These policy changes have been coupled with the drive from the nursing profession to raise awareness of personal accountability for practice through the updating of the Code of Professional Conduct (UKCC, 1992a) and the expansion of this through the scope of professional practice (UKCC, 1992b), allowing nurses the opportunity to develop their clinical practice, leadership and management skills.

Against this high expectation of nursing provision, it is important to investigate how community nurses use their knowledge and skills to ensure that individuals, families and the wider community receive the appropriate care from the person or team best able to provide it.

Defining teamwork

The word teamwork may be broken down into two aspects, team and work. Team may be defined as 'a group of people who make different contributions toward the achievement of a common goal' (Pritchard and Pritchard, 1994, p. 13), while work may be defined as 'physical or mental effort directed towards doing something' (Collins Concise English Dictionary, 1992). Some people use the words team and teamwork synonymously. This misunderstanding fuels some of the confusion that encompasses the idea that simply to call a group of people a team does not automatically mean that it will function as such without any further effort.

In reality many teams exist in name only and are passive and empty vessels. As Harding reported in 1981, successful teamwork needs more than an agreement to work together (DHSS, 1981). True teamwork demands active participation, commitment, cooperation (to unite for common effort), communication, coordination (to bring into order as parts of a whole), and collaboration (act jointly), all of which are time consuming.

The word team conjures up a variety of notions such as a set of players in a sports team, quiz teams or project teams, each requiring its participants to fulfil a defined role with a given set of parameters. This analogy of a football team, although a familiar one, provides a valuable introduction into some of the characteristics, which are fundamental components of team membership. The football team is more than a group of people with a common interest; it has a set of rules, predetermined number of players, each with defined roles, which although overlapping provide continuity for the game with each player working within recognized boundaries. Teamwork is the link that transforms the set of individual players into a team that functions as a whole, involving regular coaching which requires the activity and energy needed in order to provide foundation for success.

These general characteristics were also identified by Gilmore *et al.* as long ago as 1974, when looking into the work of nursing teams in general practice. Gilmore *et al.* (1974) highlight the need for members to 'share a common purpose which binds them together and guides their action, to clearly understand individual contribution recognising similarities and differences, pooling knowledge, skills and resources and sharing responsibility for the outcome' (p. 6). These characteristics are still recognized today as fundamental attributes of successful teamwork, although the reality of achieving these has in the main remained an illusive ideal.

Type of teams

The type of teams community nurses may participate in fall into three main categories, as identified by Ovretveit (1993) as 'clients team, network association teams and formal teams'. It is useful to define these types of teams further.

The clients team is convened by bringing together an appropriate group of people that may be from different disciplines who function as a team solely for the purpose of that client intervention. They may not actually meet each other, but need to communicate if they are to work toward providing the optimum care for that client. The major difference in this team is that the membership is not static and is continually responding to client need; therefore it is dynamic in orientation. It may be suggested that this should not be deemed to be a team, but this could be defended along the lines of it being a flexible approach to teamwork and all those involved are working toward the same common goal, that of the care of that individual client.

'Network-association teams' may be defined as 'a voluntary association of service providers, relating to cross-refer, or to co-ordinate work with a client' (Ovretveit, 1993, p. 63). They exist on the one hand purely as a referral network, for the purpose of referring a client to another professional, or on the other hand as a forum to meet to exchange referrals and discuss ideas for developing aspects of the service. The major difference in this team is that the membership is of a voluntary nature, without specified rules or a recognized leader (Ovretveit, 1993).

'Formal teams' may be uniprofessional or multidisciplinary in nature and may be defined as 'a working group with a defined membership of different professionals, governed by an agreed and explicit team policy, which is upheld by a team leader' (Ovretveit, 1993, p. 64), e.g. primary health care teams. Formal teams are the teams that community nurses may be most able easily to identify with, in name if not in either experience or reality.

Team membership and size

As the main focus of this chapter is the primary health care team it is relevant to mention the specific membership of this team and make some comments about optimum size of the group. Many articles use the Harding committee definition of primary health care team, which provides a good basis for discussion: 'A primary health care team is an interdependent group of general medical practitioners and secretaries and/or receptionists, health visitors, district nurses and midwives who share a common purpose and responsibility, each member clearly understanding his or her own function and those of the other members, so that they all pool skills and knowledge to provide an effective primary health care service' (DHSS, 1981, p. 2).

This definition identifies what may be called 'core team' members, but omits to include practice nurses, as this definition precedes the enormous growth in practice nurses employed in general practice, following the implementation of the GP Contract in 1990 (DOH, 1989c). Other team members are also excluded, these being those who are attached to or relate to several teams or geographical boundaries, e.g. school nurses, community psychiatric nurses, learning disabilities nurses and social workers. Immediately one will notice that the notion of membership of primary health care teams is a rather flexible concept.

Teams vary in size dependent on the general practice population the team is supporting; this may range from very small 'core teams' of five to rather larger teams in excess of 30, including the wider team members. Poulton (1995) in her study on effective multidisciplinary teamwork found that out of the 68 primary health care teams she collected data from, the average team size was 18, but those teams with 14 members or less interacted more frequently and participated more in team decision making. Poulton's findings are supported by the work of Belbin (1981) who found that teams of six are effective and Heron (1973) who felt that six was the minimum size with 12 being the optimum size for group participation.

Historical overview

It would be helpful at this stage briefly to set in context the historical development of the primary health care team. This particular team had a long and chequered history, and has some significance because it has become the foundation on which the concept of teamwork has been built.

Prior to the inception of the National Health Service (NHS), it was common for general practitioners (GPs) to work alone in single-handed practices providing services according to their perceptions of what their patients required or reacting to need, thus providing rather unfocused care (Baggott, 1994). In 1920 the Dawson Committee (Ministry of Health, 1920) suggested that a more coordinated service could be offered to patients if health professionals worked in multidisciplinary teams from primary health centres. The professionals identified in the report were GPs, dentists, pharmacists, nurses, health visitors and midwives. This proposal was somewhat ahead of its time and the GPs were reluctant to give up their independence, preferring to work as they always had.

The next initiative which encouraged closer team working occurred some years later and was suggested by a sub-committee of the Gillie Committee, which was looking into the future scope of general practice (Central Health Service Council, 1963). The initiative was group attachment in which community nurses, mainly district nurses and health visitors, were attached to a particular general medical practice. After an initially slow start, group attachment has now become the favoured modus operandi with many community nurses and associated teams based within general practice premises.

Following the inception of the NHS in 1946 nurses working in the community were managed and organized by local authorities (Baggott, 1994). This arrangement seemed to alienate the nurses from the doctors with whom they were meant to be liaising closely. Structurally it was difficult for the nurses to meet their professional colleagues within the practice setting. However, in 1965 as group attachment was gaining momentum health centres were being built which encouraged interprofessional partnership and contact (Hicks, 1976). In 1965 the GPs recognized that there was great potential to improve the services which were provided by them for their practice populations. The *Charter for the Family Doctor* (BMA, 1965) brought about a re-negotiation of the GPs' contract with the NHS. This led to many changes being made, including improvements to surgery premises to make them better environments in which to work and for patients to visit. The concept of group practice was further promoted to encourage GPs to pool their skills (Gilmore *et al.*, 1974). The Charter also brought in new arrangements for fee payments to GPs. One example was 70 per cent reimbursement of salary costs for two whole-time equivalent staff per principal GP in the practice. Although many GPs used this incentive to employ secretaries and reception staff, nurses were also employed to work in practices alongside their GP colleagues. Thus practice nurses were increasing in numbers and becoming valued members of the team. The practice nurse as we shall see later has become a pivotal member of the team, carrying out many aspects of care which are now seen as essential for the practice population.

In 1974 the NHS was reorganized, and the involvement of local authorities in health care provision was restricted to environmental services (OHE, 1984). This brought community nurses into the management and organizational structure of the NHS, under the auspices of the Area Health Authority. GPs remained as independent contractors to the NHS but the reorganization was another milestone in the emergence of primary health care teams, as it removed another obstacle from their path. Community nurses were now able to have more contact with their professional colleagues especially GPs and practice nurses.

Following the 1974 reorganization of the NHS there have been further major revisions in the management structure of the NHS which have impacted on service provision across the board. Probably the greatest challenge to be met by primary health care teams was the advent of the NHS and Community Care Act in 1990. The implementation of this Act has had implications for the primary health care team as it reached into every aspect of community nursing and general practice provision, sparking off a cascade of change which has shaped the primary health care team into what it is now.

The next section of this chapter will look at the reality of teamwork and then focus on two areas for further discussion, these being first the development and potential of the new Specialist Practitioner Programmes for community nurses alongside the ongoing multidisciplinary workshops that seek to advance the notion of effective teamwork and second the process and utilization of skill mix within the team.

Reality of teamwork

Many people comment on teamwork although not many of these comments relate to successful team working. The Audit Commission (1992) outlined some of the barriers to effective teamwork in the primary health care team. These are separate lines of control or accountability, as supported by Waine (1992), and diverse objectives. For example, Community Trusts employ district nurses, health visitors, mental health nurses, learning disabilities nurses, school nurses and children's nurses; yet practice nurses and practice managers are employed by the GP, who is contracted to the Family Health Service Authority (FHSA) to provide health services for the practice population. Social workers are still being employed by the local authority. Different payment systems, also cited by Waine (1992), have led to suspicion over motives and resentment, e.g. GP service payments. Professional barriers are initiated through lack of common elements of training, e.g. separate training for community nurses, GPs and social workers. This is further perpetuated after registration with few examples of shared learning being evident, and perceived inequalities in status, e.g. the power and control the GP is deemed to have in comparison with the nurses.

The Audit Commission go on to identify rigidity as another aspect detrimental to teamwork: 'Rigidity within teams with members adhering to narrow definitions of their roles, preventing the creative and flexible response required to meet the variety of human need present. They are also likely to have lower morale. For nurses working under such circumstances efficient teamwork remains an illusive ideal' (Audit Commission, 1992, p. 20).

This report has been further supported by the work of Wiles and Robinson (1994), who studied nurses' views of teamworking in 20 practices and exposed problems which reiterate the findings of all those before, namely a wide variation among team members in their feelings of integration into the team, different perceptions of shared philosophies of care, disagreement over roles, and the feeling that traditional roles had been eroded.

These findings support the experiences of many members of the primary health care team in acknowledging that teamwork was more complex in reality than most people were led to believe and is founded upon the failings of the organizational system, lack of shared learning opportunities leading to role protection and professional rivalry and lack of understanding of each other's roles.

It is with these particular problems in mind that the chapter will explore the need for shared learning through education both in preparation for specialist community practice and through specific team-building workshop programmes for primary health care teams.

Multidisciplinary teamwork

Hennessey (1994) cites Vanclay's (1994) definition of shared learning as 'any form of interacting between two or more persons from different or social care professionals. This is to improve collaboration, communication and mutual respect between members of different professions in the belief that this will lead to improved services'.

The continued call for shared learning between primary health care team members may be facilitated by the new Community Specialist Practitioner programmes (UKCC, 1994), and the ongoing work of the Health Education Authority (1995) through their multidisciplinary workshop programme for primary health care.

Community Specialist Practitioner programme

The new Community Specialist Practitioners programme, has brought eight branches of community nursing together for preparation for community practice at degree level; these branches include General Practice Nursing, Public Health Nursing (Health Visiting), Community Nursing in the Home (District Nursing), Community Mental Health Nursing, Community Mental Handicap Nursing, School Nursing, Community Children's Nursing and Occupational Health Nursing (UKCC, 1994).

This is an exciting opportunity for educational institutions to provide courses which are flexible, adaptable and appropriate, which support the need for specialist practitioners 'to exercise higher levels of clinical decision making and will be able to monitor and improve standards of care through the supervision of practice: clinical audit; the provision of skilled professional leadership and the development of practice through research, teaching and the support of professional colleagues' (UKCC, 1994, p. 3). The course is required to provide students with common core modules and specific specialist modules.

This affords the institution the opportunity to act in a pro-active way in promoting shared learning between the eight branches of the course. Although this may be criticized as being too little too late, as this is a post-registration preparation and excludes other primary health care team members such as GPs and social workers who currently have separate schemes for their professional education, it is nevertheless a commendable start in trying to explore the fundamental aspects of role definition, role boundaries and initiating groupwork, inviting GPs and social work colleagues to participate. Hopefully, in years to come, specialist community practitioner courses may extend to common modules for all members of the primary health care team and could even progress to pre-registration nurse education.

Although shared learning could well be promoted through these educational programmes, it is currently hindered by the lack of equal opportunity of funding for all branches, as both practice nurses and occupational health nurses predominantly work outside the NHS, so therefore do not attract regional funding for course fees and money toward replacement salary costs. So despite these nurses at last gaining recognition as specialist community practitioners, the reality of attending these courses may be hindered by course fees being too expensive for them to pay. On the other hand the GP may be willing to pay but unable to release the practice nurse from work for study time. This is more problematic for these two groups of nurses than their trust counterparts as many still work alone.

Multidisciplinary workshops

Lack of shared learning opportunities between GPs, nurses, social workers and other team members have been apparent for some time, although it is acknowledged that there has been increasing activity in creating opportunities for team-building workshops through the health education authority programme for primary health care (HEA, 1995).

This multidisciplinary, multiprofessional initiative began in 1987, providing an opportunity for primary health care team members 'to reflect on their current health promotion and disease prevention practices and subsequently develop plans and strategies to enhance their activities' (HEA, 1995, p. 5). The organization and delivery of the workshops has been through local organizing teams (LOTs) comprising representation mainly from FHSAs, trusts, health authorities, general practice, higher education, and occasionally social services and voluntary organizations.

These workshops are designed to encourage participants to use a problem-solving approach, that will be continued by the team back in practice. Spratley (1989) found in evaluating the workshops that they enhanced communication, teamwork and practice organization, and helped participants to clarify their roles and responsibilities in primary health care.

Skill mix

Skill mix is a concept which has a direct bearing on teams working in the community. It is a subject which appears to raise more questions than it is able to answer. Skill mix was bound to become an issue in nursing, when the government of the time decided to reform the NHS with a view to running it on business lines, where market forces are allowed to set the pace especially in relation to cost of services; increased accountability for nurses and GPs was also a feature (DOH, 1990). One aspect of allowing market forces to drive the service is the need to improve productivity which goes hand-in-hand with managing resources effectively and ensuring value for money (Audit Commission, 1992). One strategy which has been suggested as helpful in ensuring that resources are used effectively, especially the staff resource, is skill mix reviews or re-profiling.

What is meant by skill mix and what are its features? A useful definition of skill mix is provided by Sturdy (1991), who says it is the balance between trained and untrained, qualified and unqualified, supervisory and operative staff within a defined service area, as well as between different staff groups. This needs to be differentiated from grade mix which refers to an assessment of mix of grades of staff in a particular working environment (HVA, 1992). It is important to note that grade mix does not directly correlate with skill mix nor does it equate to competency (Lightfoot et al., 1992). The principal difference between these two approaches is that while skill mix is an attempt to promote the flexibility and creativity for a cost-effective service grade mix tends to support existing demarcation lines within a service, and inhibits a flexible approach to practice (Gibbs et al., 1990; Sturdy, 1991).

How can skill mix be operationalized in the practice setting? There are several options which can be used by the stakeholders but there is no set formula available which can accurately determine the appropriate skill mix for all clinical settings (RCN, 1992).

The skill mix activity which was suggested by the NHSME (1992) was simply to have an observer watch the activities carried out by nurses and to record these activities on a hand-held computer. The resultant data were then analysed and set against the expectations of nurses in relation to which nurse could carry out the said task.

This method has advantages in terms of economic activity. The task can be reduced to the lowest common denominator, that is, which lowest grade of staff is able carry out the task. This obviously appeals to managers who are increasingly having to provide a service which meets quality standards but at the lowest possible cost. The problem with this approach is that there is no acknowledgement of the knowledge base used and the decision-making skills being utilized to determine the tasks to be performed and the outcomes which may be expected as a result of the input. When the NHSME report (1992) was published, the reaction from community nursing staff was swift and positive: they saw it as a direct attack on their jobs and felt it could cause long-term and irreparable damage to the infrastructure of the community nursing service (Cowley and Mackenzie, 1993).

While the method outlined above has its uses, there has to be an approach which is more adept at identifying the needs of the community and then marrying up the skills of the workforce to meet identified need. Skill mix exercises cannot be carried out in a vacuum; they have to reflect other activities and initiatives which have been implemented such as *The Patient's Charter* (DOH, 1995), and the *Health of the Nation* (1992). Bevan *et al.* (1991) suggest that skill mix should ideally:

- start by defining the client group in question;
- identify what health care services these individuals require;
- define what work needs to be done to provide this service;
- determine what responsibilities and what tasks must be done to perform the work well and economically;
- define what mix of general skills and competencies is required;
- specify job descriptions and good personnel procedures;
- manage and achieve change to current structures.

This is a much more sophisticated approach to skill mix than the previous example and addresses many of the issues and anxieties which were identified by the profession as a result of the NHSME report and the findings of the Audit Commission in Homeward Bound (1992). Although Bevan *et al.* (1991) have given the profession a usable framework, as Littlewood (1995) points out this approach has rarely been attempted in community settings due to the perceived complexity of carrying out such a study, the strength of different professions involved and their restricted vision, as well as the difficulty of defining the client group, its needs and the service it requires.

It is important that when skill mix activities are taking place in a unit or locality the staff concerned are involved and are kept properly informed of progress and the likely outcome (RCN, 1992). Bottom-up approaches, i.e. those in which the workforce are included from the beginning and in which they have a role to play in the discussions and the decisions to be made, are more likely to be accepted and implemented successfully than those which come from a top-down or higher management perspective (Wright, 1986).

So what part can the individual practitioner play in skill mix activities?

BE PREPARED

- Even if skill mix activities are not affecting one's team directly it is prudent to be as well-informed as possible by reading material which is provided by employers and professional organizations such as the Royal College of Nursing.
- Discuss skill mix activities with colleagues and try to build alliances within the team which demonstrate commitment to delivering high quality patient care.
- If possible get involved with steering committees or project groups on behalf of colleagues, or nominate the member of the team with the most appropriate skills to take part.

NEGOTIATE

- Work with management to identify the purpose of the skill mix exercise for the team.
- Articulate the philosophy of care that is adopted by the team to ensure it is not undermined by the skill mix exercise.
- Examine the standards which have been set for the team to ensure these are not compromised.
- Assess the possible need for skills development and attendance on courses as a result of the identification of unmet need in the patient/client population.

GET INVOLVED

- Ensure that a sufficient period of time has been allocated to the exercise which reflects the true activity levels of the team.
- Make sure that the personnel collecting the data are well-informed about the level of knowledge and skill required to meet the needs of the patient/client groups and that they are aware of the level of decision making involved and that they appreciate the other activities that have to be fulfilled to meet the needs of patients/clients, such as attending meetings and being involved in special project groups.
- If appropriate challenge the data collectors to ensure they are being as thorough as possible in their task.

ANALYSE THE DATA AND IMPLEMENT THE RECOMMENDATIONS

- Ensure that the team are informed of the results of the skill mix exercise and are supported in case of adverse results.

- If possible question the data analysis, who did this and how the data were processed.
- Are there meaningful conclusions drawn from the data and can the team support them?
- Once the changes are implemented ensure there are plans for a systematic review of the exercise and standards will be monitored.
- If there are savings to be made as a result of the exercise ask how these will be reinvested in the service in the future.
- Find out what redress there is if the skill mix exercise proves to be unsatisfactory. (RCN, 1992)

Conclusion

If you take the changes discussed above in isolation, the effect is not as great but together they provide the long-awaited chance for community nurses systematically to assess the health needs of the local population, to assess their own abilities as a team player and finally to identify individual and team skills that are required to provide innovative services for the identified population.

To have a truly primary care led NHS (DOH, 1994), activity must focus on three aspects: organizational structure, efficient and effective teamwork and knowledgeable, skilful, innovative and flexible practitioners.

To continue to have primary health care team members working within an organizational structure that clearly does little to facilitate its existence is sheer lunacy and does nothing to support all the health policy advocating teamwork. The only light at the end of the tunnel was the merger of DHA and FHSA in April 1996 into health commissions (DOH, 1993). Perhaps this is the precursor to enabling all primary health care team members to work under one umbrella.

Community nurses should take advantage of the new educational developments and participate in the team-building workshops offered by the health education authority and other organizations. They should also think about how they may further develop their own skills using their practice base as centres for learning in order to 'work together, learn together, engage in clinical audit of outcomes together and generate innovation to ensure progress in practice and service' (NHSME, 1993, p. 17).

Although *New World, New Opportunities* was published in 1993 it clearly guides the primary health care team toward establishing their professional responsibility to teamwork (NHSME, 1993) and states that 'Good teamwork will be facilitated by developing written contracts and agreements and holding regular meetings between all team members to review outcomes measured against established objectives and the processes used to achieve those outcomes' (NHSME, 1993, p. 37).

Points to consider

1 What evidence is there in your primary health care team of a systematic approach to teamwork?

2 Skill mix is fundamental to a primary care-led NHS. How can you ensure your role is developed?

3 How innovative can you be in your role? Are there any role boundaries or territorial behaviours which would prevent you from being pro-active and innovative?

4 What skills do you have which are unique to your specialty? How could you sell your unique skills to appropriate purchasers?

5 How can you strike a balance between the need to provide skilled care against the battle of finite resources?

References

Audit Commission 1992: Homeward bound: *A New Course for Community Health.* London: HMSO.

Baggott, R. 1994: *Health and health care in Britain.* Basingstoke: Macmillan.

Beardshaw, V. and Robinson, R. 1990: *New for old? Prospects for nursing in the 1990s.* Research Report 8. London: King's Fund Institute.

Belbin, R.M. 1981: *Management teams: why they succeed or fail.* Oxford: Heinemann.

Bevan, S., Stock, J. and Waite, R. H. 1991: *Choosing an approach to re-profiling and skill mix.* Brighton: Institute of Manpower Studies.

BMA 1965: *Charter for the family doctor in documents on health and social services 1834 to the present day (1974).* London: Methuen and Co. Ltd.

Central Health Service Council 1963: *Fieldwork of the family doctor. Report of the sub-committee of the standing medical advisory committee of the central health service council (Gillie committee).* London: HMSO.

Central Statistical Office 1992: *Social trends 22.* London: HMSO.

Collins 1992: *Concise English dictionary* (3rd edition). Glasgow: Harper Collins.

Cowley, S. and Mackenzie, 1993: Nursing skill mix in the district nursing service. *District Nurse Association,* Newsletter, **10**, 1, 22–3.

Department of Health 1989a: *Working for patients.* London command 555. London: HMSO.

Department of Health 1989b: *Caring for people, community care in the next decade and beyond.* London: HMSO.

Department of Health 1989c: *General practice in the NHS. The 1990 GP contract.* London, HMSO.

Department of Health 1990: *The NHS and Community Care Act.* London: HMSO.

Department of Health 1991: *The patient's charter.* London: HMSO.

Department of Health 1992: *The health of the nation.* London: HMSO.

Department of Health 1993: *Managing the new NHS.* London: DOH.

Department of Health 1994: *Developing NHS purchasing and GP fundholding. Towards a primary care led NHS.* London: HMSO.

Department of Health 1995: *The patient's charter and you.* London: HMSO.

Department of Health and Social Security 1981: *The joint working group. The primary health care team. (Harding report).* London: HMSO.

Department of Health and Social Security 1986: *Neighbourhood nursing – A focus for care.* Report of the Community Nursing Review. London: HMSO.

Gibbs, I., McCaughan, D. and Griffiths, M. 1990: *Skill mix in nursing: a selective review of the literature*. Discussion Paper 69. Centre for Health Economics, University of York.

Gilmore, M., Bruce, N. and Hunt, M. 1974: *The work of the nursing team in general practice*. Edinburgh: CETHV.

Health Education Authority 1995: *Multidisciplinary team workshop programme*. London: HEA.

Health Visitor Association 1992: *Skill mix in community nursing centre circular*. London: HVA.

Hennessy, D. 1994: *Changes in primary health care clinical education*. South Thames Regional Health Authority.

Heron, J. 1973: *Experiential training techniques*. Human Potential Research Project, University of Surrey.

Hicks, D. 1976. *Primary health care. A review*. London: HMSO.

HM Treasury 1992: *Public expenditure analyses to 1994–1995: statistical supplement to the autumn statement*. London: HMSO Cm 1920.

Lightfoot, J., Baldwin, S. and Wright, K. 1992: *Nursing by numbers? Setting staffing levels for district nursing and health visiting*. Social Policy Research Unit and Centre for Health Economics, University of York.

Littlewood, J. 1995: *Current issues in community nursing primary health care in practice*. Churchill Livingstone, Longman.

Ministry of Health 1920: *Consultative council on medical and allied services (Dawson report)*. London: HMSO.

NHS Management Executive Value for Money Unit 1992: *The nursing skill mix in the district nursing services*. London: HMSO. No. 5 May, pp. 166–8.

National Health Services Management Executive (1993) *New world, new opportunities*. London: HMSO.

Office of Health Economics 1984: *Understanding the NHS in the 1980s*. London: OHE.

Ovretveit, J. 1993: *Co-ordinating community care. Multidisciplinary teams and care management*. Buckingham: Open University Press.

Poulton, B. 1995: *Effective multi-disciplinary teamwork in primary health care*. Unpublished PhD Thesis, Institute of Work Psychology, University of Sheffield.

Pritchard, P. and Pritchard, J. 1994: *Teamwork for primary and shared care*. Oxford: Oxford University Press.

Royal College of Nursing 1992: *Skill mix and reprofiling: a guide for members*. London: RCN.

Spratley, J. 1989: *Disease prevention and health promotion in primary health care*. London: HEA.

Sturdy, C. 1991: *A guide to skill mix for managers*. Human Resources Directorate, North West Thames Regional Health Authority.

UKCC 1992a: *Code of Professional Conduct* (3rd edn). London: UKCC.

UKCC 1992b: *The scope of professional practice*. London: UKCC.

UKCC 1994: *The council's standards for education and practice following registration*. Registrar's letter co/1994. London: UKCC.

Vanclay, L. 1994: *Definition of shared learning*. In Hennessy, D. *Changes in primary health care clinical education*. South Thames Regional Health Authority.

Waine, C. 1992: The primary care team. *British Journal of General Practice*, 498–9

Wright, S. 1986: *Changing nursing practice*. London: Edward Arnold.

WHO 1974: *Expert committee. Community health nursing*. Copenhagen: WHO.

WHO 1978: *International conference on primary health care. Alma Ata*. Geneva: WHO.

Wiles, R. and Robinson, J. 1994: Teamwork in primary care. *Journal of Advanced Nursing*, **20**, 324–30

10 Quality in community nursing

Milly Smith

As a receiver of health care each one of us would probably like to think that the service being provided was one of quality. The concept of quality suggests reliability, goodness and best practice, but what does quality really mean and how can it be achieved in community nursing? The purpose of this chapter is to develop the whole concept of quality, look at it in its fullest sense and discover the complex and many faceted issues that are embodied in the meaning of the word 'quality'. The issues that are explored in the chapter are concerned with understanding the concepts and definitions of quality. The discussion also considers where to look for quality within health care. To be able to determine levels of quality there must be some form of measurement. The chapter addresses some of the considerations that need to be made when attempting to assess quality. Tools that are available that assist in measuring the quality of health care are analysed for their suitability and value. The aim of this chapter is to identify for the reader a breadth of knowledge that demonstrates the complexity of what is being attempted in everyday practice: to measure quality in community health services.

Quality in community nursing

Quality must be the watchword of the 1990s. Not only in the health service but throughout the public and private sectors, people are claiming to give quality services or make quality products. In order to establish their claims about the product or service attempts are being made to measure quality. Measurement is easier for a product than it is for a service, as a product is generally more amenable to testing by objective methods. Health care falls into the service category and is less easy to measure. The methods used for measuring quality in health care have subjective elements and though it is essential to capture this evidence, it tends to carry less weight than objective information. Establishing quality in health care is not an easy task.

A favourite adage in nursing that could be attributed to the quality of care is 'if the care that nurses give to patients would be acceptable for their own nearest and dearest, then it is likely to be of a suitable quality'.

Though the sentiments of this statement are fine in principle, the naivety is easy to determine as many variables could come into play in any judgement of quality. In community health care issues such as individual standards of nursing, the level of expertise of practitioners and the expectations of the patient all play a part in determining what the community nurse perceives of the quality of care provided and what the patient/client perceives of the quality of care received. Added to this is the availability of resources, for example, nursing equipment, which supports quality care as does the availability of other services from the public, private and voluntary sectors. Any judgements on the quality of care provided by community nurses could involve some or even all of these variables. To be able to make effective evaluations of any service the indicator of a quality service needs to take into account a range of measurements and not isolated measurements that in themselves have little value because they illustrate only one part of a much larger issue. The need to address a range of measurements in order to be able to make a sound judgement on the quality of a service is probably the most fundamental point in this chapter.

The subject of quality care is not a new phenomenon. The Bibliography of Nursing cites 32 papers on the subject between 1932 and 1987 (Kitson and Harvey, 1991). Quality has always been an essential part of health and nursing care and a feature of all health professionals' duties and responsibilities. The United Kingdom Central Council (UKCC), which regulates the practice of nurses, set a Code of Conduct and issue guidelines for professional practice (UKCC, 1992). Nurses are bound to work within these regulations and there are severe penalties for those who break the rules. Other health professionals have similar codes of practice and duties of care. The regulation of professional practice therefore provides a standard of quality, as all community nurses must be on the UKCC professional register; this in itself is an indicator of quality.

Quality needs to be established, maintained and improved. Although each individual practitioner has responsibility for their standard of practice, responsibility also rests with all the members of an organization from the lowest to the highest and, rather like an orchestra, the members of the organization need to be in unison to make their individual contributions come together for the person who is receiving the service. Quality is therefore something that happens at both individual and organizational level. In community nursing it can be observed through the support afforded by the NHS Trust to the nurses who are providing patient/client care.

This paper will examine the concept of quality, the differing perceptions of quality and the measurement of quality and will attempt to determine the complexities that are involved in assuring quality nursing and health care in the community.

The concept of quality

Some definitions of quality are now offered; the fundamental issues that are embodied in the wording should emerge from the ideas expressed by different people.

Quality

'The totality of features and characteristics of a product or service that bare on its ability to satisfy explicit and implied needs' (British Standard, 4778: 1987).

Lohr and Harris-Wehling (1991) describe health care quality as the degree to which health services for individuals and populations increase the likelihood of desired health outcomes taking into consideration the state of current professional knowledge.

There are those who hold the view that quality is indefinable. Shaw (1986) felt that attempting to develop a watertight definition of quality was 'too elusive to merit the time of practical people'. An interesting and not dissimilar observation from Aukett (1990) suggests that 'to attempt to pin down what a person actually means when they use the word (quality) is to try to capture a ray of light in a glass bottle' (p. 7). Examination of the above quotes suggests that there are two distinct camps: those who feel that it is a definable but complex concept and those who accept the notion of something that is more fluid and in a state of constant change. These quite different views have implications for quality assurance. If the concept of quality is impossible to hold because it means different things to different people at different times, then it could be argued that it is not feasible to measure the quality of a service. If that is so, people are wasting their time by trying to encapsulate meaningless measurements. Perhaps the compromise view would be that any methods that are instigated to measure the quality of community nursing need to be regularly reviewed to take account of changing circumstances and are fluid enough to accommodate developments in practice.

There are further considerations that require mention in order to present a balanced picture about the quality issue. The way in which people use the term is worthy of examination. A quality product or service can suggest a standard of excellence, for example Rolls Royce have long been associated with the production of a quality car. The quality of service given in private hospitals may be claimed as higher than that of the National Health Service, the association of quality with degree of excellence is therefore acknowledged. Quality can also be used in a comparative sense; one community nursing team compares the quality of its patient care to others in the area. The comparative use of quality can also be observed in Government publications, where league tables are given in order that one organization can compare itself with others that are offering similar services

(DOH, 1995). This method is frequently used in the presentation of heath service data and is heavily criticized for oversimplification of the issues.

Juran (1988) describes quality as 'fitness for use'; this terminology suggests that a product or service must be good enough to fulfil the purpose for which it was intended and should be held at that point, as investment in further development of quality would be unnecessary. The idea of fitness for use can be observed in most purchases. A washing machine in a certain price range will offer very similar operations and will have a life expectancy that is equal to its rival products. It will do the job as stated in the guarantee but will do no more than that; it is fit for the purpose for which it was made. It appears that people may use different perceptions of quality and the particular use of the word will have implications as to how each person perceives the quality of any service. Clarification of the use of the concept appears to be an important starting point as the results of any measurements taken need to be judged around criteria that have previously been established. For community nurses this means that the decision about the level of quality of care that is to be striven towards, excellence or fitness for purpose, is required to be taken before decisions can be taken on the achievements made.

To add to the dilemma, Donabedian (1988a) identifies that the assessment of quality should take place at several levels if a balanced picture is to be achieved. The levels suggested by Donabedian are those of practitioner, patient, a caseload of patients, the whole institution and the geographical area of care. A similar notion is stated by Rutgers and Berkel (1990); they use the terms micro, meso and macro levels to illustrate the range of measures that need to be taken to establish the quality of a service. This implies that in the community one source of information on the quality of services would be the receiver of the service, the patient/client, and this would take the form of an individual or personal view. A different perspective would develop from a group of people and their combined opinions would indicate the general standard of service provided. The satisfaction or dissatisfaction expressed by a group of patients/clients would offer stronger indicators of feeling than would the opinion of a single individual.

Measures taken across the organization would illustrate comparative standards throughout a unit, NHS Trust or GP practice and could also indicate the equity of services within one organization. An example of this type of measurement could be made of the length of time that patients were on the community nursing books. This would enable comparisons to be made across similar teams and would help to determine efficiency and effectiveness which Maxwell (1984) considers are indicators of quality. Quality measurements from all the health services in an area would provide information on the standard and range of services that are provided to a geographical population; this type of indicator is necessary as it provides information on the equity of service across the trust. It is possible for the provision of community nursing services to vary within the same trust which advantages some people while disadvantaging others. Maxwell (1984) suggests that accessibility and equity for all patients/clients who require a service are indicators of quality. The need for a representative view supports the value of a number of measures to be taken around the full range of quality issues.

Donabedian (1988a) offers some thoughts; he discusses the need to assess two distinct parts of the health care provision: the technical systems and the interpersonal process. Donabedian suggests that it is possible for technical care to fail because the interpersonal process has failed. A prescribed treatment might have the potential for being effective but fails because the patient's part in the regimen has not been effectively communicated to him/her. The interpersonal process in some instances is the treatment as in some psychiatric interventions.

Perceptions of what constitutes quality will vary. Patients are likely to look for caring behaviours and professionalism (Carey and Posavac, 1982), while community nurses are likely to look towards being able to provide standards of care that are professionally acceptable and managers may consider efficiency, economy and effectiveness as measures of quality. These are three sets of people with valid, if different, perspectives on what constitutes a quality service. The question that emerges from this and must be asked is do all carry equal weight in the assessment of quality to ensure a balanced view or are some stronger than others? If power within an organization is examined, it is said to be held in different ways; certainly budget holders have power through resources but it is also held by people who hold high positions within an organization, by professionals who have expert power and a few individuals who are lucky enough to possess personal power through charisma (French and Raven, 1959, cited in Handy, 1985). There is real possibility for conflict in organizations between professional requirements and management objectives and these are likely to filter through into the quality debate. It is therefore essential that professionals understand quality issues in order that they can influence the development of programmes for the assessment of the quality of services.

Health care quality defined

It is acknowledged that determining the quality of health care is fundamentally different from the type of quality assessment that is made in production industries (Ovretveit, 1992). The argument that is made around this claim relates to the nature of the customer and the nature of the public service. It claims that the concept of the customer is complex because there may well be two customers, the patient and the purchaser, and they are likely to have different needs. The public nature of the service has implications for funding in that it largely comes from the public purse, is finite, but has to support demands that are essentially infinite. The nature of the health service and the implications that this has for assuring quality are fundamentally different from a manufacturing service in that the variables are less controllable and hence the service itself may vary because it is given by people, who are all different, to people, who are also different; therefore there may be different outcomes from similar services.

Some indications of the nature of issues that could come into judgements of the quality of community services were offered earlier in the chapter and these have been defined by several people. Maxwell (1984) determined the following dimensions of health care quality: access to services, the relevance of services to the needs of the whole community, the effectiveness of the service for individual patients, equity in services and service provision, social acceptability, efficiency and economy. The Joint Commission for the Accreditation of Hospitals Organizations (JCAHO) include the same criteria as Maxwell and add two further dimensions, those of the efficacy of the intervention and continuity and progress of care (Wilkinson, 1990). Both lists demonstrate well that quality has different connotations and is about far more than the quality of care that a patient receives directly from the community nurse. The range of considerations that come into play in assessment of quality range from individual patient care to issues that affect the health care of the whole society. The work of Maxwell (1984) and the JCAHO provide insight into the type of areas that should be receiving scrutiny in assuring quality in community nursing.

The quality of a service is not simply determined by taking measurements of the end product. It is more concerned with building quality into the system and this involves consideration of the service from design to development, through to implementation and evaluation. Quality involves such issues as expertise, education of staff, purchase of appropriate equipment and the time to carry out the work effectively. It is the integration of all these aspects that produce a quality service and they all require examination. Some organizations consider the notion of quality running through every function to be so fundamental that they use a system of management that is known as 'Total Quality Management' (TQM). The philosophy of this system is that quality is everyone's responsibility and is built into every part of the organization. An appreciation of the concept of TQM is fundamental to a fuller understanding of the achievement of quality within an organization. The work of Oakland is a valuable source of information on the subject of Total Quality (Oakland, 1993).

Donabedian (1981, 1988a, 1988b) offers some valuable advice on the ways in which quality issues can be broken down for the purpose of examination. This work is well known and frequently used to examine quality in health care but it is often not well used and is prone to the problem of producing unsound data by unsound means. The work of Donabedian offers the facility to examine care by using the structure, the process and the outcomes as three avenues that can be explored to help to form a judgement on the quality of care. The Donabedian triad recognizes these influences on the delivery of care and their interrelationships. In community nursing an example of issues would be the composition of the primary health care team, the level of expertise of staff, the availability of nursing equipment, the nature of the local area could be considered as structural and having influence on how the service is provided. The process element is the provision of the service; this may be influenced by the knowledge base of the community nurse, the degree of experience in dealing with the situation, the individuality of the patient. The outcome of care concerns the effectiveness of what has been done and this needs to take into account many other considerations; for example, outcomes may be influenced by other contributors to care, differing psychological responses of patients, or the patient's lifestyle. The three avenues that are used are thought to be dependent on each other for the provision of effective care, for instance it of care may not be effective if the structure that facilitates it is not in place. Equally the outcome of care may be influenced by the structure and/or the process. Use of the triad helps any breakdown in quality to be identified at its source. This model is not without its critics. Donabedian himself points to limited evidence to support the relationships between the structure and the process of care; how much the structures that support care influence the outcomes is therefore debatable. There is stronger evidence to support the links between the process of care and the outcomes though Bunker (1988), cited in Donabedian (1988a), observed that the usefulness of much clinical practice has still to be substantiated. These sceptical comments serve as a reminder that measurements taken should be made from scientific evidence. This will ensure that the results of the quality assessment have come from the interventions that have been made and not by chance or through default.

The measurement of quality

That the assessment of the level of quality provided in a service is a complex matter has now been established. Measurements are constantly being made of the services that are providing health care and more importantly the measurements are being published and interpreted as an indicator of quality. There is a need to consider what is being measured and what is actually measurable in health services that truly indicate their level of quality.

A look at the data required by the Department of Health (1995) that is often used as an indicator of quality suggests that it is mostly quantitative. Examples of this type of data come in the form of increased numbers of patient contacts made by community nurses, reduction in the length of stay in hospital and reduced waiting list numbers. Although this type of data may be useful in a comparative sense, it is highly criticized for presenting a distorted and oversimplistic picture. Coote and Pfeffer (1991) draw attention to the dangers of the scientific approach with a reminder that it is unilateral and not open to dissent. It is devised by experts who decided what constitutes quality and it is normally concerned with output. Government statistics fit into this category. Data of this type is, however, objective and it is a representation of one part of the picture, it provides evidence of the availability, access to and economy of care, but it does not say anything about acceptability and effectiveness. Other less objective methods need to be drawn on to illuminate the starkness of quantitative information and provide a richer balanced picture. It does matter for instance that people who are discharged early from hospital have appropriate support through to recovery and are satisfied with the quality of the service provided from the start to the finish of the intervention. Information collected about the full episode of care would provide much more useful data about the quality of the service than is provided by figures on length of stay on hospital wards alone.

A rounded assessment of the quality of a service must draw on a range of different measurements, some objective and some subjective. Scientific principles should be applied to the collection and measurement of the qualitative data. Ellis and Whittington (1993) suggest that the decisions on method can be taken around the questions what is to be measured and how can it be measured? A further point is to consider the quality of the instrument used for data collection. A range of qualitative methods are available and choosing a suitable method is extremely important. An inappropriate method may result in much time and effort being spent providing information that is of little value. Donabedian (1988a) provides a few key considerations that should be examined when making assessment tool choices: the relationship of the measurement to the causal validity, the relevance of the measurement to the objectives of care, the degree of specificity of the tool, the inclusivity of the system, its timeliness, the availability of the information, the accuracy of the measurement and the cost involved. These issues draw on much of what has been discussed in this paper and serve as a concise reminder that quality is an involved topic.

Having spent some time examining the issues that are involved in the assessment of quality it is appropriate that the next point for consideration should focus on the tools available for measuring quality. Ellis and Whittington (1993) provide a useful list that demonstrates the range of available quality assessment tools under the general categories into which they fall. Examples are given by each category that illustrate the type of tool that is attributed to the category.

Quality assessment categories	Example
Professional standard systems	Codes of conduct
Comprehensive review systems	Dynamic standard setting system (Dyssy)
Case selection techniques	Occurrence screening
Local problem identification techniques	Quality circles
Process measurement techniques	Monitor
Outcome measurement techniques	Pain measures
Consumer involvement techniques	Patient surveys
Records techniques	Historical reviews
(Ellis and Whittington, 1993)	

There are other tools and techniques that are commonly used in industry that illustrate a steady state in the quality of a product or identify potentially problematical changes, some of which may well have value in the health service. Oakland (1993) provides a comprehensive list, which includes scatter diagrams that illustrate the relationships between factors and histograms that show the overall variations. The latter may appear quite different from the categories suggested by Ellis and Whittington (1993) but they have an equally valuable role in highlighting variations in the quality of the service. This type of statistical evidence provides at a glance evidence that could give good diagnostic information about quality issues. A scattergram, for instance, could pick up variations in caseload dependency levels that could affect the quality of care across the whole span of patients/clients on the caseload.

Force field analysis (Lewis, 1951) is another tool suggested by Oakland (1993); this highlights the strength of the need for change in the provision of a service and diagnoses the factors that will facilitate or hold back the changes that are necessary. Oakland further suggests benchmarking as a tool that has particular merit. Benchmarking involves a service comparing itself to a centre of excellence in a similar field. This allows comparison to be made with 'the best' and can act as a useful quality measure and provide an updating experience in the field of care.

The tools that are available to measure quality vary considerably and they are not all sophisticated or designer made. Simple methods that occur as part of everyday practice such as evaluating patients care plans are just as important as an audit using one of the comprehensive review systems; each has a part to play in contributing information. It is the range of measures available that provide the choice that is necessary to develop a rounded quality assurance programme. If chosen with care a package of measures can be devised that takes into account an effective broad view of the quality of a service. There needs to be good knowledge of the capability and validity of the tools. The requirement of the package of measurements is that it should provide a comprehensive picture of the quality of the service; that can only be achieved if the results portray an accurate and comprehensive picture.

There are frameworks that help decisions to be made on the approach that is to be taken for the quality assurance programme (Marker, 1976; American Nurses Association, 1982; Green and Lewis, 1986; Parsley and Corrigan, 1994). The nature of frameworks is that they provide a systematic approach to the problem and act as a step-by-step guide. As quality assurance programmes are complex a framework is valuable in the development, implementation and monitoring of the system. The process of assuring quality is represented in all the frameworks as a cycle of events that generally involves assessment of the situation, setting acceptable standards that are to be achieved, devising a number of measurement strategies that will provide a picture of the quality of the service, assessing the quality of the service against the standards that have been set, taking action to improve aspects of the service that do not reach the required standard, and returning to the beginning of the cycle to continue to improve the service provided. The emphasis is on the continual striving for improvement.

As with any system that is set in place it must not run indefinitely without being monitored for its effectiveness. There needs to be evaluation of the system to be sure that it is measuring what it set out to measure and that the measurements taken still have value within the system. The term auditing the audit is used by Ishikawa (1985) who suggests that audit is required in the areas of quality control to ensure that the systems that are in place are effective. Ishikawa envisages this as being an audit that studies the entire management system. He also suggests that there should be both internal and external audit and includes customers in the external audit.

Conclusion

The services that are provided for community health care are many and varied and to be effective they must be coordinated. The resources for these services are people, equipment and time; these provide the inputs to each service that is offered to patients and clients. The activities that take place in each service between the resources and the patients/clients result in the output of the service. There should be a measurable difference from the input stage to the output stage and the difference will indicate the quality of the service. To use such a simple analogy suggests that this is a simple process but this paper has illustrated just how difficult it is to measure the quality of health care services.

It is difficult because of the very nature of the service, with individuals involved with both the administering and the receiving of the services; it is difficult also because of the nature of public services that must be provided within tight budgets. To add to the complexity, quality in any service does not stand in isolation; even at the micro or individual level there is an interplay of events, the practitioners must perform adequately and the resources must support the practitioner. If either the practitioners or the resources do not come up to standard, the quality of the service may suffer. The resource issues have implications for the organization that must provide them, thus the assurance of quality is inclusive of but also higher than practitioner level. Health service quality does not only apply at practitioner and organizational level, it also needs to be considered from the wider aspects of accessibility and equity to whole communities, to ensure that a fair distribution of acceptable services are available to all who require them.

Neither is measurement easy; many of the tools that are available take subjective measurements but these are essential because they provide richness to the data that is not present in purely quantitative evidence. No one tool can provide all the answers and the success of each quality assurance programme heralds from the careful selection of tools that are right for the job and are carefully selected to measure the things that have to be measured. Thankfully there are many every day aspects of care that provide indicators of quality and they can be a part of the general assessment of the quality of care provided. Measurement of the quality of community nursing services will provide information, however that in itself will not improve quality, it is the actions taken that improve quality.

Points to consider

1 If quality means different things to different people, what are the implications that this has for community nurses?

2 Who are the other contributors to the quality of community nursing in your area of work?

3 What are your responsibilities to quality?

4 How may quality be built into community nursing services?

References

American Nurses Association 1982: *Nursing quality assurance management learning system*. Kansas City: American Nurses Association.

Aukett, J.W. 1990: *Quality assurance in health education: myth or reality*. MSc Health Education Thesis. London: Kings College.

Bunker, J.P. 1988: Is efficiency the gold standard for quality assessment? In Donabedian, A. (1988), The quality of health care, how can it be assessed. *Inquiry*, **25**, 51–8.

British Standard Institute 4478. 1987: *Quality systems part 1: specification for design, production, installation and servicing*. Milton Keynes: British Standards Institution.

Carey, R.G. and Posavac, E.J. 1982: Using patient information to identify areas for service improvement. *HMC Review*, **7**, 2, 43–8.

Coote, A. and Pfeffer, N. 1991: *Is quality for you?* Social Policy Paper No. 5. London: Institute for Public Policy Research.

DOH 1995: *Health and personal social service statistics for England*. London: HMSO.

Donabedian, A. 1981: Criteria, norms and standards of quality: what do they mean? *American Journal of Public Health*, **71**, 409–12.

Donabedian, A. 1988a: The quality of health care, how can it be assessed. *Joint American Nursing Association*, **260**, 12, 1743–8.

Donabedian, A. 1988b: Quality assessment and assurance: unity of purpose diversity of means. *Inquiry*, **25**, 173–92.

Ellis, R. and Whittington, D. 1993: *Quality assurance in health care, a handbook*. London: Edward Arnold.

French, J.R.P. and Raven, B.H. 1959: The bases of social power. In Cartwright, D. (1968), *Group dynamics research and theory*, Tavistock (3rd edn). Cited in Handy, C. (1985) *Understanding organisations* (3rd edn). Harmondsworth: Penguin.

Green, L. and Lewis, F. (1986) *Measurement and evaluation in health education*. Palo Alto, California: Mayfield.

Ishikawa, T. 1985: *What is total quality control?* London: Prentice-Hall Business Classics.

Juran, J.M. 1988: *Juran on planning for quality*. New York: Free Press.
Kitson, A. and Harvey, G. 1991: *Bibliography of nursing quality assurance and standards of care, a handbook*. London: Edward Arnold.
Lewis, K. 1951: *Field theory in social science*. New York: Harper and Row.
Lohr, K.N. and Harris-Wehling, J. 1991: Medicare: a strategy for quality assurance. *Quality Review Bulletin*, **17**, 1, 6–9.
Marker, C. 1976: The umbrella model for quality assurance: monitoring and evaluating professional practice. *Journal of Nursing Quality Assurance*, **1**, 3, 52–63.
Maxwell, R.J. 1984: Quality assessment in health. *British Medical Journal*, **228**, 1470–7.
Oakland, J.S. 1993: *Total quality management*. Oxford: Butterworth Heinemann.
Ovretveit, J. 1992: *Health service quality: an introduction to quality methods for health services*. Oxford: Blackwell.
Parsley, K. and Corrigan, P. 1994: *Quality improvement in nursing and health care: a practical approach*. London: Chapman and Hall.
Shaw, C.D. 1986: *Introducing quality assurance*. London: King's Fund Project paper 64, King's Fund.
Rutgers, M.J. and Berkel, H. 1990: New concepts in health care: some preliminary ideas. *International Journal of Health Planning and Management*, **5**, 215–20.
UKCC 1992: *Code of Professional Conduct*. London: UKCC.
Wilkinson, R. 1990: *Quality assurance in managed care organisations*. Chicago: Joint Commission for the Accreditation of Health Care Organizations.

11 Managing change in the community

Paul Parkin

This chapter explores the process of managing change in the contemporary climate of community health care.

While stressing the challenge and difficulty of successful change management, it considers the following aspects:

- *At the 'macro' level, what change is, why and how it occurs, the changing climate of organizations and the influence of post-Fordism and the quasi-market,*
- *At the 'meso' level, the importance of taking account of organizational and professional cultures in any change effort,*
- *At the 'micro' level, it focuses on the more interactive aspects of change, details a set of questions to consider in the preparatory phase and outlines a range of strategies to use in the change process,*
- *It concludes that practitioners should behave as newcomers to each situation, to question habitually and think critically about their work in order to develop professionally and master their practice.*

'All is flux, nothing is stationary' (Heracleitus *fl* 513 BC)

'One should bear in mind that there is nothing more difficult to execute, nor more dubious of success, nor more dangerous to administer than to initiate a new order of things' (Machiavelli, 1513)

'The reasonable man adapts himself to the world; the unreasonable one persists in trying to adapt the world to himself. Therefore all progress depends on the unreasonable man' (G.B. Shaw, 1903)

'All change for the better comes about by dialogue' (Aung San Suu Kyi, July 1995)

Introduction

The deliberate choice of historical quotations aims to show a number of introductory but key points regarding the phenomenon of change. First, and rather obviously, change is not new. The factors which create and facilitate social change have been exercising philosophers', politicians' and managers' minds and skills for generations, yet the process of introducing innovative methods, systems or products does not appear to be any more understood or any more successful today (West, 1989).

Secondly, change is not exclusive to nursing. This also is not in any doubt. Change is recognized as a constant feature of modern organizations and institutions, however, in the last few years a number of policy documents from official nursing bodies have alluded, in their opening paragraphs, to the many and significant changes occurring in nursing (e.g. UKCC, 1990, 1991, 1992; NHSME, 1993; DOH, 1994; Queens's Nursing Institute, 1994).

Additionally, and focusing on the individual, the 'ability to manage change' has been identified by the English National Board as one of its 10 'key characteristics' of nurses, midwives and health visitors in the context of its Higher Award (ENB, 1991). Characteristic 10 states that practitioners should have 'The ability to initiate, manage and evaluate change in practice to improve the quality of care' (ENB, 1991).

The strategic report *New World, New Opportunities* (NHSME, 1993) also stressed that all primary health care nurses should participate in continuing education that 'is based on, and set in the clinical practice arena where new knowledge can be generated to *bring about change in nursing*' (italics added) (p. 40).

In contrast, the 1994 Primary Health Care Conference entitled 'Meeting the Challenge of Change in Primary Health Care' (Smith, 1994) focused mainly on how community nurses can respond to and cope with the health policy changes which are occurring; few sessions focused on how to initiate and manage change in the community, a gap this chapter aims to address. This omission may seem at odds with the volume of job applications in the nursing press, often for posts in the community, for nurses who are 'innovative' and have the 'ability to manage change' (e.g. *Nursing Times*, 1991, 1992, 1993, 1994), evidently written by managers who value this particular skill as, significantly, it is frequently separated from other, equally valid and relevant skills.

Thirdly, not all nurses are, can be or want to be 'change agents'. Charisma, communication skills and a good idea are not enough to be successful at implementing change. There are certain qualities and skills required that integrate notions of power and status; leadership, motivation and tenacity; high levels of communication, empathy and conflict management; characteristics of foresight, creativity and planning as well as knowledge of research, evaluation and politics; and the obligatory practice of questioning the habitual and familiar.

Managing change is first and foremost a management ability and as such requires the deft and dextrous hand of political and organizational manoeuvrings, where 'political' is used in the sense of having to deal with the vested interests of powerful individuals or groups and cope with tactics of coercion, domination and delay in the decision-making process. Many of these issues will be discussed and developed in this chapter.

The final and perhaps most important point to make in this introduction derives from Machiavelli's 'The Prince' (1513). Managing change is difficult and messy, is fraught with problems and is often unsuccessful or at best short-lived. It is difficult because it implicitly challenges conventional ways of thinking and behaving and this leads to patterns of resistance from those affected. It conveys a feeling of 'your practice is wrong, out-of-date, traditional – whereas my idea (or whatever) is better, up-to-date, research-based'. Machiavelli went on to argue that introducing change makes enemies of all those who benefited from the old system and produces only lukewarm allies who may benefit from the new. Machiavelli was a cunning and cynical statesman (change agent) who discussed ways that rulers can advance their own and their state's (organization's) interests often through amoral and unethical manipulation of other people. The point is that if an authoritarian ruler like Machiavelli found managing change difficult, how much more so do community nurses with relatively little power and status (Parkin, 1995).

These introductory points beg some questions. What is meant by change? Why does change now appear to be endemic in health work? Why is the requirement to innovate being institutionalized in course learning outcomes and in job descriptions, sometimes at E and D grade level? Is it merely rhetorical managerialist-speak, coded language for being knowledgeable and up-to-date or a genuine wish to employ staff who may upset the status quo and create organizational discord? What happens to those staff who are unable or unsuccessful in their attempts? By what criteria are change attempts evaluated? If community nurses are required to manage change, just how do they proceed? In attempting to consider these questions this chapter is divided into three main sections: the first section entitled 'Analysis' argues for the need to consider at the *macro level*, what change is, how and why it occurs, and why it is currently so prevalent in health care; at the *meso level* to consider how management practices are changing and the critical need to account for the organizational culture in any change effort; the *micro level* applies some aspects identified in these levels and focuses on the more interactive aspects of change (see Table 11.1). The second section, 'Action I' outlines a set of questions that must be asked if change is to be implemented, while the final section, 'Action II', considers a range of strategies that may be drawn on to facilitate the process of change and summarizes ways and means of making change more acceptable. This approach has been derived mainly from Baldridge and Deal's (1975) assertion that three main areas are needed to understand change in organizations:

1 a comprehensive organizational perspective entailing an understanding of the organization's subsystems

2 strategies used to cause and support the changes

3 practical experience of the dynamics of change.

Table 11.1 Levels of units of analysis of change events

Levels of change events	Units of analysis
Macro level	Social/political systems Economic policies Environmental issues Globalization Cultural beliefs Health policies Demography Education policies Health care professions
Meso level	Organizations/institutions/companies Employment practices Management styles Corporate missions Contractual obligations Professional groups Health centres/clinics GPs surgeries/primary health care teams
Micro level	Individual practitioners Interactions, meanings and perceptions Managers' styles Teamwork/leadership skills Team's aims and objectives Multiprofessional interactions Professional role beliefs

Regarding the 'practical experience' in point 3 above, readers are encouraged to reflect, as they read the chapter, on their own wide experiences of the process of change. These experiences may include managing a change project, or having a change event imposed on them. This process of reflection will assist in appreciating the phenomenology of change.

Analysis

WHAT IS CHANGE?

Change can be seen as a value-free or neutral concept. It is not value-laden in the same way as 'progress' or 'development'. The philosopher Bertrand Russell (1950) argued that there can be no debate about whether change has occurred; it is scientific and irrefutable, however 'progress' is ethical and is a matter of debate and controversy depending on perspective. Change may occur through evolution or adaptation where it is assumed that it equates to progress; it may occur through diffusion where ideas spread through contact between different individuals and cultural groups; or it may arise from revolution when a whole social or political system is subverted and replaced by new leadership, principles and governance. Much change in health care comes via government legislation, policy initiatives, technological developments and employment changes. Such approaches may align broadly to functionalist, conflict and symbolic interactionist explanations of social dynamics. Parsonian functionalism (Parsons, 1951) sees society as an organic whole with interdependent parts which function together, generally through consensus on norms and values, to maintain stability. From this perspective change is seen as evolutionary, the constant pursuit of stability, balance and equilibrium whereas conflict is viewed as dysfunctional. Using this definition of social dynamics, it is difficult to explain how radical change occurs, and it tends to reduce, to a certain extent, the role of human actions and meaning and the conflictual nature of much social reality. In contrast Marxist conflict theory conceives change not as the striving for consensus but rather as the consequence of political dissent and coercion of one group or person to gain advantage over another (Dahrendorf, 1985). It emphasizes the role of power and control in maintaining social order. Hence change may be progressive and constructive but equally can be regressive and destructive. Symbolic interactionism, which Giddens (1989) states is concentrated on the 'face-to-face' contexts of social life, claims that people act towards change through the meanings and interpretations it holds for them and these meanings are mediated via social interactions and relationships with other people (Blumer, 1969; Goffman, 1969).

Brooten *et al.* (1978) define planned change as a 'deliberate and collaborative process involving a change agent and a system' (p. 81). This definition is helpful as it stresses that managing change has to be based on a conscious plan (it is not simply 'reactive'); it emphasizes collaboration as planned change will only work (if it is to work at all) with the involvement of all interested parties (it recognizes the potential of conflict); it focuses on the 'change agent' as someone drawing on a body knowledge for change; and it includes a system – this may be a client, group or team, agency, organization or social system. Whichever of these, the preparatory rigour, commitment and managerial work is similar.

SOME THEORETICAL COMMENTS

Far from being exclusive to nursing, much of the theory on aspects of change derives from the three diverse social science literatures of social psychology, occupational psychology and sociology (West, 1987).

There are many theories of change and many of which were developed some years ago. Even recent publications, for example Lancaster and Lancaster (1984), Sullivan and Decker (1992) and Andrews (1993), cite the classic works of Lewin's (1951) 'Force-Field Model' and Lippitt *et al.'s* (1958) 'Phases of Change Model'. These models are functionalist in that they emphasize what should be done in order to effect change. Kinnunen (1990) argues that this approach does not explain why some organizations find it difficult to change. More recently anthropological paradigms emphasize cultural and symbolic approaches and management texts draw from systems theory (McCalman and Paton, 1992; Mabey and Mayon-White, 1993). Baldridge and Deal (1975) however, stress that there are 'no valid, tested scientific principles of change' as much is based on intuitive strategies. Pinto and Prescott (1987) argue that 'critical success factor frameworks' are conceptually based and there is no agreed set of factors seen as critical to implementation success. McCalman and Paton (1992) state that 'no single school of thought holds the answer to change management' (p. 19). Georgiades and Phillimore (1975) suggest that 'most of the theories in the field of change are attempts to explain the unknowable in terms of the not worth knowing'. Part of the difficulty is that much of the literature focuses on the individual seen as an innovator (Sullivan and Decker, 1992) rather than the organizational structures and roles which have greater potency and forcefulness to resist change than the individual has to promote it. The debate regarding the relationship between human action and social structure is ongoing. On the one hand structuralists such as Durkheim (1982) claim that society (or an organization) has dominance over individuals, coercing their actions through the influence of social norms and values. On the other, symbolic interactionists argue that society (or an organization) is created by individuals who decide to behave in certain cultural ways. Writers such as Silverman (1970) and Handy (1985) attempt to synthesize these approaches in terms of analysing change, where individuals are seen as social actors and are able to initiate change.

The tacit (and unrealistic) expectation of training programmes, study days and chapters such as this is that individual practitioners can follow a set of guidelines or a procedure – this may involve analysing a problem, producing a plan of action to solve it, showing it to a manager, discussing it with staff and colleagues, setting an implementation date and on that date the change occurs. The inference is that from that point on everyone works happily in a new and harmonious fashion, decided by the change agent who, because s/he has used the correct process, has been successful in implementing the required change. This process is a fantasy. Georgiades and Phillimore (1975) label this the 'myth of the hero–innovator' because the process ignores the strength and power of the organizational culture which has the force to overcome even the well planned efforts of the creative and charismatic individual. It also neglects the interrelationships between individuals and groups within the organization. The myth of the hero–innovator is described thus:

> the idea that you can produce, by training, a knight in shining armour who, loins girded with the new technology and beliefs, will assault his organisational fortress and institute changes both in himself and others at a stroke. Such a view is ingenuous. The fact of the matter is that organisations such as schools and hospitals will, like dragons, eat hero–innovators for breakfast. (p. 315)

To enable practitioners to respond realistically to job adverts, later sections develop some possible approaches, but to summarize: there is no agreed formula for managing change; implementing change is hard managerial work; it can be painful, it is messy; there is no guarantee of success, and it can make adversaries of peers, colleagues and managers. Stocking (1988) asserts that bringing about change requires not only clarity and analysis but also energy and persistence and Pinto and Prescott (1987) claim that 'The project implementation process is complex, usually involving simultaneous attention to a broad variety of human, budgetary and technical variables' (p. 328). Yet, McCalman and Paton (1992) state that change occurs continuously, has numerous causes and needs to be addressed all the time.

HEALTH CARE AND POST-FORDISM

An earlier question asked why change seems endemic in health care and why there is now organizational pressure on community nurses to be innovative. Recent analyses (Loader and Burrows, 1994; Jessop, 1994; Walby and Greenwell, 1994) have traced the socio-economic, political and managerial changes in health and welfare through a model of Fordism to post-Fordism. At risk of oversimplification, Fordism (about which there is little agreement) can be represented by the rigid assembly-line style of mass production and mass consumption of (usually) standardized consumer durables within a national economy. Demand is regulated by the supply of goods. Work is structured around inflexible times, tasks and routines. Organizations and institutions are frequently large, hierarchical and bureaucratic and are unable to respond quickly to different needs. Workers are subjected to tight and detailed controls by employers in order to improve the level of output which is based on economies of scale (Jessop, 1994). Tasks are broken down into smaller specialized units requiring specifically trained sub-occupations. Walby and Greenwell (1994) note evidence that the National Health Service in general and nurses in particular are organized along Fordist principles in order to maximize productivity through universal provision of a uniform service. Thus hospitals as bureaucracies signify routines, rules, regulations and rigidity that are hostile to change and 'seem to militate against innovation' (Carrier and Kendall, 1995, p. 25).

This bureaucratic rigidity has been systematically dismantled by successive health reforms, culminating in the National Health Service and Community Care Act (DOH, 1990) which aimed to introduce a more flexible approach to provision based on a model of private sector enterprise culture. This has meant separating into a quasi-market the purchasers of health (GPs and health authorities) from the providers (NHS Hospital and Community Trusts), requiring competitive tendering and contract-based financial relationships, basing health provision on the identified needs of the population and recognizing the consumer as a central focus of service specification.

The leitmotif of 'flexibility' in these changes reflects the more general social change to post-Fordism. Jessop (1994) sees post-Fordism first as a labour process of flexible production based on flexible systems with a flexible workforce; secondly as a mode of economic growth requiring economies of scope (rather than Fordist economies of scale), increased demand for differentiated goods, services and forms of consumption and consequently a need for constant and permanent innovation; and thirdly as a mode of economic regulation involving a shift from hierarchical, well-staffed, bureaucratic structures to leaner, flatter and more flexible forms of organization. Jessop concludes that profits of enterprise will depend on the capacity to design flexible service delivery, accelerate product and process innovation, improve quality and individual performance and rapidly respond to customers' needs through 'customization', as competition will turn on these 'non-price factors'.

Williams (1994) cautions against seeing the NHS and Community Care Act (DOH, 1990) simply as a policy shift to post-Fordist conditions. However the themes of diversity, differentiation, and flexibility are sufficient to see why there is organizational pressure for community staff to be innovative. Community Units which are able continually to reposition and quickly respond to GP fundholders' needs with services which are tailor-made, more cost-effective and higher quality than the next, will win in the competitive market, particularly if niche markets can be developed.

Smart (1993) has linked these themes to the 'post-modern' condition when we now live in the time of:

> a cult of the new, a social and economic context in which innovation and novelty have been promoted, their virtues extolled, often through implied associations with ideas of progress and development. (p. 14)

The institutionalization of innovation, when change is perpetually demanded, may lead to a relentless proactive, conflict approach where it is pejorative to be still, to be stable is to backslide, to be in equilibrium is to regress. In short, not to change is to lose.

The organizational context

Even though 'managing change' has become one of nursing's articles of faith and because managers and educators value and desire practitioners who are innovative, it can not be assumed that innovation will be the hallmark of their work. It has already been noted that to manage change is difficult. There are other contradictions. At the meso level, Walby and Greenwell (1994) argue that traditionally nurses have been managed in a Fordist-type regime using scientific management techniques. This has emphasized task certification (for every new skill a certificate is required), procedural and rule-bound actions, use of coercive threats, tight and direct control of personal work life and a hierarchical structure. Whereas this approach is not so marked in the community as in hospital, writers such as Owens and Petch (1995), Parkin (1995) and particularly Witz (1994) have noted nursing's general lack of autonomy and power:

The change agent who asserts her right to make decisions about patient care, has to challenge, or operate within, sets of existing power relations that have been shaped as much by gendered patterns of dominance and subordination as they have by bodies of medical knowledge. (p. 37)

May (1992) also notes that a range of 'inhibiting factors' inherent in the organizational context, such as workload and work organization, place limits on the level of control and autonomy that could be exercised by nurses.

New management strategies such as human resource management, ushered in by the major Griffiths changes (DHSS, 1983) tend to encourage experiment and to foster entrepreneurship. This emphasizes responsible autonomy, identification with the overall company goals and looser work-supervision via the granting of authority, status and responsibility. These qualities are simply not ingrained in the culture of nursing, neither is the structure nor the managerial trust in evidence to support them. As Walby and Greenwell (1994) state, 'Nurses lack the important characteristics of autonomy of decision making which is such a key feature of new wave management' (p. 136).

There are clear contradictions in stimulating an enterprise culture within an authoritarian and hierarchical system that itself exists in a macro-system moving towards post-Fordism. The very ethos of quality controls, auditing practice, outcomes of care, charter standards and fulfilling contracts (not to mention timed visits and appointment systems in district nursing) militate against work innovation and change.

Organizational and professional culture

Any change effort in the community, whether it be altering work patterns, introducing a new record system or quality controls or simply changing a patient's treatment involves disturbing the normal, habitual way of behaving; the 'accepted' culture of the place. Sathe (1983) has argued that culture is a fuzzy and elusive concept which plays a subtle and pervasive role in organizational life. It can be based on what is directly observed about members of a community but is more likely to be what is shared in member's minds. He defines culture as 'the set of important understandings (often unstated) that members of a community share in common'. The fact that understandings are 'unstated' makes them invisible to observers or to those not part of the organization. Professions or occupational groups such as district nurses, health visitors, practice nurses, community psychiatric nurses, general practitioners and managers all develop their own sub-cultures within the broader culture of the National Health Service (see Table 11.2).

Furthermore 'locational subcultures' will develop within different health centres, clinics and GP practices which will differ from other clinics, etc. in

Table 11.2   'Invisibles' that make up the organizational culture

Beliefs basic assumptions about the world and how it works
Values similar to beliefs but contain an 'ought to' element
Identity set of shared understandings about objects or situations, such as commitment to team-work
Climate shared understanding about what it is like to work in the organization
Pivotal value the most important corporate value, often enthroned in the mission statement. All other values revolve around this value
Norms standards of expected behaviour, such as presentation, uniform, attendance at meetings etc.
Ideology the dominant set of interrelated ideas that explain and justify why the major shared understandings 'make sense' to those who work in the organization

Source: From Sathe 1983. Adapted and reprinted by permission of publisher, from *Organizational dynamics*, Autumn/1983 © 1983. American Management Association, New York. All rights reserved.

the same health authority or trust. These sub-cultures are made up of 'invisibles' derived through 'occupational socialization' processes (Melia, 1984) of training, education and occupational norms passed via socializing agents such as peers, Community Practice Teachers and 'professional' tutors and managers. In the health professions, cultural values are internalized primarily in the training ground of the hospital which is organized hierarchically, and these values are transferred into the community, although this may alter post Project 2000 (UKCC, 1986). The strength of culture can lead to 'shared programmes of behaving' (Fabrega, 1979). Hence 'invisibles' are likely to be held strongly within occupational groups but may cause friction, misunderstanding and conflict between different groups specifically because they are invisible. Kinnunen (1990) suggests that sub-cultures are learnt spontaneously and unconsciously. Furthermore 'professional socialization takes as axiomatic that one of the tasks of professional education is to give future practitioners a strong identity and confidence' (Carrier and Kendal, 1995, p. 31). This is evident in Kinnunen's (1990) study of the occupational groups of doctors, managers and nurses within a large (over 700 employees) primary health care organization. Kinnunen developed a range of 'basic assumptions' similar to Sathe's beliefs and values and compared the content of the sub-cultures of the three groups against the assumptions. The content of the work and organizational sub-cultures of the doctors and managers emphasize paternalism, dominance and loyalty to authority. In contrast, the nursing sub-culture stresses participation, traditions and 'symbiotic harmony' in their relations within the work organization. Considering the conflict that is frequently present in implementing change, these findings, if consistently held, do not bode well for nurses as change agents. Melia (1984) found that student nurses learn to 'fit in', especially with those in authority; there is no point in trying to change routines. Eight years later, Mackensie (1992) still found that student district nurses also have to fit in with their Community Practice Teachers, not ask challenging questions or challenge ideas about practice or work organization. These findings appear to agree with Kinnunen's notion of the need to maintain 'symbiotic harmony' which in practice will conflict with the imbalancing effects of change.

Crucially, Kinnunen (1990) found that each sub-culture holds the same view about mutability, that is that in their own group, members are seen as mutable but they doubted others. Hence, if practitioners wish to 'cross-boundaries' and influence or alter the work organization/patterns/ structure of other or 'out' groups, the task will be more demanding and the strategies used to manage change have to be carefully considered. Interprofessional issues are currently developing their literature base (Howkins, 1995; Owens et al., 1995) but it should not be forgotten that in-groups (and all health-care professionals are members of in-groups be they district nurses, health visitors, social workers or general practitioners) need an opposition group for their 'self-identity, cohesiveness, inner solidarity and emotional security' (Bauman, 1990). Bauman goes on to argue that all groups must postulate an enemy to draw and guard their own boundaries and to secure loyalty and cooperation. As will be discussed in the next section this has important implications for practitioners attempting to manage change.

The strength of in-group culture is such that Coulter (1991) has pointed out that effective collaborations between multidisciplinary teams are relatively rare in Britain, due in part to mutual suspicion of each other among practitioners of the different disciplines and in part to organizational fragmentation. Owens and Carrier (1995), though stressing the positive aspect of changing ideologies in interprofessional collaboration, argue that 'altering roles and boundaries is not easy to achieve without a slow and sensitive period of re-education' (p. 2). Pugh (1993) states that 'organisations are coalitions of interest groups in conflict' (p. 109).

Action I

It has been argued that change can be reactive in response to forces external to the organization or be imposed, perhaps by delegation, by senior managers on workers, in which case the greatest degree of negative feedback will be generated (McCalman and Paton, 1992). Change can also be pro-active where practitioners may see an opportunity for improving practice through the processes of monitoring, evaluation, reflection, education, research or discussions with colleagues. To enable practitioners to go some way to addressing the requirements of the English National Board (1991), the National Health Service Management Executive (1993) and the job adverts identified earlier, it is this pro-active aspect of change that this section will concentrate on. It is therefore aimed at the micro, interactional level rather than considering practitioners' roles at the meso or organizational level (see Table 11.1) although in practice these areas are not clearly differentiated.

QUESTIONS TO ASK IN THE PRE-CHANGE PHASE

Walton (1984) produced a short typology of questions to consider when managing change. After running numerous workshops with all levels of community staff over a 10-year period, these have been expanded by the author and are shown in Fig. 11.1. First, practitioners need to be clear in their own minds exactly what the problem/need/opportunity is since they will be the initiators and responsible for seeing the project through. Lewin (1951) suggests that change agents may use tactics to raise the level of awareness or discontent about a situation. This may be a conscious act to determine what others think and feel or to 'get people on their side' and which increases the motivation for change. It is possible that the need for change has been recognized intuitively before the conscious decision to do something about it has been taken. Committing the problem to paper aids the clarification phase, especially if it can be contained within a short,

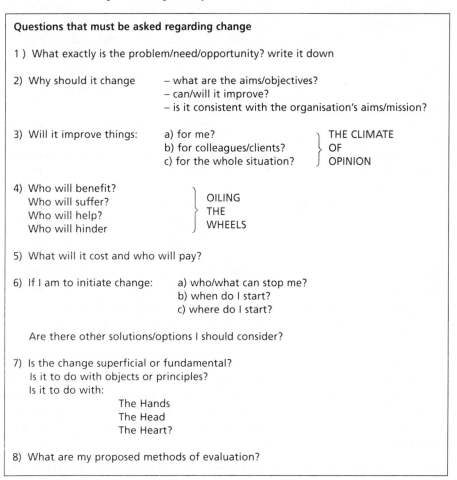

Questions that must be asked regarding change

1) What exactly is the problem/need/opportunity? write it down

2) Why should it change   – what are the aims/objectives?
                           – can/will it improve?
                           – is it consistent with the organisation's aims/mission?

3) Will it improve things: a) for me?   THE CLIMATE
                              b) for colleagues/clients?   OF
                              c) for the whole situation?   OPINION

4) Who will benefit?
   Who will suffer?   OILING
   Who will help?   THE
   Who will hinder   WHEELS

5) What will it cost and who will pay?

6) If I am to initiate change: a) who/what can stop me?
                                  b) when do I start?
                                  c) where do I start?

   Are there other solutions/options I should consider?

7) Is the change superficial or fundamental?
   Is it to do with objects or principles?
   Is it to do with:
                    The Hands
                    The Head
                    The Heart?

8) What are my proposed methods of evaluation?

Figure 11.1   Questions that must be asked regarding change (from Walton, 1984, adapted and used with kind permission of the author).

succinct paragraph, although McCalman and Paton (1992) advocate 'diagramming' to create a sense of logic and structure. This can then be mulled over, discussed with colleagues and firmed-up and improved in the light of this process. The second phase is to be clear about the goals of change (Baldridge, 1975) and practitioners should question whether change is appropriate, whether the situation can be improved and what are the more specific aims and objectives.

West (1989) asserts that the change agent will need a clear and well-developed vision of the purpose and outcome of the change. Pinto and Prescott (1987) note in their study that a project's mission statement was the single most critical factor across all stages of the project life-cycle (from conception to termination) suggesting that key objectives should be adhered to. As Pugh (1993) states, 'Don't only think out the change, THINK THROUGH IT' (original capitals).

Formulating aims and objectives will also assist in the process of communicating ideas which is critical in discussing the terms of reference with peers and colleagues. Practitioners must ensure that the change is reasonable and practicable, that the system can be changed and they are not attempting to impose a favourite theory or 'hobby-horse' since there will be cost implications of materials, time and manpower. The organization's mission statement is crucial to success; if the proposed change shares common themes there is more chance of agreement from senior managers if scarce finances must be committed.

The aims should be limited to changing and improving the identified problem. There may be a temptation for colleagues to say 'and while we are about it why don't we'. This should be resisted.

Thirdly, the scope of the change effects should be assessed, although no-one can foresee all the ramifications (Pugh, 1993). Stocking (1988) describes this as the 'climate of opinion' and suggests that careful thought should focus on whether the time is right for change. Baldridge (1975) states that any serious change must benefit the client as this is the only goal worth fighting for. It is not enough to argue that what is good for the practitioner has to equate to being 'good for the client'. Furthermore, change which only benefits a few individuals is unlikely to gain managerial support. McCalman and Paton (1992) state:

> If the problem owner can reach a point at which all those parties with a vested interest in influencing and possibly determining the outcome of the proposed change view it in such a way as to see common objectives and mutual benefits, as well as understand or at least recognise the conflicting views and arguments, then a great deal of progress will have been made. (p. 23)

Fourthly, an analysis of the conflicting forces which may simultaneously drive and restrict the change needs to be carried out (Lewin, 1951). This entails recognizing the source and magnitude of power in the decision-making process. In a telling phrase Stocking (1988) states that 'sometimes the product champions just do not have enough power and influence in the system to have their ideas accepted'. In this 'gate-keeping' role, decision making may be vested in a committee or an individual senior manager to whom access is difficult. With devolved budgets it may be a line manager, but implementing change means disturbing the status quo and the implications of one group (or clinic, etc.) gaining funds at the expense of another can spread throughout an organization.

Change agents must be prepared to share their vision, communicate with all those involved, listen to their concerns and give information which counters resistance. There will be conflict and resistance and this may come from colleagues who feel threatened or feel that their own practice is being implicitly criticized. This needs to be handled with care as their support and ownership is crucial to success. However, conflict can have a positive effect in helping to question and refine ideas. West (1989) warns about cohesive groups which can make disastrous decisions as they are more concerned with maintaining group cohesion than with task excellence. West suggests creating a climate of 'constructive controversy' where opposing opinions can be explored and new practices are challenged in a constructive manner. Baldridge (1975) sees this as building a 'political base'. It is fatal to 'go it alone' whereas a committed group can exchange ideas and reinforce each other's efforts. Forces to maintain the status quo will always be stronger than forces for change.

Fifthly, the question of costs and budgets must be considered. This has already been touched on. Any change involving costs such as employing 'Bank' staff or ordering new equipment should be discussed with budget holders as they will have to identify exactly where the finances will come from and what they intend to achieve. The effort in finding out any preliminary costings will help to show the commitment to change by the practitioner(s) and assist in the presentation of the case for change. However, discussions with the budget holder need to be held at an early stage; it is counter-productive to spend hours with a keen committee developing a new idea only to have it rejected at the final phase on the grounds of cost. Furthermore, frequently the driving force behind organizational change has been cost-cutting rather than motivations of improvement to produce a quality service (Loader and Burrows, 1994) so the answer to the question of costs must correlate with answers regarding overall improvements to the service.

Sixthly, the starting point should be considered. Pugh (1993) would suggest starting with the change agent; if leaders/managers do not change, how can they expect others to? 'Timing' is more difficult; planning and liaison committees may need to be canvassed and discussions held with finance departments; it may be necessary to delay implementation until the new financial year. Preferably an implementation deadline should be set; remember 'delay is the enemy of change, deadlines are flags that help call attention to stalling' (Baldridge, 1975). Procrastination can be used by powerful others as a political weapon to undermine and subvert ideas.

The notion of a pilot project could be considered as a safe, cost-effective precursor to the main change. This would enable unforeseen problems to be considered and allow more sceptical colleagues the opportunity to 'try it out' for a specified period. The time period will need to be negotiated and be appropriate to the focus of change.

Seventhly, what is the depth of the change. Is it superficial or more fundamental? At first glance, the answer to this seems simple. If the change is to do with objects, such as having an answerphone, a desk or administrative support, it appears to be superficial. But what about instigating or attending a primary health care team meeting? What can be so fundamental about a meeting? It is merely an opportunity for communication and data exchange? Careful thought however reveals that all these imply much more. They imply that there are fundamental territorial issues which should be recognized, ownership of knowledge, space, time, equipment and resources. They indicate professional values and issues of power and status and the control of one individual or group over others and hence involve the beliefs and values discussed earlier. It is therefore worth considering all change as being fundamental to some person or group and to proceed with caution through all stages.

Finally, how will the change effort be evaluated? Implementing a strategy of evaluation research will emphasize, to managers, the seriousness of the proposed change. Evaluation seeks to measure the success of the change set against agreed criteria; however as Drucker (1967) notes 'the problem with setting objectives for innovations is the difficulty of measuring their relative impact'. Donabedian (1966) proposed that there were three elements of health care amenable to evaluation: structure, process and outcome. Structure is the resources and facilities in the organization such as money, materials, staff and time; process involves the range of activities that go on between practitioners such as meetings, negotiation and consultation; outcome is the effect or measurement of the change in terms of increased satisfaction, effectiveness and ease of use. The ultimate validator of effectiveness has to be 'do clients benefit from the change?' Successful change attempts will also assist managers in staff appraisals and can be included in Professional Portfolios.

Action II

STRATEGIES TO FACILITATE THE PROCESS OF CHANGE

Analysing the conditions for change, and formulating and asking questions are important aspects of the change process but questions are not enough. At the same time strategies must be used to communicate, initiate and manage the essential ideas of the plan. Three main strategies are commonly discussed in the nursing literature (Chin and Benne, 1976; Haffer, 1986; Sullivan and Decker, 1992) which reflect issues of power and status described earlier. The strategies are generally separated for the sake of clarity and analysis but elements of each can and should be used as appropriate to each situation. Each strategy is underpinned by an assumption about the way people change their behaviour.

1. Strategy using power and coercion

The assumption in this strategy is that people will comply to the plans and direction of those in authority over them (Chin and Benne, 1976). It is built on the belief that people will do as they are told simply because they do not have any countervailing power. This way of making decisions is accepted as 'in the nature of things' and is more widespread than might be admitted.

Nursing is structured as a hierarchy and seniority, through either qualifications, grade or role, is power over those who are junior within an occupational relationship (Hugman, 1991). This may be within an occupation or between occupations. Power can be exercised in many ways. Haffer (1986) suggests methods ranging from force, commands, policies and laws through to moral pressure and the engendering of feelings of guilt. Hugman (1991) cautions against confusing power with authority, where authority is the exercise of legitimate command based on social status. When introducing change which involves colleagues, community practitioners are unlikely to have more power or authority than their colleagues and may find themselves in a similar position to respondents in Melia's (1984) and Mackensie's (1992) studies of needing to fit and remain 'in' the team or group. This strategy often meets with strong resistance and changes are generally not integrated if they conflict with a person's value system. Furthermore, those expected to comply will not have been involved in the change process and may be sceptical of its intentions as well as feeling undervalued as knowledgeable practitioners in their own right. This strategy may be necessary for immediate effect but since change is commonly a lengthy process it is best avoided even by senior managers.

2. Strategy using empirical evidence and rational thought (Empirical–Rational)

This strategy is based on the assumption that people are rational and will adapt to the change if it is rationally justified and personal gains and benefits can be perceived. This is founded on the 'you know it makes sense' belief of much health education that has been criticized for ignoring the structural aspects of society in influencing behaviour change (Beattie, 1991).

Methods for this strategy appeal to people's knowledge and understanding. It uses persuasion and rational argument, frequently provided in the form of scientific investigation and research evidence given by 'experts' in a 'top-down' approach. In this view knowledgeable people are legitimate sources of power and the flow of information is from 'those who know to those who don't know' (Chin and Benne, 1976, p. 39). As in outdated approaches to health education, this method fails to take into account social structure and the balances between motivation and knowledge. It assumes that judgements of what is rational are similar across time and organizations and shared by individuals. It also fails to take into account the reasons that people most often resist change: not being involved in the decision-making process.

3. Strategy using participation and professional norms (Normative–Re-educative)

This strategy is based on the assumption that patterns of action and practice are supported by socio-cultural norms and by commitment to those norms through the value systems of individuals (Chin and Benne, 1976). It is often built on a vision of the purpose and outcome of change which will be valued by those involved.

The methods focus on joint participation in identifying the problems, choosing negotiated solutions and implementing together. It uses clear and open communication, problem solving and collaborative practices which develop trust and lower status barriers. Change only occurs successfully when commitments to new normative orientations are made and this involves changes in attitudes, values, skills and significant relationships, not simply gaining new knowledge, information or intellectual rationales for practice. Haffer (1986) describes the change agent's role as falling into three areas:

- clarifying
- promoting problem-solving practices
- assuring a trusting environment.

West (1989) argues that participation in the process is the single most effective way of reducing resistance and encouraging commitment and that clarification of information helps to counter misunderstanding. As he states, change agents must 'prepare, rehearse, present, present and present' (West, 1989, p. 139).

Haffer (1986), although accepting that this strategy takes the longest, suggests that it should be used as it focuses on beliefs and values. It also promotes the view of nursing culture as espousing values of harmony and symbiosis discovered by Kinnunen (1990). In promoting participation the change agent inevitably loses some control over both the process of change and the final product. The planned end-product may be a beautiful, sleek and fast racehorse designed to win but when colleagues and managers add their own ideas and designs, the racehorse comes to resemble an ugly, lumpy camel which is slow and cumbersome and for which no-one will wish to claim responsibility.

In choosing their strategies for change, Kotter and Schlesinger (1979) identify a different set of themes. They argue that it is important to diagnose why people resist change. They see these as:

- parochial self-interest
- misunderstanding and lack of trust

- different assessments of the need for change
- a low tolerance for change.

Parochial self-interest focuses on people's own best interests and not on those of the total organization and they may raise all kinds of objections to the plan as they see themselves as losing something of value. This may be independence, autonomy and a degree of control over their work which can be seen as an implicit part of their contract with the organization. Initial questioning regarding benefits and encouraging participation should diagnose this pattern of resistance.

Misunderstanding and lack of trust is endemic in many organizations particularly between managers and employees. Rumours of the change and its effect can fuel misunderstanding and plans and progress need to be communicated at every stage. Even changes which focus on improving services to the client could be seen as a management tool for comparing the quality of one practitioner or health clinic with another and be viewed with suspicion. This point also illustrates Kotter and Schlesinger's third area of resistance – different assessments for the need for change and its costs and benefits. As Bauman (1990) describes, change can contribute to:

> the feelings of *insecurity*, generated by a drastic change in the habitual and familiar life conditions. Such a change naturally makes life more difficult. As the situation becomes more uncertain and less predictable, it tends to be experienced as dangerous and thus frightening. What people have learned as the efficient and effective way to go about their business of life suddenly becomes less reliable; people feel they have lost control of the situation. The change is therefore resented. The need to defend 'the old ways' (that is the familiar and comfortable ways) is strongly felt and the resulting aggression is directed against newcomers: those who were not present when the old ways were still securely entrenched. (p. 48, original italics)

Lastly, they suggest that people have a low tolerance for change because they fear they will not be able to develop the new skills and knowledge required. There is comfort in inertia and even when the change is rational and beneficial, the feeling that 'if it's not broken, why fix it' prevails.

Table 11.3 summarizes the main ways and means of bringing about change in an organization.

Conclusion

The substance of this paper has been to underscore the current need for and the challenges in managing change. In health care organizations however, officially accountable tasks tend to marginalize those activities which require a practitioner's individual judgement and innovation. It has been argued that social changes and the development of the competitive market has

Table 11.3 Actions to facilitate bringing about successful change

- Encourage agreement on the basic problem/need/opportunity
- Communicate this clearly and consistently to colleagues and managers
- Ensure the vision of change is consistent with the mission of the organization
- Ensure the vision of change is consistent with and develops professional ideals
- Base any actions on group decisions
- Ensure the change can be seen as raising standards
- Ensure the change benefits and can be seen to benefit client/s
- Facilitate provision for clarification and feedback
- Allow time for unnecessary fears and misunderstandings to be shared and relieved
- Enable skills/knowledge/resources to be developed to cope with new work
- Ensure that personal security is not threatened
- Listen and be seen to listen to suggestions from clients, colleagues and managers
- Remain open to revision and reconsiderations
- Strive to create an atmosphere of trust/support/confidence.

created an expectation that practitioners must be continually innovative. It has also been argued that the 'change agent' needs stamina and persistence and imagination to 'see' where change is required. There is a further element which involves those who are motivated from a professionalization perspective. Reeder and Mauksch (1979) identify three conceptually distinct 'ideal types' of nurses:

- the 'utilizer' who is engaged primarily in performing the job for wages;
- the 'traditionalizer' who feels a commitment to a personal role and legitimates nursing through sacred or secular truths;
- the 'professionalizer' who is orientated towards professional norms and collective ideals and strives for comprehensive involvement and control over practice.

Reeder and Mauksch (1979) argue that the utilizers and traditionalizers often fear the consequences of increased demands for autonomy and feel that confrontations with authority are, in some way, unprofessional. On the other hand, the professionalizers are the ones who agitate for change in practice. They are more receptive to new ideas and more likely to take on new roles and develop their practice. Continually reflecting on practice means acting as a 'newcomer' to each problem.

Newcomers are dangerous people because:

> they do not take the wisdom of our ways for granted. They therefore ask questions which we do not know how to answer, because in the past we had no occasion and saw no reason to ask them ourselves: 'Why do you do it this way? Does it make sense? Have you tried to do it differently?' The way we have lived, the kind of life which gives us our security and makes us feel comfortable, is now challenged. It has turned into a matter we are called to argue about, explain, justify. It is not self-evident and thus does not seem secure any more (Bauman, 1990, p. 59).

Despite the many and serious notes of caution, given a clear grasp of the problem of change, an intelligent control of the processes and strategies of change, a conviction to a vision and a belief that any innovation requires rigorous evaluation, there is no reason why practitioners should not successfully turn everyday limitations into opportunities to grow and gain mastery over their practice. 'Change' will always come about by evolution but Shaw's (1903) opinion suggests that 'progress' occurs through revolution. While this may seem like a daunting undertaking, it is also professionally challenging and rewarding. What nursing's professionalizers must guard against is that 'change' does not become a meaningless shibboleth for the imposing of ill considered and ill thought-out ideas.

Points to consider

1 Habitually questioning practice means seeing opportunities for change.

2 Seeing opportunities for change and acting on them means disturbing the accepted way of doing things.

3 Disturbing the accepted way of doing things implies the necessity to communicate, collaborate and cooperate with others.

4 Communicating and collaborating with others about ideas means sharing and potentially losing power and control over them.

References

Andrews, M. 1993: Importance of nursing leadership in implementing change. *British Journal of Nursing*, **2**, 8, 437–9.

Baldridge, J.V. 1975: Rules for a Machiavellian change agent: transforming the entrenched professional organisation. In Baldridge J.V. and Deal T. (eds), *Managing change in educational organisations: sociological perspectives*. Berkeley California: Cutchan Press, pp. 378–88.

Baldridge, J.V. and Deal, T. 1975: Overview of change processes in educational organisations. In Baldridge, J.V. and Deal, T. (eds), *Managing change in educational organisations: sociological perspectives*. Berkeley, California: Cutchan Press, pp. 1-23.

Bauman, Z. 1990: *Thinking sociologically*. Oxford: Blackwell.

Beattie, A. 1991: Knowledge and control in health promotion: a test case for social policy and social theory. In Gabe, J., Calnan, M. and Bury, M. (eds), *The Sociology of the Health Service*. London: Routledge, pp. 162–202.

Blumer, H. 1969: *Symbolic interactionism: perspectives and method*. Englewood Cliffs, New Jersey: Prentice-Hall.

Brooten, D., Hayman, L. and Naylor, M. 1978: Leadership for change: *A guide for the frustrated nurse*. Philadelphia: Lippincott.

Carrier, J. and Kendall, I. 1995: Professionalism and interprofessionalism in health and community care: some theoretical issues. In Owens, P., Carrier, J. and Horder, J. (eds), *Interprofessional issues in community and primary health care*. Basingstoke, Macmillan, pp. 1–5.

Chin, R. and Benne, K. 1976: General strategies for effective changes in human systems. In Bennis, W., Benne, K., Chin, R. and Corey, K. (eds), *The planning of change* (3rd edn). New York: Holt Rinehart and Winston, pp. 22–45.

Coulter, A. 1991: Evaluating the outcomes of health care. In Gabe, J., Calnan, M. and Bury, M. (eds), *The sociology of the health service*. London: Routledge, pp. 115–39.

Dahrendorf, R. 1985: Power divisions as the basis of class conflict. In Collins, R. (ed.), *Three sociological traditions*. New York: Oxford University Press.

Department of Health 1990: *National Health Service and Community Care Act*. London: HMSO.

Department of Health 1994: *The challenges for nursing and midwifery in the 21st century* (The Heathrow Debate). London: DOH.

DHSS 1983: *NHS management inquiry (The Griffiths Report)*. London: DHSS.

Donabedian, A. 1966: Evaluating the quality of medical care. *Millbank Memorial Fund Quarterly*, **44**, 166–206.

Drucker, P. 1967: *The practice of management*. London: Heinemann.

Durkheim, E. 1982: *The rules of sociological method*. London: Macmillan.

English National Board 1991: *Framework for continuing professional education for nurses, midwives and health visitors*. London: ENB.

Fabrega, H. 1979: The ethnography of illness. *Social Science and Medicine*, **13A**, 565–76.

Georgiades, N. and Phillimore, L. 1975: The myth of the hero–innovator and alternative strategies for organisational change. In Kiernan, C. and Woodford, F. (eds), *Behaviour modification with the severely mentally retarded*. London: Associated Scientific Publishers, pp. 313–19.

Giddens, A. 1989: *Sociology*. Oxford: Polity Press.

Goffman, E. 1969: *The presentation of self in everyday life*. Harmondsworth: Penguin.

Haffer, A. 1986: Facilitating change: choosing the appropriate strategy. *Journal of Nursing Administration*, **16**, 4, 18–22.

Handy, C. 1985: *Understanding organisations* (3rd edn). Harmondsworth: Penguin.

Heracleitus *fl* 513 BC. Quoted in Diogenes Laertius (Circa 3 AD) *Lives and opinions of eminent philosophers*.

Howkins, E. 1995: Collaborative care: an agreed goal, but a difficult journey. In Cain P., Hyde V. and Howkins, E. (eds.), *Community nursing: dimensions and dilemmas*. London: Arnold, pp. 66–89.

Hugman, R. 1991: *Power in caring professions*. Basingstoke: Macmillan.

Jessop, B. 1994: The transition to post-Fordism and the Schumpeterian workfare state. In Burrows, R. and Loader, B. (eds), *Towards a post-Fordist welfare state?* London: Routledge, pp. 13–37.

Kinnunen, J. 1990: The importance of organisational culture on development activities in a primary health care organisation. *International Journal of Health Planning and Management*, **5**, 65–71.

Kotter, J. and Schlesinger, L. 1979: Choosing strategies for change. *Harvard Business Review*, March/April, 106–14.

Lancaster, J. and Lancaster, W. 1984: *The nurse as a change agent*. St Louis: CV Mosby.

Lewin, K. 1951: *Field theory in social science*. New York: Harper and Row.

Lippitt, R., Watson, J. and Westley, B. 1958: *The dynamics of planned change*. New York: Harcourt Brace.

Loader, B. and Burrows, R. 1994: Towards a post-Fordist welfare state? In Burrows R. and Loader B. (eds) *Towards a post-Fordist welfare state?* London: Routledge, pp. 1–10.

Mabey, C. and Mayon-White, B. 1993: *Managing change*. London: Paul Chapman Publishing/Open University.

Machiavelli, N. 1513: The Prince. In Bondanella P. and Musa M. (eds and trans.). *The portable Machiavelli*. Harmondsworth: Penguin Books, pp. 77–166.

Mackensie, A. 1992: Learning from experience in the community: an ethnographic study of district nurse students. *Journal of Advanced Nursing*, **17**, 682–91.

May, C. 1992: Individual care? Power and subjectivity in therapeutic relationships. *Sociology*, **26**, 4, 589–602.

McCalman, J. and Paton, R. 1992: *Change management: a guide to effective implementation*. London: Paul Chapman Publishing.

Melia, K. 1984: Student nurses' construction of occupational socialisation. *Sociology of Health and Illness*, **6**, 2, 133–51.

National Health Service Management Executive 1993: *New world, new opportunities.* London: NHSME.

Nursing Times 1991: NT classified (general). *Nursing Times*, **87**, 19, 8 May, p. 66.

Nursing Times 1992: NHS appointments (community). *Nursing Times*, **88**, 19, 6 May, p. 97.

Nursing Times 1993: NT careers focus (community). *Nursing Times*, **89**, 18, 5 May. p. 73.

Nursing Times 1994: NHS appointments (community). *Nursing Times*, **90**, 19, 11 May. p. 95.

Owens, P. and Carrier, J. 1995: Introduction. In Owens, P., Carrier, J. and Horder, J. (eds), *Interprofessional issues in community and primary health care.* Basingstoke: Macmillan, pp. 1–5.

Owens, P. and Petch, H. 1995: Professionals and management. In Owens, P., Carrier, J. and Horder, J. (eds), *Interprofessional issues in community and primary health care.* Basingstoke: Macmillan, pp. 37–55.

Parkin P. 1995: Nursing the future: a re-examination of the professionalization thesis in the light of some recent developments. *Journal of Advanced Nursing*, **21**, 561–7.

Parsons, T. 1951: *The social system.* New York: The Free Press of Glencoe.

Pinto, J. and Prescott, J. 1987: *Changes in critical success factor importance over the life of a project. Academy of management proceedings*, pp. 328–32.

Pugh, D. 1993: Understanding and managing organisational change. In Mabey, C. and Mayon-White, B. (eds), *Managing change.* London: Paul Chapman Publishing/Open University, pp. 108–12.

Queen's Nursing Institute 1994: Another year of change? *Newsletter*, **4**, 1, 1.

Reeder, S. and Mauksch, H. 1979: Nursing: continuing change. In Freeman, H., Levine, S. and Reeder, L. (eds), *Handbook of medical sociology* (3rd edn). Englewood Cliffs, New Jersey: Prentice-Hall, pp. 209–29.

Russell, B. 1950: *Philosophy and politics. Unpopular essays.* London: Allen and Unwin.

Sathe, V. 1983: Implications of corporate culture: a manager's guide to action. *Organisational Dynamics*, Autumn, 5–23.

Shaw, G.B. 1903: *Maxims for revolutionists. Man and superman.* Westminster: Archibald Constable and Co.

Silverman, D. 1970: *The theory of organisations.* London: Heinemann.

Smart, B. 1993: *Postmodernity.* London: Routledge.

Smith, S. 1994: *Meeting the challenge of change in primary health care.* Conference programme. 6C and 7C October. London: Macmillan Magazines.

Stocking, B. 1988: Introducing innovation – overcoming resistance to change. In Bowling, A. and Stilwell, B. (eds), *The nurse in family practice.* London: Scutari, pp. 57–65.

Sullivan, E. and Decker, P. 1992: *Effective management in nursing* (3rd edn). California: Addison-Wesley.

Suu Kyi, Aung San 1995: *Speech on release from six years of house arrest; Burma.* British Broadcasting Corporation News, 11 July 1995.

United Kingdom Central Council 1986: *Project 2000: a new preparation for practice.* London UKCC.

UKCC 1990: *The report of the post-registration education and practice project.* London: UKCC.

UKCC 1991: *Report on proposals for the future of community education and practice.* London: UKCC.

UKCC 1992: *The scope of professional practice.* London: UKCC.

Walby, S. and Greenwell, J. 1994: *Medicine and nursing: professions in a changing health service.* London: Sage Publications.

Walton, M. 1984: *Management and managing: a dynamic approach.* London: Harper and Row.

West, M. 1987: Role innovation in the world of work. *British Journal of Social Psychology*, **26**, 305–15.

West, M. 1989: Visions and team innovation. *Changes*, **7**, 4, 136–40.

Williams, F. 1994: Social relations, welfare and the post-Fordist debate. In Burrows, R. and Loader, B (eds), *Towards a post-Fordist welfare state?* London: Routledge 49–73.

Witz, A. 1994: The challenge of nursing. In Gabe, J., Kellerher, D. and Williams, G. (eds), *Challenging medicine*. London: Routledge, pp. 23–45.

12 Marketing community nursing expertise

Anne Weeks

Confident professionals who provide a quality service must be able to sell themselves and their service in this age of market forces and competition. This chapter challenges nurses with that responsibility and highlights some of the dangers that could arise from complacency in this area.

There are three types of individuals: those who make things happen; those who watch things happen; those who wonder what happened (Anonymous).

As a consequence of the most recent reorganization of the NHS working relationships have changed and community nurses must identify and seize the new opportunities presented if they are to strengthen and develop their position as the experts in the management and provision of community-based nursing care. The value of the service must be high profile, documented, demonstrated and articulated in a business-like and acceptable format, in short – marketed. This chapter will explore these issues.

Introduction

A key aspect of the NHS reforms *Working for Patients* (DOH, 1989), NHS and Community Care Act (DOH, 1990), has been the separation of purchasers from providers of health care. All hospitals and community units are now either NHS Trusts, seeking trust status or are Directly Managed Units. The creation of this internal market has resulted in hospital and community trusts having to compete with each other to win contracts to provide services.

Having become used to the notion that fundholding GPs can now shop around between hospitals when contracting for secondary care, community nurses are having to come to terms with the implications of that freedom of choice being extended to the purchase of a community nursing service.

This new approach to the organization of health care was summarized by the then NHS Management Executive in 1990 when they circulated their working guide for trusts: trusts relate to GPs and health authorities through the contracts they make with them for the provision of services. Trusts need to work closely with GPs, health authorities and local authority social services departments to make sure that the services they provide or plan to develop meet identified needs and are properly integrated with other services (NHSME, 1990).

The creation of the internal market and the subsequent application of marketing principles and competition to provide what the customer wants at a price they are prepared to pay, can be viewed as a threat or an opportunity for both management and staff. Relationships, roles, responsibilities and caseloads are changing (NHSME, 1993) and community nurses must identify and seize the new opportunities presented if they are to strengthen and develop their position as the experts in the management and provision of community-based nursing care.

Many purchasers do not possess a great deal of market intelligence about providers (Dennis, 1993), a view shared by Goodwin (1995) who believes that not only do they not understand what community providers do but that they have neither the time nor the resources to find out. If there is a dearth of information on what providers of health care have to offer, there is no such confusion on what purchasers are seeking. The purchaser function is well documented (Spurgeon, 1993) and encompasses:

- Assessment of need in the population;
- Identification of the service to respond to the need;
- Specification of the volume of service to be purchased;
- The placing of contracts with selected providers and determination of quality standards to be applied;
- Monitoring of the subsequent delivery of those services.

There is nothing in the above which should particularly unnerve community nurses. They should, as professionals, be aware of the health status of their local population, should be working towards maintaining and improving that health status and be expert in setting standards to provide a quality service. What is required is that the value of the service provided must be high profile, documented, demonstrated and articulated in a business-like and acceptable format, in short – marketed.

Central to the process of community nursing are patients, carers and the wider community, but they do not purchase care. The purchaser of the service is the GP practice which may or may not be fundholding. The fundholding practice is one which holds its own budget and from which it both provides and purchases health care for its practice population. In some large practices, this budget may now total more than £1 million (Holliday, 1992). This facility distinguishes it from a non-fundholding practice, which still has secondary care purchased on its behalf by the district health authority. Importantly, as GPs become more involved in commissioning, whether as fundholders or through commissioning authorities, they assume wider responsibility for the care delivered to their patients.

Other prospective purchasers, who should not be overlooked, are social services departments. The White Paper, *Caring for People* (DOH, 1989) set an ambitious agenda for care in the community with local authority social services departments (SSDs) subsequently becoming the lead agencies for the development of a mixed economy of community care. Care managers are required to make assessments, plan care packages and secure services. These are predominantly for people who are disadvantaged by age, chronic ill-health or disability, users whose needs have, and could continue to be, effectively met by community teams.

The government believes that health and social services managers will see that it is in everyone's best interest to collaborate to meet the identified needs of local populations (Davis and Davies, 1991) and that the need to pursue value for money will of itself promote closer working relationships. There is, as yet, little evidence of such collaboration but SSDs are in the market for purchasing care packages and there is no reason why community trusts should not tender for such business.

Marketing is defined as 'the management process responsible for identifying, anticipating and satisfying customer requirements profitably' (Chartered Institute of Marketing, 1987). At the present time, operating for profit within the NHS is not allowed but, taking a profit and loss perspective, it is possible that those units that do not pay their way could disappear from the health care system.

Kotler (1991) suggests that the marketing planning process consists of five steps: analysing market opportunities; researching and selecting target markets; designing marketing strategies; planning marketing programmes; organizing, implementing and controlling the marketing effort.

This paper is not about putting together a formal marketing plan, a task usually undertaken by senior management. However, there are selected aspects of that process which would enable community nurses to develop strategies for marketing themselves. Thus every interaction, at whatever level, should promote community nursing as a value-for-money service which makes a significant contribution to achieving optimum health status among the population.

The marketing of services is not very different from the marketing of products, the major difference being that a service has benefits that cannot be stored (McDonald, 1989; Kotler, 1991). Services are essentially intangible and therefore purchasers will look for evidence of quality and value for money often based upon their perceptions of the people delivering the service. In the view of Kotler (1991), the service provider's main task is to manage this evidence, 'tangibilize' the intangible. This is a difficulty explored by Goodwin (1995) from the perspective of the purchaser. The use of terms such as 'empowerment', 'self-esteem', 'comfort, care and support' tell us a great deal about the intangibility of nursing care. These intangibles must be translated into measurable outcomes.

The importance and influence of field staff in promoting a service to actual and potential purchasers cannot be underestimated and this is especially true of professional services (Cowell, 1984; Kotler and Bloom, 1984), where they often perform a dual role of both performing a service and selling that service. This is something which has been addressed within the private sector, where the role of employees in optimizing the quality and provision of services to purchasers has been documented by a number of researchers (Cowell, 1984; Groonroos, 1984; Brown, 1989).

There is general agreement within the literature that marketing can be described as a matching process between the organization's capabilities and the wants of purchasers (McDonald, 1989; Kotler, 1991). It is this matching of resources to meet the demands of purchasers which is fundamental to the organization's success. The process does not take place within a vacuum but within an environment which, as has been discussed, is constantly changing. Many of these changes are outside the control of the profession; economic, demographic and technological changes are examples of variables which impinge on the organization of community nursing practice but which are beyond its immediate sphere of influence.

With this in mind, it can no longer be assumed that the traditional range of services will continue to meet the changing demands of purchasers; a status quo stance in the context of performance is no longer appropriate. Community nurses cannot know too much about the general practice to which they are attached. There is a place for intuition based on experience and observation but it must be substantiated by collating qualitative and quantitative data. This data can then be used critically to analyse the relevance of the service currently being delivered.

The first step in developing a strategy for the marketing and promotion of the service is to undertake a situational analysis. This is sometimes known as a PEST analysis and identifies and evaluates the importance of political, economic, social and technological trends and their influence on the future operation of the community nursing service. For example, political influences would encompass the reforms announced in the *Working for Patients* White Paper (DOH, 1989) which brought about a totally changed operating environment such as the separation of purchasers from providers of health care.

Working for Patients was closely followed by the second White Paper *Caring for People* (DOH, 1989) with its emphasis on social care and consumer choice and the changes in community nursing practice which were brought about by the Community Care Act are well known.

An examination of the socio-cultural environment reveals important demographic trends, particularly the ageing population. Community nurses are aware that there is scope for delaying the onset of mortality and morbidity across the life span, particularly among the elderly, and should be utilizing this knowledge to expand their role.

SWOT analysis

Once the major trends in the environment have been identified, the next step is to undertake an analysis of the capability of the team to respond. SWOT stands for strengths, weaknesses, opportunities and threats and analysis should focus on key factors only (McDonald, 1989).

Utilizing data gathered from the PEST analysis, significant opportunities and threats, those external factors which may affect the continuing success of the organization, can be identified.

Kotler and Bloom (1984) define threat as: 'a challenge posed by an unfavourable trend or specific disturbance in the environment which would lead, in the absence of purposeful marketing action, to the stagnation, decline, or demise of an organization or one of its services'. Not all threats warrant the same attention or concern. Each should be assessed according to two dimensions: its potential severity and its probability of occurrence.

As a profession, community nurses should be speaking nationally with a common voice on identified threats to service delivery. At the local level they should be able to identify changes in the organization and delivery of care which may comprise a threat. Opportunity analysis is as important as threat analysis. It is by taking advantage of the opportunities identified that the service can grow. Action to take advantage of opportunities and counteract threats should be initiated as soon as possible.

Having analysed opportunities and threats, the same process should be undertaken to identify the key capabilities (strengths) and key limitations (weaknesses) of the team. In a people organization such as nursing, strengths and weaknesses often revolve around human resource issues such as levels of knowledge and experience, qualifications, skill-mix and numbers of staff available to meet fluctuating levels, as well as types of demand. Another aspect is support for continuing education to meet the changing needs of patients, clients and carers.

Attention should be paid to distinctive competencies in which the organization is especially strong. Problems will arise when there is a mismatch between identified strengths and purchaser needs. This will involve constant re-evaluation of the team's strengths against market demands.

An example of an identified strength might be a reputation among patients and carers for providing a 'good' nursing service but the strength of the reputation of the nursing team among patients may not be enough in the future. A weakness might be that evidence cannot be produced for purchasers in terms of measurable outcomes such as health status or functional ability, again the problem of tangibles and intangibles. It is with the quality of the outcomes of nursing intervention that purchasers now seem to be concerned and upon which contracts will be awarded. An in-depth and honest SWOT analysis will aid the matching process between the nursing teams' capabilities and the wants of purchasers. Issues can then be addressed, tactics considered and objectives set to eliminate any mismatch.

The following SWOT analysis was undertaken by a practising community nursing team.

STRENGTHS

Team members come from varied backgrounds and between them have a wealth of knowledge and specific clinical expertise.

In-depth knowledge of their local population.

Strong networks within the community.

Peer support.

Expertise in caring for the terminally ill patient.

The ability to plan and focus visits effectively.

Experts in case management.

Able to help GPs.

WEAKNESSES

No overall professional leadership.

No identified leader for the team.

A lack of agreed standards of care.

No audit tool specific to community nursing.

Practice is not audited.

Do not have the resources to meet assessed need.

Splinter groups working alone, no sharing of best practice.

No flexibility allowed in the use of the nursing resource.

OPPORTUNITIES

Tendering for the meeting of hygiene needs of the chronically sick across the age range.

Tendering for teaching input to social services staff to improve the quality of care.

Tendering for personal care currently undertaken by home carers.

Taking back areas of care which have been wrongly defined as social care.

Contributing to the meeting of *Health of the Nation* targets.

THREATS

The field of practice is narrowing.

A move back to task orientation.

Workload now measured by face to face contacts and not the quality and outcome of care.

The widening definition of social care.

More onerous eligibility criteria for the provision of nursing input.

A move to multiskilling for reasons of cost-containment.

Portfolio analysis

The third step in developing a strategy for the marketing and promotion of the service is to undertake a portfolio analysis. Where there is a mismatch between the nursing teams' capabilities and the wants of purchasers there are choices to be made. Two approaches are possible: either to alter the purchasers' perceptions of their needs and wants or to change the service itself.

Kotler and Bloom (1984) could be describing community nursing within their discussion of service portfolio strategy. They hold the view that most professional organizations are multiservice operations consisting of either generalist professionals, who each provide basically the same range of services, or a group of specialists, who support and complement each other by providing different but related types of service.

Such is the case in community nursing where district nurses, practice nurses, community paediatric nurses, community psychiatric nurses, school nurses and health visitors use their generalist and specialist knowledge and skills in working with populations to generate solutions to contemporary health problems with multiple causation. Examples might include provision of primary health care services in accident and emergency departments and providing 'drop in' centres for homeless people. Regardless of the particular format of community nursing teams, the portfolio of services available should be periodically reviewed in the light of the changing needs and wants of purchasers and end-users. It is not appropriate here to give in-depth consideration to tools for portfolio analysis. However, it is useful to identify those services which should be given increased support, maintained at their present level, phased down or terminated.

Many GP practices are making considerable changes to the range of services available to their practice populations. Minor surgery, desk-top pathology and a wide range of health promotion activities are now undertaken, usually managed by practice nurses and, increasingly, nurse practitioners. Community nurses, while becoming more involved in surgery-based work, are predominantly still practising in peoples' own homes. This focus may be appropriate or it may not; it is for the profession to decide. The changing requirements of GP practices and their patients must be addressed, however, and if community nursing is to avoid becoming pigeon-holed, often by statutory and professional bodies, expertise must be developed in marketing the contribution which can be made to improving individual, family and community health.

Target markets and segmentation

The fourth step is to identify marketing opportunities more efficiently and today's organizations are increasingly embracing a target marketing approach (Kotler, 1991). An important aspect of this approach is segmentation – the process of dividing the market into groups of purchasers who might require distinct services. They may differ in their wants, their philosophy of care, their geographical location or their purchasing power.

A useful approach to segmentation is to adopt a demographic approach, one which community nurses are well qualified to undertake. Using this approach, the market is divided into groups on the basis of variables such as age, sex, family make-up, family life cycle, the employed/unemployed, religious persuasion, race and nationality and lifestyle (Titterton, 1994; Clemen-Stone *et al.*, 1995).

Such an approach can be applied to differing purchasers with differing needs such as GPs and social services departments and strategies then developed to meet those needs. Bearing in mind the characteristics of the target market, the marketing effort should focus on projecting a strong professional image grounded in a thorough knowledge of particular purchaser requirements.

Objective-setting and action plans

The fifth step in the process may be the most difficult for there is a great deal of work involved in adopting a marketing orientation. Commitment, belief and persistence are required to make the effort needed and overcome setbacks. Time expended in gathering the necessary data will be wasted without the formulation of specific objectives, stated in unambiguous and measurable form, a schedule of key tasks to be achieved within set time limits. A timetable might comprise:

PEST analysis to be undertaken

Community nursing team to discuss findings

Meeting to undertake a SWOT analysis

Data from SWOT analysis to be circulated

Meeting to discuss implications of SWOT analysis

Meeting to discuss current portfolio and identify necessary changes

Factors which can get in the way of implementation are the organizational culture, working habits, attitudes to change and team morale. When objectives have been set, however, the team will know where it wants to go. The question then becomes how best to get there.

In a service industry such as health care there are professional and ethical constraints placed upon the use of marketing and promotional methods and the view that money spent on marketing is money taken away from patient care still prevails. A case can be made, however, that promotion of the expertise of community nurses among purchasers can only benefit patient/client care in terms of quality, value for money and outcomes. Communicating the range, depth, and quality of the community nursing service to all prospective purchasers, either by word of mouth or through the use of inexpensive promotional materials is therefore acceptable.

Finally, a potent marketing tool is the constant projection of a professional image which is consistent with how the individual and organization would like to be perceived and which is congruent with the purchaser's perception of how professionals should conduct themselves. Effective marketing depends on the maintenance of a favourable image (Cowell, 1984).

Conclusion

This chapter has covered some general principles of marketing, that is the process responsible for identifying, anticipating and satisfying customer requirements.

Purchasers are looking for excellence in quality and value for money when they choose their providers. Community nurses cannot survive by simply doing a good job. It is essential that if the service is to survive within an environment characterized by financial constraints and increasing competition that everyone adopts a marketing approach that is demand led.

Points to consider

1 What are the strengths and weaknesses of your nursing team?

2 How would you segment the needs of the practice population to which you are attached?

3 How would you suggest making the value of nursing care in the community setting tangible and therefore measurable?

4 Could you justify the continuing use of the nursing resource strictly against outcomes?

References

Brown, A.B. 1989: *Customer care management*. Oxford: Heinemann.
Chartered Institute of Marketing 1987: *Marketing means business*. London: Chartered Institute to the Marketing.
Clemen-Stone, S. Gerber-Eigsti, D. and McGuire, S.L. 1995: *Comprehensive family and community health nursing*. USA: Mosby.
Cowell, D. 1984: *The marketing of services*. Oxford: Heinemann.
Davis, A. and Davies, L. 1991: In Spurgeon, P (ed.), *The changing face of the NHS in the 1990s*. Essex: Longman.
Dennis, J. 1993: NHS trusts – purchaser perspectives. In Peck, E. and Spurgeon, P. (eds), *NHS trusts in practice*, Essex: Longman.
Department of Health 1989: *Working for patients*. London: HMSO.
Department of Health 1990: *NHS and Community Care Act*. London: HMSO.
Department of Health 1989: *Caring for people – community care in the next decade and beyond*. London: HMSO.
Goodwin, S. 1995: Commissioning for health. *Health Visitor*, **68**, 1, 16–18.
Groonroos, C. 1984: A service quality model and its marketing implications. *European Journal of Marketing*, **18**, 4, 36–44.
Holliday, I. 1992: *The NHS transformed*. Manchester: Baseline Books.
Kotler, P. 1991: *Marketing management*. Prentice-Hall: Englewood Cliffs.
Kotler, P. & Bloom, P.N. 1984: *Marketing professional services*. Englewood Cliffs: Prentice-Hall.
McDonald, M. 1989: *Marketing plans: how to prepare them and use them*. Oxford: Butterworth Heinemann.
National Health Service Management Executive 1993: *New world, new opportunities*. London: HMSO.
National Health Service Management Executive 1990: *NHS trusts: a working guide*. London: HMSO.
Spurgeon, P. 1993: NHS trusts – purchaser perspectives. In Peck, E. and Spurgeon, P. (eds), *NHS trusts in practice*. Essex: Longman.
Titterton, M. (Ed.) 1994: *Caring for people in the community – the new welfare*. London: Kingsley Publishers.

13 The Experiential Taxonomy in action

Isobel M. Walker

Every community health nurse is professionally obligated to take responsibility for planning, implementing and evaluating teaching and learning activities. Whether these activities are centred on student learning, patient education or assessment of their own practice and that of others, they are more effective if the individual is conversant with a framework that addresses the total experience of teaching and learning. This paper intends to demonstrate how the educational model, 'Experiential Taxonomy' (Steinaker and Bell, 1979) can be utilized by the community health nurse as a functional vehicle which provides complete classification of both the teacher and learner activities from the moment the learner is exposed to a new experience to its highest level of completion.

The Experiential Taxonomy (ET) is used extensively by many community health nurses to plan teaching and learning activities. One of its most popular uses in the community is concerned with patient education and the formulation of health promotion packages. ET is also a valuable framework for the community health nurse who is responsible for planning and providing a learning environment for students within the context of the specialist area and to assess the student's competence to practice as a community health nurse. Within the framework of Experiential Taxonomy the community health nurse can also examine her/his dual role of teacher and practitioner. Qualified nurses can utilize many of the ideas put forward in this chapter using the Experiential Taxonomy framework and the learner nurse examples for their own learning needs.

The example outlined in the chapter is of a learner nurse who is exposed to the experience of wound care in the community and will identify and concentrate on the development of community health nursing professional practice. A step-by-step guide will inform both the teacher and learner of how any new exposure to this professional practice can be planned, with the identification of desirable learning outcomes, what teaching and learning strategies can be adopted in order to achieve the desired learning outcomes, and finally how this teaching and learning is evaluated.

An important aspect of any teaching and learning experience is for the teacher and learner to acknowledge important previous knowledge that the learner brings to the new experience. All too often this important knowledge is ignored, whether it is propositional (textbook knowledge), practical (knowledge through the acquisition of skills) or experiential (knowledge gained through direct personal encounter with a subject, person or thing) (Burnard, 1987).

Using an ET tripartite grid, both the teacher and learner can formatively assess initial levels of mastery when planning learning outcomes. With the recognition of this previous learning, expensive repetitious learning can be avoided and the new experience planned to build upon what has already been achieved. The tripartite grid is also used summatively to assess the self or learner's expected level and actual level of mastery against predetermined learning outcomes.

The notion of progression has been explicitly addressed by professional bodies responsible for nurse education. The United Kingdom Central Council (UKCC, 1994) put forward the idea of taxonomically moving through higher levels of learning, acquiring the necessary knowledge and skills for distinct areas of practice: Professional, Specialist and Advanced.

There are various models that are available to inform the development of knowledge, skills and attitudes that characterize different levels of practice. The Experiential Taxonomy (ET) is offered as a useful framework for taxonomically determining how a student or qualified nurse learns things at different levels of sophistication.

Experiential Taxonomy

Most of the competencies expected of the community health nurse are expressed in the context of the nurse acquiring or having the necessary 'knowledge, skills and attitudes'. There are various models that are quite helpful in identifying and defining learning outcomes or educational objectives. The problem is that these models or taxonomies encourage us to view learning in a fragmented way.

Although it is acknowledged that the nurse needs to have the necessary knowledge, skills and attitudes, educational psychologists such as Bloom (1956) described learning as taking place through three domains:

- Cognitive Domain of Learning (Knowledge)
- Psychomotor Domain of Learning (Skills)
- Affective Domain of Learning (Attitudes).

The cognitive taxonomy of Bloom (1956), the psychomotor taxonomy of Harrow (1972) and the affective taxonomy of Krathwohl *et al.* (1968), although extremely useful, are all responsible for describing learning as if it happens in isolated taxonomies. According to Steinaker and Bell (1979) experience or learning cannot be fragmented or understood in isolation. Experience is a whole entity, not a cognitive, psychomotor or affective response.

The learner nurse for example who is exposed to a new learning experience, wound care, in the community, will in this instance be required to attain a knowledge of wound care which involves the cognitive domain. The learner will develop the kinetic skills needed for dressing wounds such as bandaging techniques (psychomotor domain) and at the same time will interact with the client and carers using interpersonal skills that demonstrate appropriate attitudes (affective domain).

Steinaker and Bell (1979) suggest the need for a more broadly based taxonomy rather than using three or more taxonomies as models for planning. They respond to the need by developing a gestalt taxonomy that could speak to the totality of an experience. ET has five basic categories:

1 Exposure
2 Participation
3 Identification
4 Internalization
5 Dissemination.

These five basic categories have a natural logical progression leading towards the planned outcome, namely learning. An individual such as the learner nurse will move through the new experience, for example, wound care, from exposure to dissemination. This new learning is planned to take account of the total experience which embraces all three domains of learning. Planned learning should have a definite outcome and these outcomes can be planned, implemented and evaluated through the Experiential Taxonomy.

Descriptions of learning processes for each ET category

It would be useful at this stage to orientate readers with ET's categories and sub-categories (after Steinaker and Bell, 1979).

The learner nurse is about to be newly exposed to wound care in the community. What will the learner need to know (cognitive)? How skilled does the learner need to be in dressing techniques (psychomotor)? What interpersonal skills does the learner need to demonstrate (affective)? How will this new learning affect the learner (affective)?

1. EXPOSURE

Exposure is the awareness of an experience and has three sub-categories.

1.1 Sensory

The learner is exposed to the possibility of an experience, for example, wound care in the community. Awareness will be through all five senses. Initially the community health nurse who is responsible for planning the experience will provide external motivation and organize a real or simulated experience, such as the presentation of epidemiological data specifically concerned with the incidence of leg ulcers, or illustrated examples of various stages of wound healing. The learner will be seeing, hearing and using other senses where appropriate.

1.2 Response

The learner can either reject or accept this new experience. The community health nurse needs to focus the learner's attention by directing the learner's observation. Obviously this new learning needs to be relevant for the learner but equally important is the way in which the experience is organized. All the principles of adult learning should be considered when planning for and during the experience so as to avoid unnecessary anxiety for the learner.

1.3 Readiness

Usually this stage assumes the experience has been accepted and the learner is ready for the next stage of Participation. The key characteristics of exposure and its sub-categories are that the learner becomes aware of the experience. As a result of this consciousness and an understanding of basic concepts of wound care, the learner will have moved from isolation to readiness where some of the indicators of this process may include:

- feelings of anxiety
- awareness of lack of knowledge and skills
- apprehension
- difficulty in conceptualizing
- asking naive questions
- volition (exercising the will)
- non-verbal gestures e.g. head nodding, eye contact
- viewing demonstration
- reciting fact and principle
- any evidence of attending.

2 PARTICIPATION

Participation denotes a conscious decision to become involved further and meaningfully to explore the experience. Participation has two sub-categories.

2.1 Representation

The learner now has the opportunity to rehearse the experience in a protective environment. The learner will reproduce the information/knowledge encountered both covertly and overtly. Covert representation means that the learner will probably read more widely around the topic of wound care, appreciate the research conducted in this area, mentally rehearse for a classroom test, for example, what are the physiological manifestations of infection? Overt representation may be facilitated by the community health nurse through clarifying, supporting and supervising the learner's assessment of a client with a venous leg ulcer.

2.2 Modification

This may involve the integration of new learning with previous learning. This is closely regulated by the learner's feeling and search for cognitive verification. Knowledge of wound care developed previously, for instance in the hospital setting, may need to be integrated into a new order which may necessitate giving up on modifying both previous or new learning in order to minimize cognitive dissonance.

The key characteristics of participation and its sub-categories are to create a process of discovery (representation) of new learning and the subsequent verification thereof.

At the participation category the learner may:

- continue to show some anxiety
- begin to be clear about concepts and skills of wound care
- show recall of ideas and concepts (identify stages of healing)
- engage in mental and physical rehearsal
- engage in explorative activities
- engage in trial and error activities (simulated)
- begin to feel interested and integrated with the experience.

3 IDENTIFICATION

The identification process has four sub-categories:

3.1 Reinforcement

After modification the experience is repeated through various teacher and learner strategies. The learner will probably at this stage be selectively reinforcing the experience through assessing, planning, implementing and evaluating care for patients with various wound care needs. The more this experience is facilitated the more it is retained.

3.2 Emotional

The reinforcement and retention involves a conscious selection of those aspects of an individual's experience that easily harmonize with their perceptions, existing schema and personality. For example, an individual may experience this harmony when identifying with research undertaken to establish the stages of wound healing, and find this congruent with their current practice and experience. This then may lead to emotional fusion, hence, 'my experience'.

3.3 Personal

Once emotional fusion (identification) has taken place, the learner may also move towards personal intellectual identification with the experience. Attachment (identification) with the experience such as the research into the stages of wound healing will become more meaningful, organized, understood and more appropriate as the individual uses this to underpin their professional practice.

3.4 Sharing

Due to the meaningful nature of the experience the learner may readily engage in sharing this experience with others. The learner may for example design a health promotion package for clients with healed venous leg ulcers. The package would include information which would enhance the client's understanding of the importance of exercising the calf muscle to assist venous return, the importance of weight control and support hosiery to avoid the re-occurrence of venous leg ulcers.

Sharing symbolizes the true emergence of informed decisions, clearer understanding of guiding principles and acceptance of values and attitudes implicit in the experience.

It is at this stage (3.4) that the learner will have achieved the learning outcome planned.

Learning outcome

The learner will perform holistic assessment of patients' nursing needs, demonstrating the ability to use research to plan, implement and evaluate concepts and strategies leading to improvements in care.

The key characteristics of identification and its sub-categories are that the learner

- may show ownership of concepts and skills
- shows deeper insight of concepts and skills
- shows high level (rational) discrimination
- appreciates practical application
- appreciates the general utility of the experience
- creates and justifies hypotheses
- appreciates own strengths and limitations
- may seek further involvement with the experience
- engages in the classifying, associating, applying and
- evaluates of data relevant to the experience
- highlights personal meaning
- shows high appreciation and minimal anxiety.

4 INTERNALIZATION

This involves the crystallization of identified experience so that it becomes almost second nature on the learner's part. The experience begins to affect the whole lifestyle through the internalization of values, attitudes, knowledge and skills selected at identification. The process of internalization takes place through two sub-categories.

4.1 Expansion

As above, this denotes how the experience extends to other aspects of the learner's life. It is common for such an expansion permanently to change the learner's whole outlook including beliefs, philosophies and priorities.

4.2 Intrinsic

When expansion occurs to the above degree it changes motivation, lifestyle and values. At this point experience becomes much more than mental and physical, it becomes continuous and enduring. The learner by this time has met all the learning requirements and will be working autonomously as a community health nurse.

The key characteristics of internalization and its sub-categories are the learner

- shows confidence in own activity
- is able to think at a higher cognitive level
- can apply acquired knowledge to new situations
- shows creativity and individualism
- presents own interpretation and own hypothesis
- is capable of analysis and synthesis
- shows ability to extrapolate (calculate from known terms a series of other terms which lie outside the range of known terms).

5 DISSEMINATION

This level is much higher than the sharing that started at sub-category 3.4. Dissemination is also higher than internalization and has two sub-categories.

5.1 Informational

The learner (community health nurse) seeks to stimulate others to engage in a similar experience, for example, supervising pre-registration nurse learners in carrying out key procedures concerned with wound care. There is a readiness to share information and gain deeper insights.

5.2 Homiletic

The community health nurse now acts as a role model. He/she sees the experience as imperative for others. At this stage the nurse may well be a member of a wound care association or research group. Activity may well be centred around influencing health trust protocols, with the formulation of up-to-date policy for wound care based upon credible research findings.

The key characteristics of dissemination and its sub-categories are that the new role model

- shows a willingness to teach others
- debates, campaigns, defends, promotes, encourages others and so on
- acts as a role model
- shows a willingness to share
- designs and produces own learning strategies.

A checklist of words and phrases that denote feelings, thoughts and behaviours characteristic of each ET category is presented in Table 13.1.

Table 13.1 Checklist of characteristics for each ET category

Exposure		
asking questions	becoming aware	observing/seeing
attending	listening	having anxiety
apprehension	doubt	reading/studying
simulating	eagerness	having confusion

Participation		
exploring relevance	gaining insight	explore by reading
role play	explore meaning	begin to understand
discovering	participation	use of other sources
requiring guidance	interested	gaining confidence
remembering	feeling happier	needs encouragement
clarifying	making effort	comparing with the past
fitting together	appreciating	comprehension

Identification		
understanding	applying	sharing
reporting	distinguishing	interpreting
analysing	acknowledging	demonstrating
explaining	investigating	selecting
willingness to use	choosing	compare and contrast
debating	experimenting	making own choice
challenging	hypothesising	accepting

Internalisation		
feeling confident	change of attitude	expansion of experience
personal value	feeling satisfied	adopting new philosophy
creative/innovative	change of practice	carrying out enquiry
improving standards	co-operation of new values	

Dissemination		
influencing practice	demonstrating	teaching others
campaigning	publishing	influencing policy
advising	assisting others	advertising
evaluating	conferencing	organising workshops
representing	criticising	organising seminars

Source: Revised (Nyatanga, 1990a, pp. 16–17); revised (Walker, 1993a, p. 113)

Evaluation

According to Steinaker and Bell (1979) ET has real usefulness for the teacher and learner who are serious about self-evaluation as well as professional development. Research conducted by Steinaker and Bell (1979) to test the existence of ET teaching strategies that are conducive to desirable learning outcomes, infers that as teachers progress through ET categories, so do the learners.

Steinaker and Bell (1979) see teacher self-evaluation as a key not only to mastering the ET process but also to ensuring quality of the learning environment. It is assumed that self-evaluation helps the teacher move from one ET category to the next in a way that is reciprocal to learner movement within the categories (Nyatanga, 1990b).

The tool to record evaluation is the tripartite grid developed by Brooke *et al.* (1989). According to Brooke *et al.* (1989) the ET grid seems to be the quickest and most useful way of fulfilling three most important educational requirements:

- assessing the learner's initial level of mastery
- anticipating learning outcomes by stating expected level of mastery
- establishing the actual level of mastery (learning outcome).

INITIAL LEVEL OF MASTERY (ILOM)

Operationalization of the grid supports the belief that the community health nurse should start where the learners are. ILOM encourages the learner to assess themselves. This formative assessment intends that the learner and the community health nurse decide upon the learner's initial level of mastery with respect to the particular topic being taught, for example, health promotion. The learner places a cross or (I) on the grid (Fig. 13.1) against the appropriate ET category that best describes their present or initial level of mastery based upon a reflection of previous experience.

EXPECTED LEVEL OF MASTERY (ELOM)

In many professional courses, the expected level of competence is determined by professional bodies, for example the English National Board Higher Award (ENB 10 key characteristics, 1990), and this is used as an example in Fig. 13.1.

This does not mean that the learner does not participate in agreeing the expected level of mastery. If the learner is familiar with the competency and has had previous valuable experience, then they are in a position to negotiate with the community health nurse for the level they would expect to achieve. As a result a cross or E would be placed on the grid at the level they would expect to achieve.

It is important to remember that when summative assessment takes place to establish whether the learner has achieved the learning outcome expected, the minimum level or standard that is acceptable is the ET category of identification (see sub-category 3.4, Sharing).

ACTUAL LEVEL OF MASTERY (ALOM)

The tripartite grid facilitates summative assessment whereby the community health nurse and learner can evaluate the actual level of mastery. It should be possible to establish whether or not the learner has achieved the expected level of mastery or, as is the case for many learners, may have exceeded this and can demonstrate a more sophisticated level of mastery, say at internalization or even dissemination. Following summative assessment an A or cross is placed on the grid to denote the actual level of mastery that the learner has achieved.

An example of the professional nature of community health nurses is given in Fig. 13.1. The key characteristic number 6 of the ENB Higher Award programme is used as an example to illustrate how the ET grid facilitates the learner's assessment and progress.

Learning outcomes	E	P	I	I	D
The learner must be able to demonstrate the ability to:					
Discuss and teach clients, carers and team members concepts of health promotion, health education, prevention and health protection	I			E	A
Understand and apply the principles and practice of health promotion in the practitioner's work setting.	I			E	A
Facilitate client's responsibility and choice for healthy living. and the ability to determine their own lifestyle.	I			E	A
Create, maintain and take responsibility for a healthy environment within their own work setting.	I			E	A
Encourage health promotion activities with clients, colleagues and carers.	I			E	A
Develop and implement strategies for health care following recognition of health trends and their impact on the cost and other resources of care.	I			E	A

Code
I (ILOM) Initial Level Of Mastery
E (ELOM) Expected Level Of Mastery
A (ALOM) Actual Level Of Mastery

E Exposure
P Participation
I Identification
D Dissemination

Figure 13.1 Professional nature of community health nursing. Key Characteristic 6 (ENB Higher Award, 1990)

ET as a tool to determine taxonomically levels of learning

Recent developments in the United Kingdom (UK) of post-registration continuing nurse education include the perceived need to provide a coherent and comprehensive structure for continuing education beyond initial registration. The need to rationalize the present system is acknowledged by the profession.

Evidence has been provided by major reviews of the organization and provision of continuing education. Both the UKCC in their Post Registration and Practice Project (1990), and the ENB in their Project Framework for Continuing Education (ENB, 1990) express concern for the present system of continuing education that has evolved from years of expensive repetitious learning.

Individuals have been denied the opportunity to progress academically due to the lateral development of post-registration courses in nursing. The UKCC (1990) states:

> At present, practitioners can accumulate more than one learning unit of precisely the same level: for instance, two first level registered qualifications followed by two national board approved courses. As a result current learning patterns within Nursing, Midwifery and Health Visiting need radically re-evaluating to encompass the idea of movement, upwards and onwards. (p. 52)

The notion of progression has been explicitly addressed by the UKCC (1994). The idea of taxonomically moving through higher levels of professional practice is exemplified by acquiring the necessary knowledge and skills consistent with the distinct areas of Professional practice, Specialist practice and Advanced practice.

Students learn things at different levels of sophistication. Nyatanga (1990a) suggests that ET can be applied at different levels of study and once that level is established horizontal progression (HP) is possible. Before looking at examples of teaching at different levels of learning it might be useful to define what is meant by 'levels of learning'. A typical pattern for a three-year degree course is:

Year 1 equates to level 1 (Certificate of Higher Education)
Year 2 equates to level 2 (Diploma in Higher Education)
Year 3 equates to level 3 (First Degree)

Subsequent postgraduate studies equate to level 4 or Master (M). In the nursing profession, there is a general lack of description and precision of knowledge, skills and attitudes that characterize each academic level (Fox and Nyatanga, 1991). ET would appear to be a useful model for taxonomically determining levels of learning.

All community health nurses are required to plan learning experiences not only for themselves but for their students in the practice placement. The team leader is also responsible for the skill mix in the team and to develop the individual members' potential for professional development. It is essential that the community health nurse has a sound understanding of the level of learning required for professional development reached by the team member or learner.

There is a growing movement for community health nurses to define the theoretical principles which underpin their practice and widespread commitment to the organization of community health nursing work that is tailored to the individual client, the family and the wider community needs. Through the powerful nature of role modelling and a knowledge of ET the community health nurse team leader can assist team members and learners in developing an understanding of how the development of nursing theory has been influenced. By providing a nursing climate that is conducive and committed to patient-centred care the community health nurse in the role of teacher and leader will promote the individual's advancement through higher levels of professional practice. Examples of learning outcomes at level 1, level 2 and level 3 are illustrated in Figs 13.2, 13.3 and 13.4. The

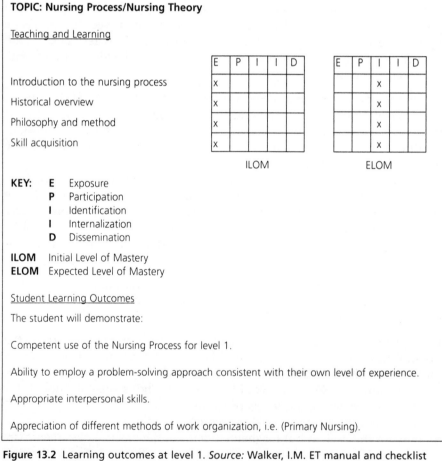

Figure 13.2 Learning outcomes at level 1. *Source:* Walker, I.M. ET manual and checklist (Walker, 1993b)

TOPIC: Nursing Process/Nursing Theory

<u>Teaching and Learning</u>

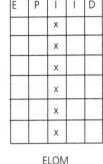

	E	P	I	I	D		E	P	I	I	D
Re-exposure to the nursing process	x							x			
Influence of North America, WHO, GNC	x							x			
Epistemology of nursing knowledge	x							x			
Nursing theory/models	x							x			
Analysis and evaluation of nursing theories	x							x			
Testing the utility of models	x							x			
			ILOM						ELOM		

<u>Student Learning Outcomes</u>

The student will:

Use an informed approach regarding appropriate Nursing Theory/Conceptual Models.

Be aware of a variety of tools of intervention.

Identify with the development of nursing knowledge.

Critically analyse and evaluate the claimed utility of nursing theory for practice.

Demonstrate what has influenced their own personal perspectives and approaches to nursing intervention.

Act as an adequate role model.

Figure 13.3 Learning outcomes at level 2. *Source:* Walker, I.M. ET manual and checklist (Walker, 1993b)

example shown is related to the Nursing Process and Nursing Theory. The team member or learner in this instance will be newly exposed to level 1 and could progress horizontally (HP) from the initial level of mastery through to dissemination. The shift from level 1 to level 2 is a vertical progression (VP). The learner will be re-exposed to the Nursing Process and Nursing Theory at a higher level of sophistication; this is known as regressive progression (RP).

The Nursing Process and its problem-solving approach is fully internalized at level 1 and the use of the process disseminated into clinical practice. Re-exposure at level 2 facilitates the study of several nursing theories that will inform the process of nursing intervention (Nursing Process). Level 3 study is intended to extend the team member or learner's knowledge in relation to nursing theory acquired during previous study or experience. This extension will progress from a level of appreciation of the construction of nursing theory (and use of theoretical models) towards a

TOPIC: Nursing Theory

Teaching and Learning

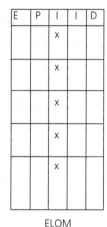

	E	P	I	I	D		E	P	I	I	D
Analysis of theoretical dimensions of nursing knowledge	x								x		
Evaluating theory/perspectives underpinning nursing models	x								x		
Examine value systems and attitudes within current nursing practice	x								x		
Theory practice gap	x								x		
Reviewing empirical evidence to support or refute nursing models in practice.	x								x		

ILOM   ELOM

Learning Outcomes

The student will be able to:

Critically analyse the diverse value systems inherent within different theoretical perspectives and their implications for care.

Reflect upon their own professional experiences in terms of the knowledge used to support their care practices, using this as a basis for the art/science debate.

Appreciate the changing and evolving nature of nursing knowledge and the potential role of research within this.

Exploit the knowledge base developed in the study of nursing theory at level 3 to facilitate the compilation of a research proposal in readiness for the completion of the Honours dissertation.

Figure 13.4 Learning outcomes at level 3. *Source:* Walker, I.M. ET manual and checklist (Walker, 1993b)

fuller, critical understanding of the complementary and competing nature of underpinning value systems, which are derived from their philosophical origins.

Conclusions

This paper has given examples of how Steinaker and Bell's (1979) Experiential Taxonomy can be used to plan, implement and evaluate teaching and learning activities.

Table 13.2 Summary of learning principles, teaching strategies and assessment techniques

Taxonomic level	Learning principle	Teacher strategies	Assessment
Exposure	External motivation Focusing attention Anxiety level	Demonstration Directing Presentation of ideas Problem identification	Observation of student reaction
Participation	Initial guidance Meaningful exploration Chance for success	Recall Clarifying, supporting and supervising Promoting Practice placement Role model	Observation of student performance Discussion and questioning Signal of understanding
Identification	Personal interaction Knowledge of results Reinforcing	Meeting students needs Promoting additional experience Reinforcing Peer teaching providing feedback	Checklists Observation Assignments Self-evaluate
Internalization	Overlearning Intrinsic transfer Differentiated output	Increasing problem solving Expanding skills practice Promoting creativity	Interviewing Observing Assignments Comparing with role model
Dissemination	External transfer Reward Internal motivation	Seminars Corrective feedback Student initiated projects Negotiated learning	Observing Self-assess and evaluate Display of total competence

Source: After Steinaker and Bell (1979)

Steinaker and Bell's (1979) work has been summarized to give a brief description of the learner's experience with an orientated walk through the five ET categories. Table 13.2 supports this orientation with a summary of learning principles, teaching strategies and assessment techniques.

According to Steinaker and Bell (1979), any effective taxonomy of educational objectives pre-supposes and possesses an intrinsic and functional evaluation system. The ET tripartite grid assists the teacher and learner to assess and build upon important previous learning and experience. For each objective written, both partners can agree an expected level of mastery. Evaluation and assessment techniques used will be appropriate to the category of ET and the learning outcome. Carefully selected strategies will best help the teacher to know the actual level of mastery that the learner has achieved.

The more one uses ET the more utility it seems to offer. ET can be used superficially as well as in depth, allowing students to learn things at different levels of sophistication. Nyatanga's (1990a) theory of regressive progression is illustrated with the development of simple units of learning at three academic levels of learning. This approach to describing knowledge, skills and attitudes at each academic level will surely be useful to the nursing profession in the verification of distinct areas of Professional, Specialist and Advanced practice.

This paper only serves to give a few examples of ET in action. The reader is advised to consult Steinaker and Bell's original work for a more in-depth discussion of teaching and learning strategies. Another useful source is Kenworthy and Nicklin's (1988) *Teaching and assessing in nursing practice: an experiential approach.*

The reader may consider using the Experiential Taxonomy as a framework for teaching and assessing. Whether one uses the model for health education, teaching and assessing learners or self-evaluation it is important to remember that teaching is a core component of the community health nurse's role and one which requires a knowledge base of how people learn and the optimum strategies that can be employed to ensure success.

Points to consider

1 What framework do you currently use to inform your role as teacher and assessor?

2 Before you read this paper what do you think your initial level of mastery was in relation to ET?

3 Could you use the ET tripartite grid as a tool for self-evaluation?

4 What do you think your level of mastery is now in relation to ET?

References

Bloom, B.S. 1956: *Taxonomy of educational objectives.* Handbook 1. The cognitive domain. New York: David McKay Inc.

Brooke, P., Nyatanga, L. and Walker, I. M. 1989: Facilitating the self care concept. Using the Experiential Taxonomy: Part 2. *Senior Nurse,* **9,** 1, 8–9.

Burnard, P. 1987: Towards an epistemological basis for experiential learning in nurse education. *Journal of Advanced Nursing,* **12,** 189–93.

English National Board for Nursing, Midwifery and Health Visiting 1990: *A new structure for professional development: the framework for continuing professional education and the ENB higher award for nurses, midwives and health visitors.* London: English National Board for Nursing, Midwifery and Health Visiting.

Fox, J. and Nyatanga, L. 1991: Organisational factors in APEL. *Senior Nurse,* **11,** No. 2.

Harrow, A. J. 1972: *Taxonomy of psychomotor domain*. New York: David McKay Inc.

Kenworthy, N. and Nicklin, P. 1988: *Teaching and assessing in nursing practice. An experiential approach*. London: Scutari Press.

Krathwohl, D. R., Bloom, B. S. and Masia, B. B. (eds) 1968: *A handbook of educational objectives: the affective domain*. New York: David McKay Inc.

Nyatanga, L 1990a: *An investigation through inter-rater reliability of the hypothesis that students' own personal learning transcripts match descriptors of the categories of the Experiential Taxonomy (ET)*. Unpublished MSc Thesis, Wolverhampton Polytechnic.

Nyatanga, L. 1990b: The ET penumbra. *Senior Nurse*, **10**, 7, 12–14.

Steinaker, N. and Bell, R. 1979: *The Experiential Taxonomy. A new approach to teaching and learning*. London: Academic Press.

United Kingdom Central Council for Nursing, Midwifery and Health Visiting. 1990: *The report of the post registration education and practice project*. London: United Kingdom Central Council for Nursing, Midwifery and Health Visiting.

United Kingdom Central Council for Nursing, Midwifery and Health Visiting. 1994: *The future of professional practice*. The Council's Standard for Education and Practice following Registration. London: United Kingdom Central Council for Nursing, Midwifery and Health Visiting.

Walker, I. M. 1993a: *Development and formative evaluation of a criterion referenced rating scale*. University of Wales, Cardiff.

Walker, I. M. 1993b: *Experiential Taxonomy manual and checklist*. University of Central England in Birmingham.

14 The reality of clinical supervision

Maggie Dickerson

This chapter explores the challenges that clinical supervision make to community nursing. It reflects on the emergence of a variety of interpretations of clinical supervision.

The chapter takes the reader through issues linked with clinical supervision in community nursing from the NHS Management Executive (1993) concept of clinical supervision as a 'formal professional support structure for competence and accountability and the development of practice and enhanced consumer protection' (p. 41), to an evaluation of ideas from prior experience in supported community nursing practice. The reader is offered a reflective view of how ideas of supervision from past practice help to underpin current developments.

The concluding sections of the chapter attempt to provide a realistic framework for clinical supervision in community nursing by identifying the need for a comprehensive approach that is built upon the practitioner's individual need. The focus of the final section suggests ways forward for the underpinning structure of clinical supervision.

The chapter attempts to identify where clinical supervision came from, why it was introduced and the effect it will have on practitioners working in the community. The chapter also examines the ideas and policies surrounding evolving patterns of clinical supervision and the implementation of clinical supervision in NHS trusts in the UK since 1990.

The Oxford Dictionary (1984) defines the word supervision 'to direct, oversee or inspect the performance or operation of an activity or process'. The definition of clinical is interesting: dispassionate, coldly, detached, related to the patient in bed. This definition supports a notion of clinical supervision in terms of performance and activity.

Definitions and developments

In the spring of 1994, the *Nursing Standard* carried an article highlighting a debate between the nursing professionals and Health Service/trust managers about the introduction of clinical supervision for nurses (Scott, 1994). This debate indicated a tension between the financial cost of clinical supervision and the professional driving force behind the implementation of clinical supervision for registered nurses. Who would clinical supervision be controlled by, management-led budget holders or developed educationally by the professionals working in the wards, units and the community?

Exactly a year later in March 1995 the *Nursing Times* carried two articles (David, 1995; Reid, 1994) examining the support available for nurses who move from the acute sector to community nursing services; clinical supervision did not feature prominently in the articles. The profession and community nurses appear confused about the issues surrounding clinical supervision and it is not surprising given the variety of experiences gained in clinical supervision between and across the profession. Bower (1994) highlights this confusion by offering definitions of supervision from the simple, an exchange between practising professionals to enable the development of professional skills, to the more complex, a meeting between two or more people who have a declared interest in examining a piece of work.

Supervision of performance and process has existed as part of managerial and strategic coordination in industry and organizations for some considerable time. There have been supervisors on the factory floor and within department stores, since Taylor published his work on scientific management in 1967 in which the supervisor had an important role to play bridging the gap between management and the workforce. More recently, supervision has been expanded to include monitoring and profiling staff performance and development needs. This has occurred in many organizations including local government where the development of the role of the supervisor would now be regarded as a middle management initiative which emerged during the 1990s. It could be linked with independent pay reviews and performance related pay awards.

The Department of Health report *Vision for the Future* (1993) formalized the thrust by the NHS Management Executive to introduce clinical supervision to the workplace stating in Target 10 that the concept of clinical supervision should be further explored and developed. Discussions should be held at local and national level on the range and appropriateness of models of clinical supervision and reports made available to the professions within the year.

The document describes clinical supervision as a formal process of professional support and learning which enables individual practitioners to develop knowledge and competence, assume responsibility for their own practice and enhance consumer protection and the safety of care in complex clinical situations. It is possible to argue that for some community nurses, district nurses and health visitors, this definition aptly suits the function of the period of supervised practice that has traditionally been located at the end of programmes of education for practitioners qualifying in community nursing. This is where some confusion about the term clinical supervision emerges; the historical development of supervision in the different specialisms in community nursing may influence perceptions of what the reality of clinical supervision is. For example, community psychiatric nurses may have a different concept of clinical supervision; their experience has generally been located to a supportive, counselling role that focuses on the development of clinical practice. Community psychiatric nurses may focus on counselling in supervision, while health visitors might locate the development of their experience of supervision in an educational frame.

However, a general acceptance of clinical supervision is presumed in a *Nursing Times* editorial (1994) 'Clinical supervision is here to stay. Do not miss the opportunity to say how it should be developed'. Olgier and Cameron-Buccheri (1990) indicated the positive benefits in terms of job satisfaction when linked with a period of supervision. They stress that the importance of an appropriate supervisory style cannot be overemphasized. This is particularly necessary if entrants are to be attracted into nursing and experienced nurses supported through the many changes that are taking place. Olgier and Cameron-Buccheri (1990) also suggest that this will help nurses remain in nursing. They consider that this applies to both learner and qualified nurses. Supervision encourages the individual to develop into a thinking, caring person rather than a conforming drone and this is essential.

The supportive style of clinical supervision is emphasized by Kohner (1994), when discussing the implementation of supervision in a unit described as 'the Cinderella of the mental health services' (p. 13). It came from the need to innovate and to pay attention to the needs of staff. By addressing personal and professional development the organization was able to demonstrate an investment in staff and that staff were valued.

Post-registration community nurse education may have helped set the scene for a focus on supportive clinical supervision since a number of models of supervision were available across the community nurse specialisms. Mental health has traditionally provided support for practitioners in the form of clinical supervision (Bodley, 1992), while health visitors and district nurses have supported community practice in education with taught and supervised practice (ENB, 1991). The fact that a variety of options in terms of supervision existed through community nurse education and training suggests that community nurses may find concepts of clinical supervision confusing. It may be difficult to fit these established concepts of support with clinical supervision of practice in community nursing.

The history and development of supervised practice in community nursing has much to offer in helping practitioners and policy makers to develop a model of clinical supervision for the future. The time spent in supervised practice offered the community nurse the opportunity to reflect on ideas and concepts related to nursing practice and the development of nursing strategies, specifically linked with the allocation of resources in community nursing. This notion of reflection seems apt to any formulation of a model of clinical supervision. Reflection should include a consideration of issues that are associated with the provision of an effective, efficient and economically sound clinical practice. The United Kingdom Central Council for Nursing, Midwifery and Health Visiting (UKCC) has recently published a statement that argues that clinical supervision is not the exercise of managerial responsibility and managerial supervision nor is it a system of formal individual performance review intended to be hierarchical in nature (UKCC, 1995).

There is a possibility that through misinterpretation of the term, clinical supervision could be used in a simplistic way and, as such, it might be at risk of providing a back-up role for managers to identify under-performance in practice. An example of this might be if the UKCC (1995) guidelines on preceptorship were to be implemented for the wrong reasons. It is possible to argue that much of the statistical interest related to community nursing services focuses on the number of visits made, the length of time spent with the patients and a coded number of activities or diagnoses. In this way clinical supervision could be inappropriately developed as a management tool for measuring and comparing output, rather than as a supportive tool for promoting quality patient care.

Clinical supervision should be designed as an extension to community nursing practice providing new experiences for practitioners, helping them to meet competencies as well as to provide opportunities for self-assessment and peer assessment of practice. Butterworth and Faugier (1993) suggest there has been little recent publication in the nursing literature that did more than enshrine clinical supervision in sentiments appropriate for 'motherhood' and 'apple pie'. These sentiments imply that clinical supervision is something that nurses should favour. However, comfortable or uncomfortable this definition feels, it is time that community nurses formulated very clear ideas about the current concept of clinical supervision.

As previously suggested the variety of meanings given to the term supervision by professionals in community care may confuse the issues. The social work profession also has problems with the word supervision and has relinquished the term, replacing it with the title assessor of practice (CCETSW, 1992). This change represents an interesting twist to events. In community nursing the reverse has occurred and the term supervision has replaced assessment of practice. It could be argued that neither term is suitable and that the language and terminology employed to indicate the nature and purpose of clinical supervision are crucial to the way in which it develops.

Ideas related to supervision of practice published in an HMSO Report (Mental Health Review Team, 1994) on collaborative approaches to care by the Mental Health Review Team suggest that clinical supervision takes a variety of guises and that these depend on the philosophy and style of the intervention being offered. This report states that all clinical supervision can be underpinned by a number of fundamental principles:

- Skills should be constantly redefined and sophisticated throughout life.
- Critical discussion about clinical practice is a means to professional development.
- Introduction to the process of clinical supervision should begin in professional training and continue thereafter as an integral aspect of professional development.

- Clinical supervision requires time, energy and commitment: it is not an accidental activity and must be planned and effectively resourced.

Models and frameworks

Bodley (1992) also indicates a process of clinical supervision for psychiatric nursing, that moves from purpose of the interview through observation, assessment, content, impressions and finally evaluation. This process would allow the clinical supervisor to design and develop individualized programme of clinical supervision to meet the specific needs of students and practitioners in the community. It may be possible to develop a flexible model of clinical supervision for all practitioners in community nursing.

Evans (1990) suggests that 'live' supervision has four main phases: pre-interview, interview, time-out, and post-interview. The purpose of such a structure according to Evans is to maximize the student's learning through active participation in the preparation, input and feedback of the experience in some settings such as residential and day care. This approach can make supervision more spontaneous and less formal, with discussions before and after contact with the clients.

This perspective of supervision in social work is different from experiences of clinical supervision in mental health nursing. However, the variety of experiences documented suggest that flexibility of approach should remain firmly in mind since nursing in the community can be an isolating experience. Practitioners work alone in the patient/client's home and as the nature of community nursing is infinitely variable, a fixed framework may not be suitable for all practitioners.

Community nurses do not have the ward environment or the ward team support at their finger-tips and therefore clinical supervision may provide the support and development that is much needed in community nursing. It is important to acknowledge that the organization, management and delivery of community nursing services continues to change. Subsequently, education, including the practice element, also continues to change and it is possible to argue that the role of the community practice teacher/supervisor of practice will be different from the traditional model utilized in community nurse education in the past. The future role may be more akin to a system of mentorship, utilizing student-focused learning experience documented through reflective writing.

At the same time, it is important to acknowledge that this type of support and development is essential for nurses who are newly qualified and for nurses who are changing their area of work. In 1991 the English National Board for Nursing, Midwifery and Health Visiting (ENB) commissioned Fish and Purr to research teaching, support and supervision on Branch Programmes of Project 2000 courses. The main thrust of the findings suggest that support for practice-based learning was inadequate and that preparation for those nurses involved with assessment of practice was inappropriate. The report argues that a nationally recognized course should be developed to replace the ENB 997/998, in order to prepare qualified practitioners for their role in support for Project 2000 students in the practice setting.

The findings in the ENB publication suggest that support for Project 2000 students should include the practical techniques of debriefing and reflection during assessment of practice. Since the problems indicated above appear to have existed in pre-registration education for some considerable time, it may be possible to argue that a suitable model for this support exists, somewhere between the notion of clinical supervision and the model of support provided for post-registration students of community nursing.

In this way, any period of clinical supervision might be regarded as an important element of pre- and post-registration support in community nursing since it reflects the requirements indicated above by the ENB. Careful management of the process of clinical supervision would be essential to avoid the problems identified by the ENB, relating to the confused and haphazard levels of support for students during education and training. The guidelines for clinical supervision might revolve around issues related to individualized needs, identification of strengths and limitations plus support for the reflection on and development of community nursing practice.

At the same time, the UKCC (1995) states that clinical supervision will play an increasingly important part in ensuring safe and effective standards of clinical care. They suggest that clinical supervision will link practitioner responsibilities as an accountable professional to everyday clinical work. It is possible to draw from the ENB (1991) and UKCC (1995) publications a conceptual model for clinical supervision in community nursing, which may be more appropriate for the 1990s within the changing nature of community health and social care. This model might include the following:

- an aspect of self-assessment related to previous experience in practice and identified needs;
- a clinical supervisor's diagnostic assessment of need;
- guidelines relating to accountability and responsibilities specific to community nursing practice.

Subsequently, it would be important for the practitioner to complete a reflective account of clinical supervision, as a means of evidencing experience relevant to the support given in practice. Johns (1994) indicates that one way of reflecting and sharing experiences during clinical supervision is in groups. Furthermore, clinical supervision is advocated as a means to ensure practitioner development of effective practice. Thus the reflective record of nursing activities might include aspects of the following:

- an observation of community nursing practice;
- a period of supported community practice;
- independent practice evidencing confident accountability.

Each of the elements of clinical supervision indicated above might take account of three very important elements of community nursing practice: the appropriate knowledge, skills and attitudes to support confident accountability.

Clinical supervision in community nursing

Community nurses experienced a continuous process of change during the late 1980s and early 1990s until the present time. These changes included dramatic changes in government policy, health service management styles and changes in the definitions of skills required to provide nursing services for the local community. Many of these changes will be specific to each community trust rather than developed within a 'national' framework. Subsequently, the reality of clinical supervision for community nurses will vary from trust to trust. This means that unless community nurses take the initiative themselves and, more importantly, share their experiences with other community nurses, the 'reality' of clinical supervision in community nursing will be fragmented and outside of their influence.

Work experiences in community nursing will also affect the 'reality' of clinical supervision. Several of the attempts to set up structures and processes for clinical supervision in community nursing are still in their infancy. However, the work experiences mentioned above might include the amount of time a nurse spends working alone, the differences between a corporate caseload (shared by the team) or an individual nurse's caseload (individual nurse responsibility) and the size of the caseload and geographical area covered. All of these factors will influence the reality of clinical supervision for individual nurses and should be taken into consideration within the day-to-day reality of the work experience. At the same time the general practitioner, who controls a budget and opts for employment or contractual arrangements for community nurses, will influence developments in practice. The NHS Management Executive Report, *New World, New Opportunities* (1993), supports this view by recognizing that many GPs, as small employers, may not have the range of skills and resources required to give staff proper training. The report endorses the move of many FHSAs to take steps to ensure the provision of training and support for primary health care nurses employed in general practice.

Clinical supervision will take time and effort on the part of community nurses and it may be the case that contracts of employment will influence opportunities for clinical supervision. Wiles (1994) comments that the attitude of GPs appeared to account for community nurses not feeling part of the primary health care team. The nurses interviewed for this study of teamwork in primary health care, inferred that leadership was defined in terms of power and status, with over half of the sample placing team leadership with the GPs. These attitudes will clearly influence experiences in clinical supervision since patterns of employment in some community trusts appear to be transferring hiring and firing of community nurses to GPs. The expectations that general practitioners have of community nurses and their role within the primary health care team may influence developments in clinical supervision.

Allocation of resources to support the implementation and development of clinical supervision will be related to caseload management and skill/grade-mix within the community nursing teams and employment patterns within community health services. One bonus of clinical supervision within the community nursing services is that it may provide the opportunity to examine patterns of sick leave and stress-related absence. Clinical supervision may also offer the opportunity to address some of the problems encountered in the delivery of community nursing services.

Community nursing services may also be affected by other issues, some social services departments have experienced major problems related to contracting and costs in providing services for groups of patients (Flynn *et al.*, 1995). This is particularly the case for the long-term sick or disabled and those who require complicated and expensive packages of care. Subsequently, assessment and delivery of community nursing care may be compromised by events in other departments/units providing community care and, in turn, any model of clinical supervision introduced to the community setting will be influenced by these factors.

However, it may be the case that community nurses will grasp the opportunity to utilize clinical supervision in a positive way. Hennessy (1994) makes an interesting point in a study related to education. The collapse of the nursing hierarchy in community nursing has introduced supervision at field level when, in the past, this responsibility traditionally rested with the nursing officer or manager. Clinical supervision may be the only way forward in community nursing, given the changing nature and structure of the community nursing services.

Clinical supervision in community nursing may have a number of important roles to fulfil in the future, helping nurses maintain their registration and providing support for practitioners on a contractual basis. This may be outside community health trust responsibility in both formal and informal settings. The word formal is used here to represent the way in which a clinical supervisor could provide support for practitioners working through preceptorship, maintaining their registration and working to quality specifications. The word informal represents the range of possibilities within the clinical supervision framework to reflect on practice and work towards self-assessed goals, within a team setting, peer support or practitioner-centred experience.

It is important to develop a flexible approach to clinical supervision in community nursing. This should take into account the independent and autonomous nature of community nursing practice. The attitudes and values of those involved, whether patients, clients, families, friends, community health care nurses, trust managers or GPs need to be considered. Clinical supervision should be implemented in a flexible and comprehensive way, focused through issues related to working towards quality specifications linked with patient/client care and job satisfaction for those involved with delivering community nursing services.

A further strategy that demonstrates flexibility is long-arm clinical supervision. This may be implemented between nursing teams or community units providing opportunities to build networks of professional support. These may include:

- Self-assessed or peer-assessed needs.
- Shadowing or observation.
- Independent or supported practice.
- Review and reflection in practice.
- Record of experience within clinical supervision.
- Accountability in practice.
- Care and programme management analysis.
- Clinical practice leadership.
- Research and development in practice.

However, it is possible to argue that any development of support systems for nurses who work in the community should include the existing options of:

- Supervision of research projects undertaken as part of research and development in community nursing;
- Taught and supported practice during the assessed 50 per cent practice element of educational programmes for community health care nurses;
- Clinical supervision through preceptorship, accountability and peer support in practice.

The careful implementation of the three aspects of supervision in community nursing listed above should provide a comprehensive and flexible framework of support for practitioners in community nursing services during the challenging aspects of community health care nursing in the future. At the same time it is important to note that community nursing services continue to change and subsequently concepts of clinical supervision change.

Points to consider

Could clinical supervision be utilized as an anchor for community nursing practice during periods of change as a means to promote and develop quality patient care and confident accountability through:

- Identification of individual needs in observed and supported practice?
- The recording and review of a period of community nursing practice?
- Clinical practice leadership?
- Peer support in community nursing practice?

References

Bodley, D. 1992: Clinical supervision in psychiatric nursing: using the process record. *Nurse Education Today*, **12**, 148–55.

Bower, H. 1994: Watching me, watching you. *Practice Nurse*, 1–31, July, 67.

Butterworth, T. and Faugier, J. 1993: *Clinical supervision: a position paper*. School of Nursing Studies, University of Manchester.

Central Council for the Education and Training of Social Workers 1992: *Education regulations*. London: CCETSW, p. 24.

David, A. 1995: The shift to community. *Nursing Times*, March, **91**, 12, 39.

Department of Health 1993: *A vision for the future*. London: HMSO.

English National Board for Nursing, Midwifery and Health Visiting 1991: *Education guidelines*. London: ENB.

Evans, D. 1990: *Assessing student's competence to practice*. London: CCETSW, pp. 42.

Flynn, R., Pickard, S. and Williams, G. 1995: Contracts and the quasi-market in community health services. *Journal of Social Policy*, **24**, 4, 529–50.

Hennessy, D. 1994: *Changes in primary health care clinical education*. Oxford Health Care Management Institute, pp. 23.

Johns, C. 1994: The growth of management connoisseurship through reflective practice. *Journal of Nursing Management*, **2**, 253–60.

Kohner, N. 1994: *Clinical supervision in practice*. London: King's Fund Development Unit, pp. 13.

Mental Health Review Team 1994: *Working in partnership*. London: HMSO, pp 20.

NHS Management Executive 1993: *New world, new opportunities*. London: HMSO, pp. 41.

Olgier, M. and Cameron-Buccheri, R. 1990: Supervision: a cross cultural approach. *Nursing Standard*, 25/4, number 31.

Reid, P. 1994: Editorial. In *Nursing Times* September 28, **90**, 39.

Taylor, F.W. 1967: *The principles of scientific management*. New York: Harper and Row.

Scott, G. 1994: Clinical supervision: the big issue. *Nursing Standard*, **8**, 33, 7.

UKCC 1995: *Clinical supervision for nursing and health visiting*. Registrar's Letter 24th January.

Wiles, R. 1994: Teamwork in primary care: the views and experiences of nurse, midwives and health visitors. *Journal of Advanced Nursing*, **20**, 326.

PART THREE

Developments in community nursing

The papers in Part three consider some of the future trends that are likely to influence community nursing. They raise topics that are emerging at this time and require the influence of community practitioners to mould them into acceptable, workable practices. The issues contained in this section will probably change the face of community nursing and they should be well debated by community practitioners who need to balance the need for change against the needs of the nursing profession and the purpose of nursing which still retains the requirement to care for patients.

Developments in community nursing

15 Specialist and advanced roles

Sarah Luft

The purpose of this chapter is to examine nursing development and to consider how this relates to community nursing in contemporary society. The reader is asked to bear in mind the various influences that have shaped nursing to date – these have been addressed elsewhere in this book so it is inappropriate to include them here. Arguments centre around the importance of recognizing a supportive framework for developments; this incorporates managers' involvement which becomes complex when the concept of advanced nursing is placed in the context of business. Nurses are urged to develop both personal and professional competencies in order to enhance their practice and to keep sight of their value systems in a society where technological change is constant.

The framework

Developments in nursing are most likely to emerge within a supportive framework, and that framework consists of the organizational culture and the people involved in it. Health care management structures play a crucial part in determining the culture which will in turn influence professional development. As well, the United Kingdom Central Council (UKCC, 1994) propose a model of nursing practice which refers to the newly registered nurse in primary practice, where there is a preceptorship programme for a period of time; many nurses may choose to remain in primary practice throughout their career. The UKCC sees advancement through specialist nursing practice which will incorporate both primary and secondary care settings, and where nurses will have completed further study at degree level. This qualification is recognized by the professional body for nurses working in various community disciplines, and these specialist practitioners will be able to demonstrate higher levels of clinical decision making, be able to monitor and improve standards of care, contribute to research and teaching, and support professional colleagues (UKCC, 1994). Specialist nursing practice can then be viewed as advancement. However, the Council also refer to advanced nursing practice, but at present do not clarify how this role is actually different from specialist nursing practice except to say that it will be more concerned with advancing the profession of nursing as a whole. The suggestion is that in order to push forward the boundaries of practice these nurses may have studied at Master's level, an area currently being reviewed by the UKCC. It is interesting to note that this is a suggestion rather than a statement. It could be that there is evidence which demonstrates that nurses with a Master's level qualification do not automatically work as advanced nurses. It could also be that nurses with lesser qualifications are working as advanced nurses. There is an urgent need for the profession to be more definite about identifying the difference between the three areas of practice. Managers will want to know what they are purchasing and what extra benefit or health gain will come about if advanced nurses are employed instead of specialist nurses.

Lurie (1981) recognized the importance of professional socialization and she refers to two schools of thought. The first is the Mertonian School which stresses the value of education and training and certainly the changes that have occurred in nurse education reflect this area. The other school of thought is Becker-Freidson which Lurie quotes as saying that situational factors in the work setting are crucial and that the environment in which the nurse works plays a key role in advancing professional status; this is likely to occur through interaction processes and personal compatibility. Where health reforms are providing increased flexibility, more opportunities are opening up to nurses who will have to adapt to changing circumstances. Lurie suggests that professional socialization for nurses is about acquiring skills and values and adjusting them to the demands of the work setting and this ability reflects personal competencies.

Managing care

The role of managers in health care organizations is to respond to client need in the most effective and efficient way possible. However, many service managers do not have a nursing background and clients themselves are requesting a service provision which may not require specialist expertise as such, rather a person who is able to carry out a particular skill. Managers then can employ cheaper personnel than professional nurses to carry out many routine tasks, so why should they employ more expensive specialist/advanced nurses? Calkin (1984) insists that hiring professional staff is not simply identifying tasks and employing someone to do them. Professionals bring to an organization the results of a process of formal education and socialization. They assess and intervene more from their pre-employment preparation than do practical or technical nurses. For Calkin (1984), the first step for managers when deciding whether or not to employ advanced nurses is in fact to differentiate the nature of advanced from basic nursing practice. Benner (1984) has contributed much to nursing knowledge in her examination of novice nurses compared with expert nurses and Calkin (1984) develops this theme arguing that there are three levels of practice. She identifies these as the nurses' ability to respond to the health need of the person or population. In the first instance the beginning practitioner has a knowledge and skill level which can only equip her/him to deal with a narrow range of average responses of individual patients or groups. This equates with rule governed behaviour and practice is likely to be task orientated. The second level of practitioner she refers to as experienced. This person has a capacity to sense the nature of a problematic response that goes beyond the conscious analytic diagnosis of the novice. However, Calkin (1984) argues that this experienced nurse is not able to articulate the cognitive processes that guide their actions. This experienced nurse could, however, provide sufficient expertise to be appropriate to employ in certain environments. One community setting, for instance, may be a relatively static environment which does not throw up too many different problems. Another community setting may incorporate a population which demands specialist Hospital at Home skills and potential problems here could demand a greater expertise.

If managers do not require nurses to teach or to defend the basis for diagnostic statements or provide a rationale for action then the experienced nurse provides the right fit. The implication is that some managers will not want to employ advanced nurses. For Calkin (1984) advanced nurses are those who do have increased knowledge and skills which enable them to be better equipped to meet the demand of health need. Calkin (1984) refers to advanced practice as the deliberative diagnosis and treatment of a full range of human responses to actual or potential health problems. Figure 15.1 develops Calkin's thinking by illustrating how this framework could work in the community setting.

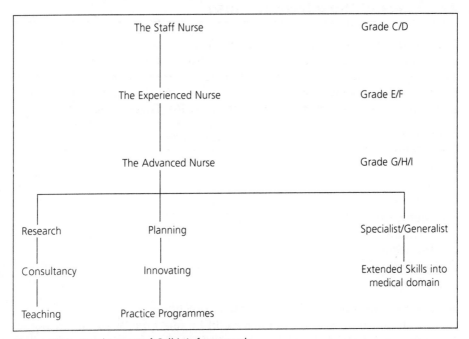

Figure 15.1 Development of Calkin's framework

The idea of the strands attached to the advanced nurse is to enable the manager to decide which area requires specific expertise so that the role can take the appropriate shape to fulfil the organizational needs. Advanced skills in communication are common to all three strands: the advanced nurse could be employed to take on a clinical teaching and research role, or if new patterns of care were emerging there may be a need for a person to be involved in the planning processes. The specialist/generalist strand is likely to be required if there is a shortage of medical cover – nurse practitioners can fill this gap by extending their skills. The type of structure could meet both professional and market needs; the model proposed by UKCC (1994) could equate with Calkin's thinking in that the staff nurses will be viewed as the newly registered nurses in primary practice, but as they gain more experience they will be used more widely. Undertaking further education will enable them to become specialist practitioners who Calkin (1984) would refer to as advanced nurses. The difference in the UKCC model lies in the fact that there is no clarification of a role for the advanced nurse although it is thought that this person will influence the profession of nursing and act as a role model for other nurses. However attractive and sensible these professional models may be, nurses cannot get away from the fact that to a greater or lesser extent the profession is market driven, and demand and supply are at the heart of this debate. Identifying whether or not there is a need will guide the managers' decision making, as employing expensive professional nurses on high grades must be justified.

Attributes of the advanced nurse

The advanced nurse will require not just experience, knowledge, skills and education, but will bring to the role personal attributes. Patterson and Haddad (1992) suggest that personal attributes are important for advanced nurses, and interviews carried out with nurses working formally as nurse practitioners supports this statement (Luft, 1996). These nurses cited:

autonomy
flexibility
openness
imagination
confidence
competence
innovation
self-esteem
assertiveness
enthusiasm

as necessary personal attributes for nurse practitioners.

The role of the nurse practitioner could be one type of advanced nurse. This list correlates closely to the concept of intelligence broadly defined by

Sternberg (1984) who calls it purposive or successful adaptation in a real-world context. Adaptation can be seen as a key component in today's management of health care where boundaries are changing and the consumer is deserving of high quality nursing.

Clarke (1994) notes that as the old command and control hierarchies are stripped away, and new sets of attitudes and behaviours emerge, so flatter structures will require greater expertise from its staff in the way of increased responsibility and accountability. Clarke records a research project carried out by the Ashridge Management College which suggests that, in future, managers will have to operate in organizational environments that are growth and customer orientated. The faster moving pace of change will demand much greater responsibility, initiative and leadership from managers at all levels of the organization. The concept of adaptation is endorsed by Naish (1995) who recognizes that in the fast changing nature of the market place, the NHS continually requires new skills and attitudes from its leaders, and that this development has exposed long neglected chinks in nursing's armour. Naish cites Steve Wright who at an RCN fringe meeting (1995) related how he had been observing people he has met and worked with; he is now co-authoring a book on leadership. Key descriptors include expertise, lateral thinking, empowering others, assertiveness, consistency, humour, sense of judgement and clarity of values. At the same meeting Naish (1995) also cites Fawcett-Henesey who declared that it is not about leading from the front any more, it is about having a value system, about being a visionary, it is about networking. For Lanara (1993) the future presents many challenges for nurses and the competencies and responsibilities for the twenty-first century are about nurses who believe in the higher values of life, who live with consistency and change and actualize this in practice. These are the nurses who will responsibly confront the ethical issues and dilemmas and be able to use the scientific and technological innovations for the benefit of society's health. Whether or not nurses are prepared to carry out specific nursing or medical procedures is not the main issue here. Fundamental to nursing advancement is the development of the professional who has the personal attributes that reflect qualities relating to leadership and vision.

The changing shape of nursing

This paper recognizes some of the influences that have shaped nursing and it is clear that to a great extent nursing has reacted to these environmental influences. However, contemporary nursing is about developing a pro-active as well as a reactive service and to achieve this aim various factors need to be in place:

- An organizational culture that values leadership and vision;
- Recognition from the professional body that advanced nurses exist;

• Personal characteristics of the nurses themselves.

To address the first point, organization cultures have been and still are in the process of change. For instance, Barker (1994) refers to the conventional paradigm, where organizations were built on a belief that the world and events could be controlled. This led to hierarchical structures, an emphasis on logical decision making and rationality. This paradigm is being replaced by a new one which characterizes the following:

mutuality and affiliation
acknowledging complexity and ambiguity
cooperation vs. competition
an emphasis on human relations
process vs. task
acceptance of feeling
networking vs. hierarchy
recognition of the value of intuition.

For Barker (1994) the last decade has seen a slow shift from centralization to decentralization, from directive decision making to participatory management, from power to empowerment and from managerial governance to self-governance. The changing nature of such a shift creates a certain amount of conflict and uncertainty and other authors such as Porter O'Grady (1994) recognize that many of the values and expectations of individuals are upset during times of significant change. This serves to underline the importance that nurses can be relied upon to hold on to their integrity and values in spite of the changing environment.

The model proposed by UKCC (1994) goes some way towards providing a structure which nurses can recognize so that they can build on their knowledge and experience. It does not, however, suggest that there should be a separate register for advanced nurses which perhaps will be addressed at a later date. The personal characteristics of nurses can be seen as constant; the character of the nurse has been acknowledged over the years and in this age of shifting values and new technology those characteristics need underlining or the sheer complexity of events could take over. Leadership attributes that link to personal values can in turn be linked to the organization. As well, visions of health and healing must predominate. For Chin (1994) it is time to turn our attention to creating visions for the foundations of future nursing practice. She insists that determining specific roles and types of nursing practice have not served us well in the past.

Chin (1994) envisages for the future interactions that nourish the human spirit and enhance peace and comfort. These are values that were in fact embodied by Florence Nightingale; the evidence is, however, more likely to indicate that the new managers will look to employing nurses who can carry out key tasks, and woolly descriptions of advanced nursing practice that fail to promote definite skills may not be helpful.

To develop a highly valued service in the community, nurses need to examine the values held by the people they serve and the organizations in which they work, as well as their own values. Nyberg (1994) cites Glenman (1985) who notes that nurses have strong professional values, but they have bureaucratic responsibilities also. They are caught in a conflict. Do they work for an organization that argues for higher productivity (consider league tables and performance indicators) or is working for the patient the prime consideration? Nyberg (1994) points out that optimal patient care and optimal efficiency do not always go hand in hand. However, she suggests that such conflict could be addressed by nurses involved in direct care, holding conferences with other disciplines clearly to identify system problems and develop alternatives that place the needs of the patient first but still meet the organization's constraints of efficiency. Such an approach demands characteristics of a nurse who is able to tread the fine balance between adjusting to a business environment while keeping patients' needs at the top of the agenda. Together with technological advances and the business market, nurses face many challenges that will exercise their skills to the full. Lessons to be learned for the nurse working in the community could be summarized as:

- The need to articulate their worth: nurses will not necessarily be employed automatically; there are others who can carry out nursing tasks.
- Understanding market forces – and making them work for patients.
- Keeping up to date with the ever increasing technological advances.
- Responding positively to increasing accountability.
- Using information wisely for the benefit both of patients and the professional.
- Welcoming the opportunity to participate in collaborative working with other health professionals.
- Working pro-actively according to the changing structure of society and their values.

The health care reforms are bringing about changes in the patterns of health care delivery with an emphasis on value for money, effective and efficient care. Innovative ways of providing that care are considered with the consumer view forming a part of the process (*Patient's Charter*, DOH, 1991). But advanced nursing practice is more than just about acquiring more skills and knowledge, even if it does move into the medical domain where skills may be considered as prestigious. It is about pride in a value system that can see further than a series of tasks. It is about developing a caring professional who is prepared to serve a population in a way that generates greater communication and cooperation. Future graduates of nursing are well placed to achieve a strengthened identity for nursing if they take on board personal as well as professional growth and respond positively to the challenges associated with current health care demands.

Conclusion

This paper raises many issues, any one of which could be explored in greater depth. It is not possible to discuss developments in nursing without addressing external factors. The sociopolitical and economic climate of the times is inevitably reflected throughout society of which nursing forms a part. The introduction of a stronger academic base for nursing can be seen as a positive step forward in that this will contribute toward personal and professional development. The registered nurse in primary practice continues to acquire sufficient skills and knowledge to carry out safe nursing. The specialist role takes this development further as it looks to adding depth and breadth to the role particularly in areas relating to research, supervision and teaching. But influencing and developing the profession will come about by practitioners who not only have skills, knowledge and experience but who have taken opportunities to achieve personal growth in order to enable professional enhancement.

Points to consider

- What do you see as the helping factors for developments in nursing?
- What do you see as the hindering factors for developments in nursing?
- Do you feel comfortable with a model of advanced practice? What do you see as the necessary requisites for this?
- As a team leader with responsibility for a budget, on what basis would you decide to employ an advanced nurse at grade G or H?
- Do you think that in your role you are working as an advanced practitioner? How do you justify this?

References

Benner, P. 1984: *From novice to expert: excellence and power in clinical practice*. California, Menlo Park: Addison-Wesley.

Barker, A. 1994: An emerging leadership paradigm: transformational leadership. In Hein, E.C. and Nicholson, M.J. (eds), *Contemporary leadership behaviour* (4th edn). Philadelphia: J.B. Lippincott Co.

Calkin, J.D. 1984: A model for advanced nursing practice. *Journal of Nursing Administration*, **14**, 24–30.

Chin, P.L. 1994: Looking into the crystal ball. Positioning ourselves for the year 2000. In Hein, E.C. and Nicholson, M.J. (eds), *Contemporary leadership behaviour* (4th edn). Philadelphia: J.B. Lippincott Co.

Clarke, L. 1994: *The essence of change*. New York, London: Prentice-Hall.

Department of Health 1991: *The Patient's Charter*. London: HMSO.

Lanara, V.A. 1993: The nurse of the future: role and function. *Journal of Nursing Management*, **1**, 83–7.

Luft, S. 1996: *The developing role of the nurse practitioner alongside the health care reforms.* University of Wolverhampton, Unpublished Thesis.

Lurie 1981: Nurse practitioners: issues in professional socialisation. *Journal of Health and Social Behaviour,* **22** (March, pp. 31–48).

Naish, J. 1995: Who are the new leaders? *Nursing Management,* **2,** 3, June.

Nyberg J. 1994: The nurse as professnocrat. In Hein, E.C. and Nicholson, M.J. (eds), *Contemporary leadership behaviour* (4th edn). Philadelphia: J.B. Lippincott Co.

Patterson, C. and Haddad, B. 1992: The advanced nurse practitioner, common attributes. *Canadian Journal of Nursing Administration,* Nov./Dec., **5,** 4, 18–22.

Porter O'Grady, T. 1994: Of rabbits and turtles – a time of change for unions. In Hein, E.C. and Nicholson, M.J. (eds), *Contemporary leadership behaviour* (4th edn). Philadelphia: J.B. Lippincott Co.

Sternberg, R.J. 1984: Toward a triarchic theory of human intelligence. *Behavioural and Brain Sciences,* **7,** 2, 269–315.

UKCC 1994: The future of professional practice – the Council's standards for education and practice following registration. Position statement on policy and implementation March. London: UKCC.

16 Assessing health needs in the community

Sue Chilton and Eileen Barnes

The aim of the chapter is to provide the reader with an overview of the process that involves identifying and assessing the needs of local populations, with the aim of developing services sensitive and appropriate to specific needs. A central focus is the involvement of consumers in the process of planning and evaluating health care provision. A range of sources of data and methods, both qualitative and quantitative, which contribute to this assessment process will be considered, highlighting both their potential and drawbacks. The role and contribution of community nurses within this process is a prime concern.

Introduction

The focus on profiling of need arises primarily from the statement of the National Health Service and Community Care Act (1990), on the need to restructure resources in a more rational manner in relation to need rather then predetermined formulae. Traditional methods of allocating resources have related to numbers and population density as opposed to the predicted or specific needs of populations or communities. The Audit Commission (1992a) identifies allocation of community nurses on the basis of numbers and not need. Deprivation indicators suggesting high areas of need bear little or no relation to the allocation of staff in community settings.

Recent foci on assessing the needs of populations, whether for local communities or for general practitioner practice populations, recognize the variation in need on a local level. The complexity of need, often linking health and social aspects, seems to be increasingly acknowledged. Profiling of need therefore demands the use of methodologies which combine to offer a holistic picture. The recent health care reforms centred on the National Health Service and Community Care Act (1990) have clearly differentiated between those who purchase health care and those who provide it. It could be argued that this separation of responsibilities creates divisions which may be accompanied by suspicions as to motives, particularly as finance impacts on every transaction.

By gathering information on health and social factors, there is the potential to make community nursing services increasingly needs led. Clearly, assessing the requirement of a local area/general practitioner practice population is a prerequisite in the development of care packages. As clinicians are becoming involved more directly in the contracting process, assessment of need is an area where purchasers and providers can collaborate in striving to deliver high quality care. Assessing need on an individual basis has long been the keynote of community nursing practice. A major concern now must be to translate those skills into a broader arena to afford a more informed awareness of the total population needs and, therefore, the employment of an appropriately skilled workforce and effective use of budget with regard to purchasing of services. The knowledge held by community nurses about the community is invaluable and must be incorporated into the policy process to both recognize its value and effectively and economically utilize skills.

Within the chapter the main approaches to data collection, that is, quantitative and qualitative methodologies, will be addressed. The utility of each approach will be discussed along with potential pitfalls and weaknesses. The perceived valuable information held by community nurses will be a factor in the overall picture and will be highlighted.

In justifying the approach of the chapter, the needs of individuals and hence of communities can only be seen as multifaceted. Clearly, the definition chosen to give to the words used has a potential to alter its interpretation. In defining need, Bradshaw (1972) explains four different types: felt, normative, expressed and comparative. A felt need is presented by community members themselves in terms of what they want, whereas a normative need is identified by the expert or professional, who may have a narrow and possibly inaccurate perspective. An expressed need is one that has become a demand and a comparative arises in comparison with another.

In the assessment of health needs, it is necessary to specify the population or community in question. A term that is commonly employed in community health nursing is 'community profile'. Again, it becomes important to clarify the meaning with regard to the community, which can represent a social structure or activity, a locality or a sentiment (Orr, 1992).

In order to depict that need, methods need to be varied and versatile. Murray and Graham (1995) suggest that a 'combination of practice based and centrally held information for the same locality would provide a more complex picture of need than either could separately' (p. 1443). The utility of varied types of data has been emphasized in terms of the general practitioner population by Azeem Majeed et al. (1995), highlighting the value of 'social, ethnic and demographic characteristics' (p. 1373) as essential for planning health services and for use in research. It needs always to be borne in mind that the collection of data, of whatever sort, is directed towards a purpose. It is a time-consuming and potentially expensive exercise. Expectations should be realistic and methodology tailored appropriately. Techniques developed should be simple, specific and easily applied to the documentation used in practice by community nurses. Counting caseload numbers on its own can be sufficient, if it meets the information need!

Factors relating to health need may have diverse origins, so there is a requirement to approach the subject from a position that is supported by as many of the relevant agencies and organizations as possible. Implications for those services that supply health and social care also need to be considered. Issues will inevitably arise that mean service providers need to question the appropriateness of their activities.

An initial exploration of the various methods that might be successfully employed in gathering information will guide the practitioners' final choice of strategies. Both quantitative and qualitative approaches to data collection provide valuable contributions to the process of needs assessment. Each has a specific focus and validity, as well as limitations. Combining the two approaches potentially provides the maximum range and depth of information.

Quantitative data

Quantitative data have much to tell us about the social world in which needs arise, describing in numerical terms the parameters of society, expressing patterns of various sorts within the population. Methods associated with quantitative approaches include amongst others:

- surveys
- interviews
- questionnaires
- observational studies.

Both epidemiology and demography focus on quantitative data and the broad profile of the population, whether the general or the at risk population.

The question needs to be asked: What sorts of 'hard' quantitative data might contribute to the identification of need and what might be the nature of that contribution? Epidemiology and demography can provide a statistical description of the disease profile, highlighting at risk groups or identifying key social indicators contributing to or indicating potential areas for targeting. The role of epidemiology is both to describe the nature, scale and potential evolution of a disease, or health problems and to explore aetiology.

A relevant example of this 'tracking' process is the clarification of the incidence of HIV from its initial appearance. Initially associated primarily with lifestyle, it has since emerged as a condition relating to transmission by known routes, and hence by specific behaviours. This refinement process, aided by epidemiological studies, has enabled the development of more appropriate and more sensitive health promotion initiatives, as well as increasing service sensitivity to the social stigma which can impact on care delivery. Both aetiology and service needs have been served.

National data

The value of the contribution of Government generated statistical data, such as census data to an information profile rests in its ability to define the scale of conditions and problems and indeed on its ability to describe, predict and reflect on the social make-up of a changed and changing society. As information needs change, so the tools for collecting that data have evolved. While the introduction of the collection of 'ethnic/race data' into the census generated some debate as to appropriateness and utility, the data once collected is utilized to highlight relevant issues for specific service groups. A word of caution which might need to be attached to the use of such data is that the use of 'race' as a category implies 'the acceptance of some notion of homogeneity of condition, culture, attitudes, expectations and ... language and religion within the groups defined' (Ahmed and Sheldon, 1993, p. 127). Such assumptions might erroneously lead to the provision of services, seemingly appropriate to need, but in fact based on a false initial premise of homogeneity.

Statistical data can provide substantial information on a range of issues relating to the health of the population. Its function is to provide and to quantify indicators of the socio-economic conditions of the health of the country and an enormous range of data is covered. The usefulness of this data is vast and varied. Epidemiological data, specifically mortality and morbidity statistics, offer an indicator for the health of the nation, or rather the ill-health. Standardized mortality rates (SMRs) in particular are a clear indicator of health and the variations in health of different areas. A high SMR relating to breast cancer, for example, may provide a starting point from which to explore the contributory factors to that higher rate. In combination with further work and research, changes in service provision may be put in place, for example, additional breast screening facilities.

The prevalence and incidence of diseases may also indicate both the present numbers of people with a specific disease or condition (prevalence) in a community and whether the number of new cases per year (incidence) is rising or falling. Hence both the size and pattern of the disease can be determined.

A key indicator often utilized to target specific areas of need is that of deprivation. Deprivation indicators, such as the Townsend *et al.* (1982) and Jarman (1983) scores, consist of a combination of variables, for example, unemployment, overcrowding, social class distribution. The census is the prime source of information 'on a range of deprivation factors and is the principal source of ecological data on social conditions' (Orr, 1992, p. 29). The Black Report (DHSS, 1980) utilizes social indicators to highlight inequalities in health and the links between deprivation and ill-health. The combining of various indicators is commonly used to explore variations in health status and the factors which contribute to this. Recent studies on unemployment, often used as an indicator for poor health, suggest that, in fact, issues such as local attitudes to unemployment may influence the impact of being unemployed (Duffy, 1993, p. 28).

Since the inclusion of race/ethnicity as a variable in the collection of census data, the consideration of ethnicity in relation to other factors has become more accessible. It would seem, therefore, that the introduction of race/ethnicity is an opportunity to explore possible connections or correlations. Bhopal and White (1993) identify the need to highlight the relationship between 'ethnicity, socio-economic deprivation and health' but there is a need to exercise caution and challenge the assumptions that are often made that 'health problems are the result of biological or cultural factors when they are as likely to have a political or economic basis' (Ahmed, 1989, p. 162).

Local data

While national and regional statistics offer very valuable data, local statistics and other forms of 'hard' data also have a key contribution to make to the profiling of need. At times the combining of national data with locally based information or with related clinical research can be significant. Suicide risk amongst older people, for example, can be indicated on a macro level by specific indicators such as increasing age and economic deprivation, while more local data would provide other relevant data relating to social isolation or service provision. The addition of individual clinical data to the broader picture completes the clinical picture. The rounded picture can facilitate the meeting of needs in a relevant and sensitive way.

The contribution of community nurses in the process of needs assessment and more immediately in the profiling of local needs is becoming in-creasingly significant and an increasingly common imperative from both purchasers and provider units. The use of profiling as a tool to generate team working in primary health care has proved to be of value in team building and expressing a commitment to quality care delivery. Shared working on GP practice profiling or locality profiling generates both a wealth of information from a variety of perspectives but also has 'spin-off' effects of an increased team focus on the specific needs of local people and specifically of patients.

As expert practitioners in the field, all community nurses have an evolving role in seeking out and identifying health needs in order to develop, with sound justification, pro-active practice development, both for their own practice area and for specific groups of patients. Recent and forthcoming developments such as the initiatives being taken for those patients with continuing health care needs (e.g. for elderly mentally infirm patients, or for those requiring rehabilitation) present an opportunity not to be ignored for the enrichment of community nursing.

The community nurse is therefore faced with two areas of 'hard data' on which to focus. The first is data relating to both national, regional and local statistics which is very attractive because of its 'availability' (Hopton and Dlugolecka, 1995). Census data in particular are easily accessible, and presented in a reasonably readable format. Owing to their inclusion of the whole population, they are also authoritative. Government collected data, while appearing to be highly reliable, can be limited both through being 'broad brush strokes' of description and because they are inevitably out of date (RCN, 1990). The census data collected dicennially rapidly lose accuracy, particularly in areas where the movement of populations can be rapid.

Locally developed systems of data collection, for example through the computerized records of general practices and the Health Authorities have the benefit of being current and frequently updated. Many general practices are now linked directly to Health Authorities' information systems and practice profiles are collated as a tool for the revision and review of service delivery as well as for other purposes. The merger of DHAs and FHSAs can only have facilitated the expansion of such information systems. Local mapping of populations is carried out using enumeration districts (i.e. the districts covered during the census by individual enumeration officers), linked with postal codes. The census data can then be expressed in approximation to the patients registered with general practices. This avoids the disadvantages of census data which are limited by being amalgamated into electoral wards.

The second element in the equation of health needs assessment can often be the consideration of data provided by community nurses themselves and gathered by their information systems. Caseload profiles, which examine in depth the referral and visiting patterns of community nurses, as well as the scope of their own caseload populations, can highlight quite dramatically issues of access to services, of uptake and hence of the equity and sensitivity of nursing services within the overall health care service.

Seeking consumer data

Among the current changes and developments in the NHS, consumers of health care remain a common, and indeed, constant factor and should be the focus of our attention, if we are not to lose sight of the purpose of our endeavours. The important role of the consumer of health care is detailed in various nursing documents (DHSS, 1986a; DOH, 1992) but it was the Griffiths Report (DHSS, 1983) that originally recognized the necessity of obtaining the experiences and perceptions of patients when planning and implementing services within a given population. Purchasers and providers alike have a responsibility to involve consumers in the assessment of their requirements of the health care system.

Professionals may have a biased, narrow and inaccurate perception of the requirements of their service users and existing methods of working may not easily facilitate a search for consumer views and opinions. It would appear that consumers are rarely permitted to take part in assessing the services they receive and such assessment tends to be insensitive and miss important issues (Pollitt, 1989).

Ong (1991) believes that it is fairly well recognized now that disease, as seen as a bio-medical phenomenon, differs qualitatively from illness as an experience and states that 'Within the context of nursing, the possible discrepancy between the professional's definition of need and that of the client has to be understood in the light of the opposition between disease and illness. The implications for the assessment of need are obvious: needs have to be defined in a co-operative manner, resulting from a dialogue between professionals and clients' (p. 639).

Patient satisfaction, according to Richardson (1990) originates from their expectations of the services, which are usually based on past experience and firmly established within their own cultural definitions of health and illness. Although acknowledging its importance, Richardson (1990) states 'It is rare to find the concept of patient satisfaction defined and there has been little clarification of what the terms mean to researchers who employ it or to respondents who respond to it' (p. 435).

Developing workable ways of seeking consumer opinion with regard to both the requirements people have of community nursing services as well as their views on outcome measurements presents community health nurses with a challenge. This type of data collection can also produce the evidence which informs contract negotiation and resource allocation.

Smith et al. (1993) identify the importance of developing information systems that capture the true essence of our work as health care professionals. As part of our evaluative practice, community health nurses should ensure that needs assessment is incorporated into activities recorded on daily activity schedules/computer systems. If this is not the case, there is the danger of needs assessment becoming another one of those hidden activities that constitute the 'invisible workload' identified by Evers et al. (1992).

Differentiation has clearly been made between a purchaser-led contracting process and an alternative approach described by Smith et al. (1993) as 'a new kind of local integration with an emphasis on provider involvement; local integration of social and health services; mechanisms for sustaining trust, morale and hence motivation to produce meaningful contracts between purchasers, front-line providers and their managers; and involvement of clients' (p. 123).

Community health nurses are in a strong position with regard to their role in ensuring quality services and positive client outcomes.

Consumer involvement can take place not only within the individual working relationship between the patient and health care professional but also on local and national levels. Ashton and Seymour (1988) describe a type of collective, pro-active and needs-led approach to the assessment of health as 'new public health'. Evaluating the quality of community health care services is complex. Patients often report higher levels of satisfaction than can be demonstrated in medical or nursing outcomes of care. So it is crucial to involve both consumer as well as professional perspectives regarding services. Richardson (1990) suggests that any study that incorporates issues that affect patients' perspectives as well professional views will be small scale and intensive. Such research will tend to use qualitative rather than quantitative data and the results will probably not be generalizable.

Clearly, the right personnel should be involved in the gathering of information and all those involved should be given equal credibility and recognition, regardless of their status in the organizational hierarchy.

When considering appropriate methods for collecting consumer views and opinions, McIver (1993) explains that cultural and language variations between a wide range of different types of people using community services leads to difficulties in constructing a single tool to elicit comments and feedback. Whilst acknowledging their strengths, she outlines the limitations of employing surveys, such as a structured self-completion questionnaire, to gain information from consumers.

Surveys gather quantitative information, such as rates or incidences of occurrence, whereas other methods such as group discussions, unstructured interviews and observation collect qualitative data. A combination of qualitative and quantitative methods will enhance the nature of the information obtained.

Research into consumers' opinions is not a new development. Although the issue was highlighted by the Government in the Griffiths Report (DHSS, 1983), studies have been conducted since the early 1960s (Cartwright, 1967; Raphael, 1969). This research has demonstrated that there are common issues of concern to patients, whichever service they are using. McIver (1993) identifies these as:

- The nature of their relationship with health care professionals, especially effective communication and being treated as a patient.
- Adequate information to decrease anxiety and promote a sense of control over their situation.
- Effective treatment and care.

A core set of questions to address the quality of the client–practitioner relationship, information transmission and treatment and care could be devised as these issues are considered to be important to patients in all service areas. Williams and Calnan (1991) support this in the summary following their large-scale study when they state that 'Our findings clearly suggest that issues concerning professional competence, together with the nature and quality of the patient–professional relationship, are consistently the most important predictors of overall consumer satisfaction with general practice, dental and hospital care' (p. 715).

Methods can be simple and developed from existing structures. For example, using the complaints procedure as a quality development tool (Audit Commission, 1992b). Other ways of encouraging user participation include quality action groups and patient participation groups, which were first developed in Oxford in 1972. The notion is endorsed by the Royal College of General Practitioners, and the DHSS (1986b) document *Primary Health Care: An agenda for discussion* describes patient participation groups as an effective method of promoting quality. There are both 'open' and 'nominated' groups. Open groups develop from open meetings to which any patient may come along. On the other hand, representatives of other community groups and associations form nominated groups.

Other non-survey methods of gaining user feedback/views include types of observation and focused group discussion. Focus group work is a method widely used in organizations such as the Community Health Council.

Obviously, an explanation of the target population helps in delineating the area of study, e.g. the GP practice population or a recognized geographical area/locality. When eliciting information from a fairly large community population a triangulation of methods may provide a more complete picture of the area under study.

Participatory Rapid Appraisal is a research strategy that produces results quickly and has participation as its central tenet, involving community members both in the research and subsequent decision making. Participatory Rapid Appraisal originated in developing countries, where it was employed to evaluate the need of disadvantaged rural populations. It has been adopted in the UK and used in deprived urban areas (Cresswell, 1992). This approach enables:

- local residents to participate in the appraisal and make their views heard. They identify their problems, needs and opportunities and so increase their ability to influence post-appraisal decision making.
- key professionals and people in the area to make their opinions heard and participate in the research process. This encourages communication with local residents and provides a more complete picture of local needs.
- information to be gathered quickly but the actual time span will depend on local circumstances.
- the inclusion of a wide range of data collection methods so that information from many sources often inaccessible to more traditional methods becomes available.

Data collection methods may include semi-structured interviews with local residents, key people and key professionals; focus group interviews with specific members of the community; written reports; field surveys; hard data of various sorts, observation and photography and video work. Findings reflect local concerns and conditions and are 'owned' by community members. As a result, subsequent action is taken by community members who have not only identified problems but also discussed possible solutions.

In a community setting, Participatory Rapid Appraisal is a strategy that can involve many local agencies and organizations in working together. Community workers cannot work in isolation. Police, school teachers, youth workers, councillors, the community health council, voluntary organizations as well as health and social care professionals need to research community health needs together. By working together with residents in an appraisal of local needs, professionals may develop greater awareness of the roles of colleagues and help avoid duplication.

Although the notion of user participation in health care is supported in theory both formally by the Government and by lay and professionals alike, there are well established organizational and cultural practices that do not always facilitate it.

Stoller (1977) suggests that there are a few changes to be made before real participation can become a reality. Two major prerequisites include, first, the need for consumers to have a group identity to match the occupational identity of the providers and secondly, the development of a sense of consumer competence and self-confidence in a relatively unfamiliar situation. The variable viewpoints of the provider and the consumer of health care need to be acknowledged and attempts made to negotiate new roles. 'The conflict that may accompany this role negotiation serves a positive function during the early history of such organizations by allowing participants to work together to construct an effective organisation' (Stoller, 1977, p. 177).

McIver (1993) suggests that initiatives such as local patients' charters, health newspapers, public meetings, exhibitions, improved complaints procedures and telephone help lines will help to move the traditional culture of the NHS towards a more participative style in which the views of consumers are valued in relation to their own health and the care delivered to the community as a whole.

Conclusion

It is important to recognize the importance of applying the principles generated from needs assessment to community nursing practice activities in the future, so that consumer questioning regarding treatment and outcomes along with other relevant data becomes an integral part of care delivery.

The inclusion of research within contracts between purchasers and providers has been recently highlighted in the Culyer Report (NHSR and DTF, 1994), which places responsibility on purchasers to support relevant research. Primary and secondary sectors, for the first time, are given equal status in applying for central National Health Service Research and Development funding. Practitioners should ensure that needs assessment appears on the agenda in contract negotiations as an integral part of their role.

Participating in needs assessment is an opportunity for community nurses to take an active role in the policy process, by identifying their contribution and commitment to the development of appropriate and effective health services.

Points to consider

1 Consider ways in which you might use consumer participation/feedback to help in the development of your practice.

2 How might you seek that participation/feedback? Which data collection method would be most effective for your needs?

3 How familiar are you with the demographic and epidemiological data for your practice? Are there issues of access or equity which would be useful to explore?

4 What factors might influence consumer participation in the delivery and planning of services?

References

Ahmed, W.I.U. 1989: Policies, pills and political will: critique of policies to improve the health status of ethnic minorities. *Lancet*, i: 148–50.

Ahmed, W.I.U. and Sheldon, T. 1993: 'Race' and statistics. In Hammersley, M. *Social research: philosophy, politics and practice*. Milton Keynes: OU Press.

Azeem Majeed, F., Cook, D.G., Polonicki, J., Griffiths, J. and Stones, C. 1995: Sociodemographic variables for general practices: use of census data. *British Medical Journal*, **310**: 1373–4.

Ashton, J. and Seymour, H. 1988: *The new public health*. Milton Keynes: Open University Press.

Audit Commission (1992a): *Homeward bound: a new course for community health*. London: HMSO.

Audit Commission 1992b: *Presentation to advisory group communicating with patients project*. London: HMSO.

Bhopal, R. and White, M. 1993: Health promotion for ethnic priorities: past, present and future. In Ahmed, W.I.U. (ed.), *'Race' and health in contemporary Britain*. Milton Keynes: Open University Press.

Bowling, A. 1992: Assessing health needs and measuring patient satisfaction. *Nursing Times* Occasional Paper: July 29, **88**, 31.

Bradshaw, J. 1972: The concept of social need. *New Society*, **30**: 640–3.

Cartwright, A. 1967: *Patients and their doctors*. London: Tavistock.

Cresswell, T. 1992: Assessing community health and social needs. In North Derbyshire, using Participatory Rapid Appraisal. *Community Health Action*, issue 24.

Department of Health and Social Security 1980: *Inequalities in health (The Black Report)*. London: HMSO.

Department of Health and Social Security 1983: *NHS management inquiry* (Chair Sir Roy Griffiths). London: HMSO.

Department of Health and Social Security 1986a: *Neighbourhood nursing – a focus for care*. London: HMSO.

Department of Health and Social Security 1986b: *Primary health care: an agenda for discussion*. London: HMSO.

Department of Health 1992: *The patient's charter.* London: HMSO.

District Nursing Association 1992: *Key issues in district nursing (paper 3) Challenges for district nursing: quality care, health needs profiling and skill mix.* UK: District Nursing Association.

Duffy, D. 1993: Preventing suicide. *Nursing Times,* **89**, 31, 28–31.

Evers, H., Badger, F. and Cameron, E. 1992: Finding the limits. *Nursing Times,* **88**, 30, 60–2.

Hopton, J.L. and Dlugolecka, M. 1995: Need and demand for primary health care: a comparative survey approach. *British Medical Journal,* **310**, 1369–73.

Jarman, B. 1983: Identification of underprivileged areas. *British Medical Journal,* **286**, 1705–9.

McIver, S. 1993: *Obtaining the views of users of primary and community health care services.* London: King's Fund Centre.

Murray, S.A. and Graham, L.J.C. 1995: Practice based health needs assessment: use of four methods in a small neighbourhood. *British Medical Journal,* **319**, 1443–8.

National Health Service Research and Development Task Force 1994: *Supporting research and development in the NHS.* Chairperson Professor Anthony Culyer. London: HMSO.

Ong, B.N. 1991: Researching needs in district nursing. *Journal of Advanced Nursing,* **16**, 638–47.

Orr, J. 1992: The community division. In Luker, K. and Orr, J. (eds), *Health visiting: towards community health nursing.* Oxford: Blackwell Scientific.

Pollitt, C. 1989: Consuming passions. *Health Service Journal,* **99**, 5178, 1436–7.

Raphael, W. 1969: Do we know what patients think? *International Journal of Nursing Studies,* **7**, 209–23.

Richardson, J. 1990: Gaining perspective. *Health Service Journal,* 22 March, 435.

Royal College of Nursing 1990: *The GP practice profile.* London: RCN.

Smith, P., Makintosh, M. and Towers, B. 1993: Implications of the new NHS contracting system for the district nursing services in one health authority: a pilot study. *Journal of Interprofessional Care,* **7**, 2, 115–24.

Stoller, E.P. 1977: New roles for health care consumers: a study of role transformation. *Journal of Community Health,* **3**, 2, 171–7.

Townsend, P., Davidson, N. and Whitehead, M. 1982: *Inequalities in health.* London: Penguin.

Williams, S.J. and Calnan, M. 1991: Convergence and divergence. Assessing criteria of consumer satisfaction across general practice, dental and hospital care settings. *Social Science and Medicine,* **33**, 6, 706–16.

17 Hospital at Home

Barbara Johnson

This chapter describes an aspect of advanced nursing care provided for patients at home in order to prevent the inappropriate admission to institutional care, through the provision of an additional resource to the primary health care team.

An experienced and skilled district nurse leads a team of carers and nurses to provide extra time and resources as well as a flexible and innovative system of practice. The service aims to offer practical and cost-effective methods of providing alternative care packages to meet patients' needs. It puts into practice a model demonstrating the shift from secondary to primary care and offers patients and carers choices about their care.

The challenges of setting up and providing new services were matched with the need to learn new skills in measuring outcomes, demonstrating value for money, cultivating partners and fighting for scarce resources.

An outline of how the project developed, its aims and results are described here as an example of an enterprising way of enhancing community nursing care and is intended to stimulate the reader into considering alternative practices.

Background

Since the well publicized Peterborough Hospital at Home scheme (which was developed 20 years ago) the whole culture of health care has rapidly developed to encourage and embrace home nursing care, as a cost-effective and realistic alternative to secondary care. The emphasis on the shift from acute hospital services to the community, focused upon the primary health care team, has been well documented in several government reports and White Papers in the last 10 years, such as *Nursing in the Community* (NHSME/North West Thames RHA, 1990), *Neighbourhood Nursing* (DHSS, 1986), *New World New Opportunities* (DOH, 1993), *Homeward Bound* (Audit Commission, 1992), have all examined the benefits and shortfalls in community nursing services. Furthermore, *Caring for People* (DOH, 1989a), *Working for Patients* (DOH, 1989b), *The Patient's Charter* (DOH, 1991) and *Health of the Nation* (DOH, 1992) have led to a series of NHS and social services' reforms, which gave an impetus to nurses in the community to refine and develop their services to meet the newly defined needs.

Taking into account these recent changes, the aim of a Hospital at Home service must be to provide care for patients in their own homes as an alternative to a hospital admission or to enable patients to return home earlier than usual after a hospital admission.

There is a belief that care at home is better for patients, particularly elderly people (Durham and Durham, 1990). They found that care at home instead of in hospital can prevent the breakdown of support networks and confusion – both very common when elderly people are removed from their familiar environment during a period of acute illness or crisis (Durham and Durham, 1990). The Hospital at Home service must take into account:

- the appropriate skills, knowledge, attitudes of current staff;
- resources in terms of manpower, equipment, training;
- training implications for existing staff;
- other professionals who may be involved in the scheme;
- the appropriateness of the scheme for the patient and their family.

Different types of alternative home nursing and therapy care provision have been developed throughout the UK and parts of Europe encompassing the following areas: orthopaedics, paediatrics, gynaecology, medicine, surgery, AIDS care and elderly care. These have all been targeted to a greater or lesser degree with different models of service. Selected examples of these are as follows:

A paediatric Hospital at Home service evaluated by Jennings (1994) demonstrated parent and child satisfaction but found that poor liaison between hospital and community services and loose medical cover compromised the success of the service,

A successful Dutch scheme has been described by Kessels-Buickhuisen (1994), which concentrates on day surgery postoperative care at home, which contributed to the targeted hospital achieving a much higher rate of day surgery than previously possible. This benefited both the patient and the organization of health care.

There must be expectations that patients receiving care through a Hospital at Home type service will be provided with a service to the same level as in hospital. The patients are also expected to receive the extra benefits to them that care in a familiar environment (their own home) is believed to bestow.

The target groups should be selected and based on the identified health needs of the local population. If a health district has a specific identified health need related to the population it may be appropriate to concentrate on that target group, however, this could be a dilemma between local health needs and central government directives (DOH, 1992). An example is in a district with a high proportion of frail elderly people it may seem inappropriate to target people with AIDS.

The Department of Health has been enthusiastic in recent years about finding alternatives to apparently expensive and perhaps unnecessary hospital bed occupancy. They have been supportive, at least in theory, of quality alternatives outside the hospital setting. NHS reforms detailed in

Caring for People (DOH, 1989a) resulted in major changes in the way that community care was to be provided.

The Peterborough scheme set up in 1978 was established to examine the complementary roles of hospital and district nursing services. Knowelden *et al.* (1991) evaluated the Peterborough service and felt that there were more patients cared for at home than would usually have been looked after by the district nursing service and that this enhancement of care could prevent terminally ill cancer patients in particular being admitted to hospital. Mowat and Morgan (1982) described some of the difficulties and advantages of being involved in this innovative new service: the need to communicate well with existing services; the need for adequate resourcing; the need for qualitative, quantitative and financial evaluation of the outcomes and the possible need to re-allocate capital to fund further schemes. The Peterborough scheme has now evolved into a well established partnership of district nurse, medical practitioner, therapist and hospital service – all working together to provide comprehensive Hospital at Home services for patients. This service covers a wide variety of conditions and diagnoses, the initial emphasis being on early discharge and orthopaedic care.

The Swindon model – the Community High Dependency Service

This substantial shift in health care culture, along with a genuine enthusiasm to develop community nursing practice and a determination to provide improved patient care and choices led to the development of a scheme with a different emphasis. The aim was to learn from the example of Peterborough and other similar services. It was important to target the people in the local community who could benefit from the scheme, and whose needs could be met by an alternative type of service. This service therefore did not target early discharge or orthopaedic patients as their care was considered to be of a high quality already. The care of the high dependent, frail and very sick people in the community was seen to be of a higher priority.

In 1993 funds were granted from the then Swindon Health Authority (currently The Health Commission for Wiltshire) to examine the possibility of providing two new experimental services linked to the district nursing services in the Swindon locality. This followed a review of district nursing services and a desire to enhance the mainstream services by providing an extra resource for the primary health care team.

The first proposal was to set up a traditional Hospital at Home service to facilitate early discharge of patients from the local district general hospital, possibly targeting orthopaedic patients and including an expanded nursing team including a physiotherapist and occupational therapist.

The second proposal was to develop a nursing Emergency Response Team in partnership with the social services to provide care for people in the community in a crisis and prevent inappropriate admission to hospital, nursing home or residential home.

After six months in operation an internal evaluation led to the two services being redesigned, renamed and amalgamated. The rationale for this was that by amalgamating the services a more comprehensive package of care could be provided and that this would avoid the confusion caused by running two services. The new service in phase two became The Community High Dependency Service and incorporated for the first time the provision of a district nursing overnight service. This provided night nursing and sitting for patients on the scheme and also care for other patients receiving district nursing and GP services. This name was chosen because it was felt to describe the high dependency rather than intensive care needs of the users. Intensive care was not considered appropriate because it is associated with the notion of high-tech hospital services. It was also felt that the service offered more than the traditional Hospital at Home type care as it included social and carer support in addition to the health care needs of the patient.

The aim of the service was to provide enhanced district nursing services to patients with high dependency needs so enabling them to stay at home instead of going into hospital, nursing home or residential home. The high dependency could originate from nursing, medical, carer or social needs and there was a wish to avoid demarcation of responsibilities. These can be a major problem in community care, when old barriers between health and social care workers may be resurrected as each compete for scarce resources (Hyde, 1995). Patients are in danger of falling between the two services and consequently may not receive any care (Calkin and Pierpoint, 1989). The operational policy and criteria for admission were left flexible to allow the scheme to develop without too many rules and regulations and the staff were employed to become jacks of all trades, providing social and nursing care as needed.

The project loosely followed the Prince project management style from the outset (NHSME, 1990). This involves the project being supported by a team composed of, in this case, senior strategic managers from health, social services, hospital and GP services. As part of the model an operational management group was also created. This was concerned with the initial recruitment, monitoring, marketing and development of the project. This group had among its members the project manager, the district nurse running the service and representatives from social services, general practice, district nursing and hospital liaison services. The Prince model provides two levels of support and supervision and these assist in the development of global and objective monitoring.

Operational policy and criteria for admission

Before the service could start an operational policy was written (see Operational policy overleaf) this detailed the criteria for admission to the scheme (see Criteria for admission below). Although there was a need to be as flexible as possible it was necessary to make clear to the referrers and the patients why it was sometimes not possible to accept certain patients for care.

Once this policy was agreed the recruitment and selection process could begin. Employment terms were a little different from the usual community nursing staff Whitley contractual conditions.

Operational policy

- The scheme would provide care based on patient and carer choice in partnership with other statutory agencies in the patient's home, including a residential home if this was the patient's home.
- It would be a complementary service to the primary health care team in a specified limited geographical area.
- The scheme could not care for maternity, acute mental health or paediatric patients – the team did not have the specialist clinical skills for these care groups.
- Care would be assessed by the scheme Sister or her relief within one hour of referral (if the admission criteria were met and there were available spaces on the scheme). Care would be available 24 hours a day, 7 days a week. Patients were expected to remain on the scheme for between 2 and 10 days depending on their care needs, however, no rigid upper or lower limits were set.
- Patients and carers should be willing to accept care, be well motivated and able to comprehend and retain information. The Sister or GP need to be contactable at all times.
- Clinical records would be kept and data would be collected on patients who were admitted to the scheme, and on those who refused admission.

Admission to and discharge from the service would be in collaboration with the district nurse, GP and social services department.

Criteria for admission

All points in the operational policy were to be observed, plus:

- Referrals could be from the primary health care team, social services staff and hospital staff at any time of the night or day.
- Patients with a chronic illness could be admitted to the scheme if they were undergoing an acute phase of illness. The scheme could not, however, take on the long-term care of people with a chronic illness or disability. This was to avoid scarce resources being tied up in long-term care, which could not be sustained and to avoid overlapping with mainstream services.
- There must be a telephone in the house. Telephones could not be provided but an extension lead could be loaned if needed. This was to help improve communications and ensure that the patient or carer could summon help.

- Requests to support a carer in a crisis situation would be accepted, for example, if a carer had a sudden illness and could not care for their relative. In such circumstances the service could replace the carer for a limited time and prevent the unnecessary admission of the patient.
- A small stock of emergency equipment could be provided immediately but most home loan equipment was to be available from our Home Loans Service.
- Early discharges from hospital would be accepted if the patient met the criteria. The Hospital Discharge Liaison Sister was the link professional to identify potential users of the services and liaise with hospital and community services.
- A limited amount of all night sitting would be available for patients who needed enhanced care overnight because of acute illness, frailty or treatment needs.

All referrals were considered on their merits and patients were sometimes accepted for care who perhaps did not quite meet the criteria. The scheme was able to offer some measure of alternative care for such patients. For example, a patient with an acute illness living alone was cared for while the relatives travelled from Lancashire to be with the patient. There were no age criteria (except for children) and no restrictions as to disease or condition. It was important, however, that the resources were not stretched too thinly, as this could lead to a lowering of clinical standards. Thus a limited number of places were available at any time (generally 6 to 9, depending on the level of individual needs). It was also important not to be all things to all men and then let patients down because of lack of specialist skills. However, this did mean that expected care outcomes were difficult to define as there was not a specific care group.

SELECTING THE STAFF

The initial attempts to recruit a district nurse, physiotherapist and occupational therapist were thwarted by the inability to attract suitable staff to join on short-term contracts. Nurses, just like other professional people, need job security and a regular income, neither of which are guaranteed with a fixed term contract. The funding for this service was only agreed six monthly and all contracts were extended on that basis. The short-term solution to this was to second a district nurse from within the standard district nursing services to run the scheme. This proved to be most successful and meant that a nurse was chosen who already knew the district and the existing care networks and was an enthusiastic supporter of the idea. Existing physiotherapy and occupational therapy services were also accessed and those salary allocations were used to provide extra care assistant hours. Three care assistant/nursing auxiliaries were employed, who between them would provide seven day a week cover from 8 am to 5 pm. The bulk of the hands on care was to be provided by support staff. The High Dependency Service District Nurse was to undertake initial rapid assessments and provide skilled nursing care in partnership with the patients' own district nursing team. Following the initial referral to the service the Sister from the High Dependency team would undertake a rapid assessment of immediate needs. Lengthy and comprehensive care planning would be the responsibility of the district nurse to whom the patient belonged. Care would be provided by a combination of the nursing team, social services care team and supplemented by the project carers.

A team of care assistants employed on bank contracts also covered a 24-hour on call rota, which enabled a carer to be available at all times. Basic induction and in-service training was provided (for example, manual handling, health and safety, clinical care, continence care, grief and bereavement). A retainer was paid for this on-call commitment and staff received the hourly nursing auxiliary rate when they were called out to provide care.

A local nursing agency service was used as a back up if the scheme was short staffed. This was the first time that a nursing agency had been used within the district nursing services. It was necessary to be very specific with the requirements as agencies may not necessarily have the same quality standards as a statutory agency. There were problems initially with a lack of appropriately skilled carers, unreliability and poor quality standards of care.

The provision of uniforms, in a different colour from those of the district nursing auxiliaries, identified them as a service extra to the regular services and helped the staff to recognize their slightly different role. The patients were able to recognize them as a nursing service and as an offshoot of the usual uniformed district nursing services.

The project managers were very keen to portray this project as an enhancement to the district nursing team, partners in care, not competitors. Therefore it was vital to communicate to the district nursing teams, particularly the sisters, that this was a project to enhance not replace their care. The service was to provide the extra resources that they had wished for in the past, when they saw their patients admitted to hospital because the level of community care was inadequate. This was easier said than done, communications were inadequate and unfortunately did not come early enough to avoid initial suspicion and scepticism. It took hasty reassurance of the teams of district nurses that this service was there not because they lacked the necessary skills or knowledge but was there to provide them with extra resources for patient care. Perhaps a better application of change theories (Bennis et al., 1976) would have made the process easier to manage for both the district nursing staff and the project team.

THE SERVICE STARTS

As part of the start up process information sheets were sent to GPs in the initial catchment area, to district nurses and to social worker colleagues. An overview of intentions and details of how to access the service was given. This was later followed up with more detailed information, outlining the criteria for admission, publicizing the overnight nursing provision. To catch the GPs' attention information was printed on very bright 'dayglo' paper.

Initially requests for the service, on both days and nights, was slow and time was needed to catch the attention of the market. Several referrals from GPs came at the outset which looked like an attempt to get rid of patients with multiple long-term problems. The scheme relied on the strong-willed, confident and assertive sister to explain that, however much she sympathized with the problem, it was beyond the remit of the scheme.

Gradually over the first three months the referrals began to increase and it was found that the service was caring for more and more of the type of patients that were being targeted. Carers were supported during crises, so preventing admission to care. Patients with pneumonia, stroke, AIDS and back injuries were nursed. Patients waiting for a hospital bed were maintained and the scheme was able to provide an enhanced level of care and support to patients with terminal illnesses. The level of referrals was and still is at the time of writing lower for patients whose needs are primarily for social care. This was a surprise as it was anticipated that the demand for social care would be high. The GP and social services colleagues gave anecdotal accounts of numerous patients being admitted to hospital, for social rather than medical care, due to the absence of appropriate community-based alternatives. Some financial support was received from the social service budget and the scheme was always considered to be a joint initiative. Despite the strategic and professional collaboration, involvement in social care has been, in the main, only a small part of care packages.

ACTIVITY AND COSTS

During the first 12 months of the projects, 98 patients were cared for and this involved 1449 contacts. Most of these patients would have been admitted to hospital if the scheme had not been available. Some of the patients may have been admitted into residential care and some would have struggled at home. Evaluation of the scheme showed that an estimated 546 hospital bed days had been saved.

In the following months the activity increased and 68 patients were cared for in just the first 5 months of 1995, with over 1095 contacts. This saved at least 414 hospital bed days.

In the first 6 months of the new night nursing service being established the nurses did more than 140 visits to patients between the hours of 2200 and 0800. This was supporting not only the Community High Dependency Service patients but also GP and district nursing patients, involving mostly acute clinical care such as re-catheterizations and terminal care. The night service had done 23 visits during January 1995 but this had increased to 89 visits by December of that year. There were more than 72 visits of over 8 hours duration (usually overnight) and more than 32 visits of over 2 hours duration between January and May 1995.

The length of stay on the scheme was expected to be between 2 and 4 days for patients with mainly social needs and between 2 and 10 days for nursing or medical needs. The scheme aimed to be as flexible as possible and assess patient and carer needs on an individual basis. This would give the mainstream statutory services time to develop care plans and long-term provision. The aim was to respond to a referral by providing an assessment within half an hour and a nurse or a carer could usually be provided for the patient within an hour.

The service seemed to offer improved value for money when compared with the cost per unit of low dependency in-patient care in either a community hospital or a district general hospital. There are no community hospitals in this trust area however. The cost on average per patient day was estimated to be around £132, compared with hospital costs of between £150 and £220. However, as this was still a project at the time of evaluation full accounting periods could not be used, as the funding included start up and other non-recurring costs.

It was suggested by the formal evaluation that the extent of wider implementation of the scheme could result in savings only if money could be released by permanent transfer of services from secondary to primary care services. This could cause a dilemma for the funders of this type of service who would really have to ensure that the money followed the patient.

Evaluation and quality

The range of conditions and diseases, the type of dependency, the initial costs were critically examined to establish whether patients were being offered a real alternative to institutional care. Although this evaluation was relatively simple it was found that the majority of patients really would have had no alternative but to go into some sort of residential care, if they had not had access to this service.

As the project developed the increasing numbers of referrals meant that the scheme became more cost effective in service delivery and was regularly providing care for up to nine patients per day. An outbreak of an infection at the local hospital trust during the winter led to the closure of several wards and a subsequent increase in the demand for our service. Hospital at Home was able to work in closer partnership with hospital colleagues to devise packages of care particularly suited to patients with medical conditions.

A formal evaluation was commissioned in 1995 by the commissioning authority to examine this and three other projects in Wiltshire with similar aims and objectives. Future funding of the services largely depended on this report which was undertaken by Lynx VOI, a private management consultancy firm. Statistical and financial information was collated and a series of interviews with providers, referrers and users of the service were conducted. Even if continued funding is not available the scheme was identified as a new and innovative idea that provided considerable benefits to the users and could be revisited in the future. The report was cautiously enthusiastic about the project. It highlighted the favourable reception for the service given by GPs and patients and identified the financial considerations that needed to be taken into account when considering setting up a new service, without re-allocation of resources. The evaluation did however identify the need for robust financial and accounting systems to support such a project and the need to set clear outcome measures at the start. Neither of these objectives could be fulfilled to our satisfaction, due to lack of resources in information technology, administrative support and lack of experience. The project as a prototype was necessarily loose which enabled flexibility and evolution but this also made it difficult at times to identify clear outcome measures.

In the summer of 1995 a multidisciplinary Clinical Audit of the service was conducted with a patient satisfaction survey. Both demonstrated that objectives were being met and that the service was highly valued by the patients and carers. The full results of the Clinical Audit was used to help plan improvements and developments in the service for the remainder of its existence. The intention of audit is to demonstrate an improvement in quality of service delivery. Doctors may talk of audit, nurses may talk of quality assurance and managers may talk of total quality management but when they come together to do the audit it means the same thing, a way of demonstrating improvement (Smith, 1992).

This service offered a new model for the development of the primary health care team incorporating health and social care in a holistic nursing framework. Multiskilled staff were able to handle the overlapping health and social care needs that are so common in clients in the community, the so-called grey area of community care. The qualified district nurse already has the appropriate specialist skills to assess and plan for the provision of these alternative, enhanced packages of care. The district nurse running this scheme had to develop more specialist management skills in order to manage and supervize a new type of nursing auxiliary. The district nurse undertook a course to be an NVQ trainer to help prepare her for this responsibility.

Conclusions and issues for discussion

Primary health care has become a focus of interest since the 1980s. The interface between secondary and primary care and the shift of care from one to the other has led to the development of innovative new models of service delivery. The Conservative government, in power at the time of writing, has initiated major health and social care reforms since 1989 – whether to improve the quality and range of care or whether to try and reduce public spending is, and should be, open to debate. These changes have, however, forced health care providers and nurses to examine different methods of delivery of their services. Hughes and Gordon (1992) in their paper for the

King's Fund explore alternatives to hospital care in London as part of the huge exercise to redeploy health care resources in the capital in the early 1990s. This issue is likely to cause controversy for a long time as some famous London teaching hospitals face closure or merger.

The original Peterborough scheme has spawned similar services all over the UK and the Peterborough scheme now seems totally established as a core community nursing service. A full range of patients needing postoperative care are now nursed, providing a much wider range of service than the original focus, which was on orthopaedic early discharge and terminal care services (Hackman, 1993; Few, 1995). All over the country services have been and are being developed to provide general and specialist nursing care for patients and their families at home. Patients that only a few years ago would have been cared for in hospitals and institutions now receive care at home.

When considering the push to provide more and more high-tech or high dependency nursing and social care in the community, commissioners of services, be they purchasers or providers, must consider the economic, social and clinical implications of changing patterns of delivery of care. Community nurses may well need to develop new and enhanced clinical skills in order to provide the sort of sophisticated care required by specialist groups of patients. In some services the nurse herself may not have the necessary skills and knowledge to provide enhanced care, for example in paediatric nursing at home. The whole issue of managing change and adapting to a new health care culture needs to be considered, with changing working patterns and practices and this is not always easy.

Future Hospital at Home schemes will be competing for resources with the traditional hospital services. Movement of money from one provider to another is most unlikely, especially when the two providers are probably NHS Trusts which are already in competition with each other and struggling with inadequate resources. Despite the apparent enthusiasm from the Government and the NHS Executive for extra community care, staff and services are expected to provide more care with no increase in resources. Hospital services will be keen to demonstrate their ability to provide outreach services into the community as a cost-effective way of providing enhanced care at home with no loss of their budget.

District nurses will need to be able to articulate their expertise and special skills and knowledge and show their ability to adapt and change as the needs and requirements of the patients change. They need to be able to demonstrate that their service offers value for money. They need to be able to measure clinical outcomes, to develop robust dependency tools and they need to reflect critically on their practical and political role in the future of health care provision. Research into the effects of nursing interventions and the contribution of nursing to health status must be integral to the philosophy of community nursing care.

Hospital at Home projects must prove themselves to be an appropriate means of delivering care and not just one of the current trendy issues in nursing or health care practice. It must be the expert in community nursing who takes these issues forward by being more skilled, knowledgeable, clinically expert and politically aware. Community nurses have a unique function described by McIntosh (1985) in being the group of nurses placed in a situation where they understand the consequences of early discharge on patients and their carers. They are the experts on the effects of nursing in deprived circumstances, of the needs of the frail elderly, of the special problems of nursing at home and of the effects of community care. The opportunity to use and articulate these special skills must not be lost.

The experience of setting up a new model of community nursing services in partnership with other agencies has highlighted the difficulties of demonstrating value for money, improved outcomes of care and changed attitudes. The Community High Dependency Service has provided at the time of writing almost two years of an enhanced model of district nursing service delivery and an alternative to institutional care. Marks (1990) suggests that Hospital at Home services should not be seen just as services to promote discharge or prevent admission. As they are unlikely to save huge amounts of money they should be seen as a final argument for providing services with humanitarian and good clinical grounds. The future of this service however seems to be in the hands of the purchasers, not in the hands of the users or the nursing profession.

Points to consider

1. What strategies should nurses use to demonstrate effective clinical care outcomes of the services that they provide? Did this project do this?

2. Why must managers/planners and providers of new services take into account management of change theories? Did this project do this?

3. Why is there a belief that patients are better cared for at home and is this belief borne out? How can community nurses influence changes in care provision?

4. If you were setting up a Hospital at Home service would you select a particular client group? If so, which group and why?

References

Audit Commission, 1992: *Homeward bound: a new course for community health*. London: HMSO.

Bennis, W.G., Benne, K.D., Chinn, R. *et al.* 1976: *The planning of change*. London: Holt Rinehart and Winston.

Calkin, C. and Pierpoint, B. 1989: A joint response. In Bernard, M. and Glendennig, F. (eds), *Community care for older people; strategies for the 1990s*. Stoke on Trent: Beth Johnson Foundation Publications in association with the Centre for Social Gerontology, University of Keele, 47-57.

DOH, 1989a: *Caring for people*. London: HMSO.

DOH, 1989b: *Working for patients*. London: HMSO.

DOH, 1991: *The patient's charter*. London: HMSO.

DOH, 1992: *The health of the nation*. London: HMSO.

DOH, 1993: *New world new opportunities, nursing in primary health care*. London: HMSO.

DHSS, 1986: *Neighbourhood nursing – a focus for care*. London: HMSO.

Durham, J. and Durham, G. 1990: Alternatives to the admission of some elderly patients to acute medical beds. *New Zealand Medical Journal*, **103**, 481–4.

Few, S. 1995: Post operative wound care at home. *Community Nurse*, **1**, 6, July, 33–4.

Hackman, B. 1993: There's no place like home. *Nursing Times*, **89**, 37, 28–30.

Hughes, J. and Gordon, P. 1992: *An optimal balance, primary health care and acute hospital services in London*. London: King's Fund Centre.

Hyde, V. 1995: In Cain, P., Hyde, V. and Howkins, E. (eds), *Community nursing: dimensions and dilemmas*. London: Edward Arnold.

Jennings, P. 1994: Learning through experience, an evaluation of 'Hospital at Home'. *Journal of Advanced Nursing*, **19**, 905–11.

Kessels-Buickhuisen, M., Wesseling, M. and Vissers, J. 1994: Home comforts. *Health Service Journal*, 3rd March, 24–7.

Knowelden, J., Westlake, L., Wright, K.G. and Clarke, S.J. 1991: Peterborough Hospital at Home; an evaluation. *Journal of Public Health Medicine*, **13**, 3, 182–8.

Marks, L. 1990: Hospital care at home: prospects and pitfalls. *Health Care UK*, 106–11.

McIntosh, J.B., 1985: District nursing: a case of political marginality. In White, R. (ed.), *Political issues in nursing, past, present and future*, Vol. 1. London: Wiley.

Mowat, I.G. and Morgan, R.T.T. 1982: Peterborough Hospital at Home scheme. *British Medical Journal*, **284**, 641–3.

NHSME/North West Thames RHA, 1990: *Nursing in the community. The Roy Report*. London: HMSO.

NHSME, 1990: *Successful project management for a resource management project*, Trio 1, General guidelines for resource management projects under Prince. London: HMSO.

Smith, R. (ed.) 1992: *Audit in action*, London: British Medical Journal.

18 Nurse prescribing

Marion Brew

Nurse prescribing became a reality in 1992 but as this chapter suggests progress in implementing it has been reduced to a minimum. This chapter looks at the political history leading up to nurse prescribing before discussing the financial review and subsequent very limited implementation.

There then follows some discussion on the reaction by the medical profession, as well as the mixed response by nurses themselves, who considered the Crown Report's recommendation to be divisive by allowing only qualified district nurses and health visitors to undertake initial prescribing from a limited nurses' formulary.

Professional boundaries are considered and suggestions made as to how professionals can overcome these.

Issues and concerns regarding how competence is assessed to prescribe are discussed fully with emphasis placed on the requirements of the Statutory Body to protect the public at all times. There is little doubt that this aspect of client care will become part of the nurse's role and it is important that nurses are not blown off course by what may seem in a few years' time as 'teething troubles'.

Nurse prescribing

'Prescribing nurses, what a preposterous idea. Physicians, pharmacists and patients of by-gone years would gasp in amazement at the very thought' (Rawlings, 1990, p. 12).

This comment could easily apply to many areas of nursing as it is practised today. Over the years, in response to a challenging health care system, nurses have developed many new approaches to practice which are designed to maximize their therapeutic role and achieve optimum health outcomes for their patients and clients. Nurse prescribing is but one of these changes and needs to be considered in the wider context of nursing as a whole. According to McMahon (1991) nursing is concerned with the provision of care which is dynamic in nature. This approach has the patient's health as its prime objective and takes account of the uniqueness of each individual in relation to issues such as self-care ability, self-esteem and self-determination. Within this context, it is argued that the ability to prescribe would allow nurses to improve the delivery of speedy and effective care within the community setting.

This chapter explores the background to the nurse prescribing debate, explains its current status and offers some pointers to the future.

Political history

Before discussing the wider implications of nurse prescribing and considering some of the issues arising out of the debate, it is useful to review the recent history relating to the political arena into which nurse prescribing was introduced, and examine some of the legal and political processes which have been involved to date. In 1986, when Baroness Cumbelege chaired a working group which was charged with examining community nursing, the Government was already in the process of reviewing the health care system as a whole. This was felt to be necessary due to the fact that the social, political and economic climate which prevailed in 1948 when the National Health Service was established, had changed beyond recognition. Thus, the analysis of community nursing services was one part of a larger exercise. Every community nurse is familiar with the report which resulted from this wide-ranging review – *Neighbourhood Nursing – A Focus for Care* (DHSS, 1986). One of the findings in the report was that time was being wasted when community nurses had to wait for prescriptions to be signed by general practitioners (GPs) before they could continue to provide appropriate treatment. As a result of this particular finding, the Report recommended that qualified community nurses should have the authority to prescribe in certain circumstances. This may go some way towards explaining the reason why the move for nurse prescribing focuses on community nursing, that is, the move emanated from, and was driven by, a review of community nursing.

Following this recommendation, the Government White Paper *Promoting Better Health* (DOH, 1987) advised that consultation between the standing medical, nursing, midwifery and pharmaceutical advisory committees should begin and members of these groups were nominated to establish a Nurse Prescribing Advisory Group, which had as its guiding principle the consideration of what is best for patient care, both in terms of clinical effectiveness and convenience for patients and their carers (DOH, 1989, cl. 1.11). The Report from the Advisory Group was published in 1989 (*The Crown Report*) and concluded that nurses had a central role in caring for patients at home, but were unable to write prescriptions for products which were essential for the care of these patients. In the Report, the Advisory Group made recommendations relating to practice, education, administration, legislation, communication and public safety, and envisaged three sets of circumstances where nurses should be able to prescribe to improve patient care. These are:

- Initial prescribing for individual patients where the nurse is the responsible practitioner;

- Prescribing for the care of patients within a group protocol;
- Prescribing for the care of patients within an individual protocol.

Furthermore, the Report recommended that only those nurses with a United Kingdom Central Council (UKCC) recognized qualification in district nursing or health visiting should be authorized to undertake the independent activity of prescribing. Other specialist nurses working in the community could, in certain circumstances, alter the timing and dosage of drugs and supply items within predetermined protocols. The rationale behind this decision was that district nurses and health visitors were the only nurses, at that time, who were required to undertake a period of further study within a higher education institution. Therefore, it would be possible for the necessary preparatory education to be incorporated into existing educational programmes. This situation has obviously altered radically at the time of writing, and raises many questions surrounding the issue of who should be allowed to prescribe. Many nurses would argue this is 'restrictive' and 'illogical' and the right to prescribe should be determined instead by the individual's role and competence.

Although this Report was published in 1989, it was not until 1992 that the legislation permitting nurse prescribing received Royal Assent through a Private Members Bill. The Medicinal Products: Prescription by Nurses Act (1992) amends the Medicine Act of 1968 and Section 41 of the National Health Service Act, 1977. These amendments, which are the main focus of the Bill, will enable retail pharmacists to dispense medicinal products listed in the nurses formulary which was devised as a result of a study of items for which community nurses generated prescriptions. These items were, in fact, often requested by community nurses and merely 'rubber stamped' by general practitioners. This legislation is necessary in order to protect the public safety and ensure that only properly educated and prepared nurses may undertake the responsibility for prescribing.

Financial review and delays

The delay which accompanied the passing of the Private Members Bill in 1992, which is also linked to the delay in the implementation of country-wide nurse prescribing, is largely attributed to uncertainty surrounding the potential costs of introducing the practice throughout the UK. In 1991, in an attempt to estimate the costs and benefits associated with implementation, the Department of Health commissioned Touche Ross to undertake a cost–benefit analysis (DOH, 1991). A preliminary assessment of the background to nurse prescribing identified that, although potential costs and benefits associated with nurse prescribing had been noted frequently, the actual costs and benefits had not. It therefore seemed reasonable to proceed with the analysis. This cost–benefit analysis concluded that the implementation of nurse prescribing would generate a net increase in prescribing at a time when prescribing costs were rising. It is, of course, true that politicians were concerned that an increase in prescribers would in turn escalate costs. Conversely, it could be argued that community nurses would be signing prescriptions which, in the past, the GP would have been asked to sign, thus only substituting prescribing rather than causing an actual increase. However, the expected costs need to be compared with the expected benefits, such as time saving for the community nurse and delivering more responsive treatment to clients and patients. In view of this, and as a result of the passing of the Bill, Baroness Cumberlege, by now Parliamentary Under Secretary for Health, announced that demonstration sites for nurse prescribing would be established by 1994, thus enabling the exploration of the clinical, managerial and financial implications of nurse prescribing. This, it was argued, would give nurses an opportunity to demonstrate how nurse prescribing could be both cost effective and provide measurable benefits in patient care.

Reaction by the medical profession

Change is often considered a slow and painful process and working patterns exist which are often long established through custom and practice. There is little evidence of the reaction of the medical profession to this fundamental shift in how prescriptions are obtained. It is possible that GPs may see this activity as an encroachment on their doctor–patient relationship since visiting the GP often results in obtaining a prescription. This is a powerful territorial issue and nurses would be politically naive to underestimate the reaction from other professionals to this issue. The limited nature of the nurse formulary agreed by the Department of Health where the committee consisted largely of doctors may have been one reason for the lack of interest by the GPs. In simplistic terms, the nurses formulary consists mainly of items used in wound care management, bowel and bladder management and simple analgesics which are all readily available to buy from the high street pharmacists. Since the original nurses formulary was published, six 'Prescription only Medicines' (POMs) have been added and one could argue that there is scope for further expansion. One current issue encouraging nurse prescribing concerns the hours and activities of junior doctors which are under scrutiny. This may provide some explanation for the Government's agreement to go ahead with the demonstration sites, since it would be feasible for some tasks to be delegated to nurses who are a cheaper form of labour than doctors.

Why limit prescribing to district nurses and health visitors?

Although the decisions discussed previously involve other professions, it is within the nursing profession itself that nurse prescribing causes the most heated debate. The importance of setting a required standard of educational competence cannot be overemphasized, and the wisdom of limiting prescribing powers to certain nurses, at this time, seems obvious. It has been argued that other community nurses besides qualified district nurses and health visitors are clinically competent and patient care would be enhanced if the nurse prescribed. Nurse-led clinics are now very much part of the work of the primary health care team. These are often run by nurse practitioners and practice nurses, some of whom have undergone rigorous training in specialties such as asthma, diabetes and women's health. It seems a natural and desirable progression for such nurses to be able to prescribe in those areas in which they are competent and have specialist knowledge. Nurse practitioners are presently a small group within the nursing profession but one which attracts nurses who are willing to challenge current issues and bring about change. One such group, working within an inner city area with single homeless people, has incorporated a list of drugs alongside a locally agreed statement which defines the standard management of certain categories of patients and conditions. These drugs can be supplied to initiate treatment for identified conditions following nursing assessment and under the direction of a doctor. Projects such as this need to work within the legal framework and confines of the Medicines Act of 1968, and involve lengthy consultation processes. Implementation requires the commitment of highly motivated and committed nurses. Lynch (1990) suggests that other community-based nurses such as community psychiatric nurses (CPN) have not undertaken a post-registration course and that as many as 70 per cent of CPNs have no additional educational preparation for community practice.

This then is the political background against which nurse prescribing is being introduced and tested. What has occurred to date is history. What is important now is that community nurses are aware of the political and economic climate in which nurse prescribing, if implemented, will be required to survive. There are many issues which arise out of the debate surrounding nurse prescribing and, like most good debates, discussion usually raises more questions than answers. The key current issues include the real costs and benefits, the notion of empowerment and control, boundaries between professionals, the anomaly of limiting prescribing rights to district nurses and health visitors and the need to respond to a rapidly changing health care situation, while dealing with a legal and political system which can involve extremely protracted processes. Radical changes within the health care system over the last 10 years, producing an entirely new range of jargon, has made it difficult to use the Medicines Act (1968) effectively. Legislation is not keeping pace with the trends and phrases in the Act are no longer meaningful, making interpretation difficult and confusing. The shift in the focus of care from hospital to community settings has altered the meaning of health care, and legislation intended for a 'hospital orientated' health service is now being interpreted locally, leading to a lack of consistency among trusts, particularly Community Trusts. There is also a considerable contrast between hospital and community practice. Patients may be 'positively inconvenienced' (Young, 1990) because community nurses have to obtain a prescription for the supply of products which a hospital sister could obtain from supplies. Certain items, particularly with regard to prescriptions for wound care items, may not be available on prescription. This may cause the patient to feel the hospital can offer a 'superior' service.

It is also important to remember that this particular development is only one initiative in an arena where the leading bodies in nursing are striving to strengthen the structure and raise the standard of post-registration education. Current educational programmes for nurses are reflecting the changing environment in which health care is delivered, and also address political developments within the United Kingdom as well as in the wider international community (UKCC, 1990). The UKCC also contends that, in order to rise above the turmoil and uncertainty in health care, nurses must be willing to change traditional attitudes in practice and so shape a future for the lasting benefit of patients and clients. This kind of 'new animal' (UKCC, 1986) needs to be acutely aware of the debate surrounding nurse prescribing in order that the profession as a whole can contribute to the outcome which best meets the ideals of nursing practice and benefits patient care.

Costs and benefits

It is stated by the Department of Health that nurse prescribing is being introduced at no extra cost to the NHS as it would be considered to be substitute prescribing and, as such, the funding is already within the NHS. This is certainly the overwhelming message from the Department of Health which agreed that demonstration sites for nurse prescribing could be set up. There is, as a result, an expectation that those nurses involved in the project will continually consider the costs involved. The Department have made the message clear that, should the exercise prove to be too costly, it is unlikely that nurse prescribing will be given the 'go ahead'.

In a recent development, district nurses in Sweden are now prescribing and, according to the Chairman of the Swedish Society on General Medicine, Dr Jonas Sjorgreen (1994), 'allowing District Nurses to prescribe will presumably lead to increased prescriptions' (p. 1077). He is also keen to point out that a prescription represents the sum of medical judgment. 'It assumes that one can examine the patient, evaluate differential diagnoses and make a correct diagnosis. Nurses are not qualified to do this' (p. 1077). Should this prescription prove to be accurate in the United Kingdom, this would provide another reason why nurse prescribing may not be implemented.

Nurse prescribing has led to the review of many existing administrative systems including budgets. Although costs should never be the only consideration when prescribing, it cannot be ignored. Information about nurse prescribing will be fed back in much the same way as it is to GPs at present.

The Prescription Pricing Agency (PPA) is a special health authority within the NHS which processes 400 million prescription items a year at a value of £3.3 (Bottomley, 1990). It makes up 10 per cent of the total expenditure of the NHS. It checks prices and authorizes payments to contractors for the dispensing of NHS prescriptions. Finally, it provides information about NHS prescribing and dispensing, excluding prescriptions, in various forms to health authorities/health commissions. The cost of the practice nurse prescriptions can be charged against the GP budget since the practice nurse is directly employed by the GP.

Of the three major information projects conducted by the PPA, the 'PACT' is the most relevant to the nurse prescriber. It will allow employers to audit prescribing trends and expenditure for individual nurse prescribers. At present, PACT information can improve GPs' services to patients, enabling them to review prescribing habits and costs and develop and monitor prescribing policies within the practice. It also allows GPs to compare themselves with colleagues in the same area and nationally. Finally, it should improve the cost effectiveness of prescribing within the practice. In order to clarify budget arrangements, the practice nurse who has a district nursing or health visiting qualification, and has undertaken training to become a nurse prescriber, will dispense items on a lilac form and district nurses and health visitors employed by a Community Trust will use green forms.

Since no precedent exists, the demonstration sites will be able to explore the best way to set contracts so that future participants in nurse prescribing can benefit from the experiences and outcomes of the demonstrating sites. As in all new developments in contracting, the data for the first contract needs to be based on historical activity. Patterns and emerging trends after the first year will provide the basis for further work in the area. In order to help set budgets for district nurses and health visitors employed by a provider unit, analysis of the caseload of current patient needs and their prescriptions will help to identify which items are from the nurses formulary. This tracking process will use different forms of data to establish the likely numbers of prescriptions generated by community nurses to enable resources to be transferred from the practice to the provider unit. Although not entirely accurate, it will provide some useful information, and as patterns are established this can be fine tuned.

In the case of community-based district nurses and health visitors, the cost of their prescriptions will need to be built into the contract which the GP has with the provider unit. This will inevitably lead to existing contracts being re-negotiated to effect a transfer of resources to the community provider. There is no easy way to calculate the appropriate level of resources to be transferred so they will have to be reviewed over time in the light of experience.

Many benefits of nurse prescribing should certainly be demonstrated as a result of the evaluation of the project. Nurses will be more familiar with the products and package size, which means that prescribing powers for nurses could minimalize waste, and should avoid practices such as requesting far more than is appropriate for certain clients in order to stock-pile for emergencies. There is a problem of use of inappropriate dressings as an immediate measure because appropriate resources are not available, leading to an extra visit being required when the correct resources do become available. Nurse prescribing should also help to stamp out another practice which clearly flaunts the UKCC Standards for the Administration of Medicines (1992a). Namely, the situation wherein urgently required items are supplied by the pharmacist before a valid prescription is presented.

Costs and benefits are, therefore, not only a matter of finance, but can introduce a variety of issues which need to be analysed more fully in order to decide the most appropriate way forward.

Professional boundaries

The impact of changes such as nurse prescribing will affect not only nurses themselves but other health professionals with whom they work. The Royal Pharmaceutical Society supports, in principle, prescribing by community nurses in appropriate circumstances, and they recommend developing professional links with the community nurse and the high street pharmacist (Gape, 1990). Over the last few years, pharmacists have been encouraged to play a wider role in health care by advising patients in the treatment of minor ailments. Thus, the question arises as to whether pharmacists should be granted prescribing rights for some products. There has been political debate in recent years as the charges for prescription items have increased. Changes in what products can be purchased 'over the counter' are seen by the public as an attempt to reduce the prescribing bill and encourage individuals to consult the pharmacist and buy proprietary products. Doctors too will be affected as, in a general practice setting, there is often an agreed list of prescribable products which allows fundholding practices to work within agreed drug budgets. It would therefore require good communication and teamwork for safe, effective nurse prescribing.

It is a prerequisite that good communication exists between nurses, doctors and their patients, and that local guidelines are laid down to include pharmacists. There must be an understanding of which records should be kept and clear protocols need to be developed for writing prescriptions. Record keeping is an intrinsic part of the professional care of the patient, essential for recalling earlier treatments and changes in the patient's condition as well as for communication with colleagues. It has been necessary to design and agree protocols covering every aspect of nurse prescribing. The protocols are essential in ensuring that the standards are followed and are within the legislative boundaries. Multidisciplinary involvement has been essential in preparing and agreeing them. GPs in particular must be prepared to recognize the role of protocols, or there may be considerable pressure on nurses to work outside their competence and the recognized guidelines.

Health care takes place within a complex environment in which many professionals are involved. Teamwork is encouraged with primary health care teams functioning as a whole to provide a more effective service for patients and clients. An essential part of teamwork involves understanding roles within the team, keeping team members up to date and ensuring that colleagues, particularly GPs and pharmacists, are well informed regarding nurse prescribing. The impact of nurse prescribing may be perceived in both positive and negative terms by those involved. For instance, on the plus side, nurse prescribing may mean that GPs save the time that they would normally spend discussing and signing prescriptions for nurses. It could mean that their job satisfaction will improve as they have more time available for patient consultations. They may, however, feel it a disadvantage as it might mean less contact with certain patients and reduce the opportunity to discuss other issues of concern with the district nurse or health visitor. In a team situation, assertiveness and negotiation regarding nurse prescribing are vital in agreeing protocols. Nurse prescribing will affect GPs, pharmacists and other nurses including specialist nurses within the team and it is important that there are highly efficient shared systems of records if nurse prescribing is to work. New opportunities will emerge for team members to work more closely together and each professional group will need to be particularly vigilant in order to ensure multiple and possible conflicting prescriptions are not issued. Careful assessment of all factors involved in the decision-making process before prescribing is essential.

Competence for nurse prescribing

Despite the fact that the issue of nurse prescribing was raised as early as 1986, it was not until November 1993 that the decision to have eight demonstration sites from the 1st September 1994 was announced, the results of the project to be evaluated and announced after one year. Almost overnight a flurry of activity was generated to move this project forward. The eight demonstration sites were selected from fundholding GP practices in each health region in England. The speed of project siting generated a requirement for an intensive training programme to achieve the required degree of professional competence. It is hoped that opportunities will be made available to enable these practitioners to reflect on their practice, and to use situations from within practice to enhance their knowledge of prescribing. Certainly nurses need some knowledge of pharmacology if they are fully to understand the implications of their prescribing and be aware of the long-term effects. The responsibility of prescribing requires proficiency in the prescriber to be able to make a differential diagnosis. Nurses may prescribe by rote unless adequate funding, adequate education and training and effective demonstration of competence and safety to carry out this activity can be assured. It will fall within the remit of the UKCC to establish and identify authorized nurse prescribers on the register and to make information from it readily available to bona fide enquirers.

The UKCC has a statutory duty to maintain standards of professional practice, and the Code of Professional Conduct (1994) constitutes strong guidance to registered practitioners. The UKCC and the National Boards have defined the standards to be achieved and thus determined the level of competence required for specific activities. Professional assessment of competence often involves undertaking an approved course, gaining individual certification for specific tasks and being entrusted to undertake this activity. This situation was radically changed by publication of the UKCC document *The Scope of Professional Practice* in 1992b. This emphasizes the nurse's professional accountability and places decisions about the boundaries of practice in the hands of the individual practitioner. This is linked to Clause 4 of the UKCC Code of Conduct (1994) which requires nurses to acknowledge the limits of their competence. Any function, including nurse prescribing, must be within these limits. In this new way of working, nurses would be responsible for assessing their competence and mechanisms such as standard setting, audits and peer review should be developed. Nursing is still very much in a transitional state in this field. The real test of the development of nursing as a profession and the scope of professional practice will be the extent to which nurses not only take on the responsibility for additional tasks, but also achieve authority over the nature of this practice. Much is written about the tendency for nurses to expand their role by assuming responsibility for many aspects of patients' management which may have been handed down by medical colleagues.

One of the key risks associated with nurse prescribing must surely be the need to safeguard the patient. The profession has chosen to record on the Professional Register those who are nurse prescribers at a time when *The Scope of Professional Practice* advocates the rejection of specific task related competencies and certification in favour of a more general individual responsibility for personal development. Knowledge of prescribing following assessment and diagnosis has traditionally been undertaken by doctors. New possibilities will be created as nurses learn to make differential diagnoses using appropriate assessment skills and tools to reach decisions regarding the practice of nursing.

As a nurse prescriber, an individual will have authority to make prescribing decisions and these will have to be justified. Accountability is at the core of nurse prescribing, and provides a new dimension in which to demonstrate awareness of the implications of nurse prescribing in terms of responsibility and accountability based on individual patient assessment and care. Nurses need to be professionally and legally accountable for their actions and knowledge of the actual product prescribed is only part of the picture. This knowledge has to be assessed in the context of the following:

- the patient's circumstances including current medication
- the patient's past medical history
- the patient's current and anticipated health status
- thorough knowledge of the item to be prescribed, its therapeutic action, side effects, dosage and interaction
- thorough knowledge of alternatives to prescribing
- frequency of use in a variety of circumstances.

Health professionals are increasingly working with a more educated and assertive population. This may result in patients asking for a prescription in a situation when a nurse prescriber may not be able to make a fully informed decision, perhaps because of lack of resources or information. Many GPs will admit that it is very easy to prescribe as it satisfies the patient's wishes. Nurses, as prescribers, may have to face the same pressures and decisions. It is important, therefore, that the patient's needs are fully assessed before any prescriptions are issued.

Assessment of competence is a debate within nursing which is ongoing. Some nurses might argue that nurse prescribing should be a developmental aspect of the role of the nurse and that the UKCC and the English National Board (ENB) have gone 'too far' in separating this activity from many others which are carried out by nurses accountable and responsible for their practice. It is no surprise, therefore, that considerable discussion involving the project planning team from the Department of Health, the medical profession, the pharmaceutical profession, the ENB and educational institutions took place. It was decided that competence could best be demonstrated by a multifaceted approach and that assessments of student knowledge related to nurse prescribing must include a formal written assessment. This could consist of short questions and answers, with a second part providing short case studies which should give students an opportunity to demonstrate the decision-making process in relation to prescribing. In keeping with most courses, accreditation points can also be considered. On successful completion of the assessment, the nurse prescriber's entry on the UKCC Register will be annotated to signify qualification to prescribe from the nurses formulary (DOH, 1989).

Nurses are trained to focus on health promotion and facilitate self-care with their patients and clients and nurse prescribing should be seen within this context. According to Smith and Ross (1992), nurses are already skilled in many other therapeutic options and the decision to prescribe should always take account of these possible alternatives. Many items included in the nurses formulary are already available 'over the counter' and it may be that, when the nurse prescribes, the public will expect safe products and will not question their suitability.

Nurse prescribing: possible outcomes

The current project has placed the eight demonstration sites within GP fundholding practices. This will provide a particular type of data, but may not acknowledge the possible advantages and disadvantages of nurse prescribing involving those clients not necessarily registered with a GP. Nurse prescribing is a new experience for district nurses and health visitors and, therefore, full evaluation of the demonstration sites will be required. It will be important to explore the clinical, managerial and financial aspects of nurse prescribing before this activity is generally adopted.

There is anecdotal evidence to suggest that prescribing nurses remain frustrated in their efforts to provide an effective service to clients. The limited nature of the nurses formulary means that the patients may need prescriptions from GPs of regular medications, as well as those prescriptions issued by the nurse for the management of other treatments such as wound care. This in effect prevents the client from gaining the full benefits of nurse prescribing, and may, in some cases, increase the administration required to receive appropriate treatment. Throughout the year of the demonstration site project, prescribing nurses have been asked by the Department of Health to draw up a 'wish list'. This will help to identify items which would have been prescribed in given situations, had the nurses been able to do so. At present, the nurses formulary is limited and clearly results in dissatisfaction. The list will inevitable extend, but how this will come about remains unclear, and the extent to which the formulary will be expanded remains to be seen.

While the idea of nurse prescribing has met with a great deal of support, it has not been universally welcomed. Some nurses and doctors alike have expressed reservations, fearing that it would in fact be counter-productive and actually take the nurse away from patient care. It is possible that time saved through nurses having prescribing powers could be taken up with extra paperwork created by its introduction. The proposed nurses formulary has been criticized in that it is too restrictive (Payne, 1994) and does not reflect the products used by nurses in practice. It will have to be regularly evaluated and monitored to ensure that the items contained within it are appropriate. Allowing nurses to prescribe may give them the political power to persuade the Department of Health to sanction the inclusion of new items. It is hoped that nurse prescribing will promote the development of a service which is more responsive to patient's needs, and that it will eventually extend to other groups of nurses.

Conclusion

Nurse prescribing is an exciting initiative which has the potential to alter practice for the benefit of patients and clients. However, community nurses need to demonstrate that they will use the power effectively and prove, beyond doubt, that the right to prescribe will result in improvements in the care of patients in the community setting. Only then will the initiative progress and be developed. The evaluation of nurse prescribing in the eight demonstration sites will provide indicators for practice, but it will be the responsibility of individual nurses within individual trusts to help shape and develop practice in response to recommendations. This will require a significant commitment from highly motivated and competent practitioners and educators.

Points to consider

1 Nurses are increasingly looking for other approaches through the use of protocols. Many community pharmacists express concern regarding the legal position raised by this approach. This expediency may weaken the issue and prevent nurses taking responsibility and accountability for their actions.

2 Consideration of not only the process of implementing this activity but explaining how the outcome will benefit the client and family as well as to the nursing profession.

3 It is important to stress that the benefits of this project should not be judged entirely by cost. Evaluation methods have a focus on the costs of the exercise: colleagues, particularly GPs, need to be supportive to ensure there is every opportunity to develop this area of patient care. Changes in attitude are required to give nurses the confidence that is required. Prejudices have to be tackled and addressed before nurse prescribing becomes a widespread reality.

4 The benefits to patients need to be highlighted and are potentially significant.

5 What are the implications of an incremental approach to implementation of this scheme? Nurses may lose out by the stalling of the politicians.

Points that had to be considered during the movement towards reality

1 Nurses may become disenfranchized by the medical lobby and politicians. This would weaken the case for nurse prescribing. The proposed nurse prescribing offers health visitors and district nurses the ability to prescribe within their own professional judgement and make appropriate decisions.

2 Nurses amongst themselves must agree that there is a need to open this activity to other groups of equally qualified practitioners.

3 In the light of evidence based practice, it has to be asked if nurse prescribing will become a reality. The benefits are difficult to measure and nurse prescribing needs to be able to meet the criteria in providing evidence that this activity will allow nurses to be more effective in meeting clients' needs, and that clients and families will benefit from a more responsive service.

Points *continued*

4 The outcome of the demonstration sites will take some time to complete. In the meantime, the initial evidence needs to be considered when reviewing whether this initiative for nurses will become adopted throughout the UK and extended to other groups of nurses. The Department of Health is being urged by particular groups of nurses, for example family planning nurses and practice nurses, to extend nurse prescribing, pointing out that these nurses influence GP prescriptions in many areas such as asthma and diabetes.

5 In January 1996 the Department of Health announced that further demonstration sites for nurse prescribing would get underway on 1st April 1996. The chosen geographical area was the Community Health Trust, Bolton, and would involve both fundholding and non-fundholding GP practices in an attempt to widen the scope of this new venture for a further 70 health visitors and district nurses.

6 Published accounts of the evaluation of the initial eight sites is not yet available. Since completion of the initial project in October 1995, the profession is awaiting a report from the University of York where the focus of the research is the cost effectiveness of nurse prescribing. Anecdotal reports suggest that there is great variations of costs on a national basis. The Government made it clear that there is no new money for nurse prescribing. The money is already in the system, as it is substitute, not new, prescribing which is advocated.

7 A qualitative research project carried out by Liverpool University will take longer to emerge and is likely to explore issues such as client/patient satisfaction with nurse prescribing as well as considering the perceptions of the GPs and nurses involved. Unofficial reports suggest that most parties involved consider that nurse prescribing is more responsive to clients' needs, provides nurses with a greater sense of professionalism and frees the GP from clerical duties.

8 Measurement of the effectiveness has yet to be demonstrated but nurse prescribers are aware that the major challenge is to prove the value of their expert contribution in the area.

References

Bottomley, V. 1990: Nurse prescribing deferred. *District Nursing Association UK*, **10**, 3, 13.

DOH 1968: *Medicine Act*. London: DOH.

DOH 1977: *National Health Service Act*. London: DOH.

DOH 1986: *Cumberlege report – neighbourhood nursing – a focus for care*. London: DHSS.

DOH 1987: *Promoting better: the government programme for improving health care*. London: HMSO.

DOH 1989: *Report of the advisory group on nurse prescribing: the Crown Report*. London: HMSO.

DOH/Touche Ross 1991: *Nursing prescribing: final report – a cost benefit study*. London: HMSO.

DOH 1992: *The medicinal products: Prescription by Nurse Act*. London: DOH.

Gape, E. 1990: The nurse prescriber and the pharmacist. *Nursing Standard*, **5**, 2, 38.

Lynch, S. 1990: Who prescribes? *Nursing Times*, **86**, 9, 16–17.

McMahon, R. 1991: Therapeutic nursing theory, issues and practice. In McMahan, R. and Pearson, A. (eds), *Nursing as therapy*. London: Chapman and Hall.

Rawlings, M. 1990: A View from the Pharmacy. *Nursing Standard*, **4**, 44, 12.

Sjorgeen, J. 1994: *Lancet*, **344**, 15 October, 1077.

Smith, F. and Ross, F. 1992: Prescribing for pain. *Community Outlook*, **10**, 4–5.

UKCC 1991: *Report of the proposals for the future of community education and practice*. London: UKCC.

UKCC 1992a: *Standards for the administration of medicine*. London: UKCC.

UKCC 1992b: *The scope of professional practice for nurse, midwife and health visitor*. London: UKCC.

UKCC 1994: *Code of professional conduct for the nurse, midwife and health visitor*. London: UKCC.

Young, L. 1990: Nurse prescribing. *Journal of District Nursing*, **8**, 9, 2.

19 Nursing in Europe

Brian Pateman

It is perhaps true that most nurses have a better understanding of American health care systems than European, despite being members of the European Union since the 1970s. It appears that nurses, in common with the general public, have little understanding of Europe or of the influence of the European Union upon nursing.

There is some evidence of change and a growing interest within the UK in European nursing matters. European concerns are now frequently discussed in nursing literature and conferences. Several European nursing networks are now in existence for clinical and professional issues.

This chapter looks at the differing organizational and philosophical approaches to community nursing throughout Europe. There are lessons to be learned which are pertinent to the UK

The main part of this paper summarizes the issues for community nurses in Europe discussed at the University of Manchester, School of Nursing Studies, 1993 5th Annual Good Practices in Community Nursing Conference. A discussion on the significance of Europe to UK nursing and the impact of the European Union on nursing follows.

Issues for community nurses in Europe

Two key papers with European community nursing themes were presented at the conference. Salvage highlighted difficulties facing countries of eastern Europe and the newly independent states following the collapse of former communist regimes, and the role of the World Health Organization in European nursing. The second, by Verheij, examined the provision and organization of community nursing in Western Europe which compared and contrasted need and provision in our neighbouring countries France, Germany, the Netherlands and Belgium. Representation from nurses in Central and Eastern Europe enriched conference proceedings.

The themes of the key papers might be seen as a tale of two cultures, poorly resourced east taking advice from well organized and lavishly funded west. However, this is not entirely the case. Hands-on patient care is much the same in any of the countries and all are going through changes because of cost containment in some form. Some solutions that are being tried in other countries are pertinent to consider in the UK as they challenge the way we carry out care. Many countries, for example, see amalgamation of social and home nursing services as the best way to give truly holistic seamless care.

Jane Salvage, Regional Adviser for Nursing and Midwifery, World Health Organization Regional Office for Europe, points out that first it is important to clarify what is meant when we talk of Europe. It is possible to consider Europe in several ways: United Kingdom's neighbours, members of the European Union or members of the World Health Organization European Region. Salvage (1993) comments that the 'new Europe' is an exciting place – so exciting that it is hard to keep up with the pace of change. 'In the World Health Organisation, new member states are joining literally month by month. WHO's European Region stretches from Kamchatka in the east to the Canary Islands in the west, from Lapland in the north to Israel and Malta in the south' (p. 1).

Destruction of the Berlin Wall in 1989 and the collapse of the communist regimes in central and eastern Europe has played a major part in the rapid expanse of the new 'Europe'. These former USSR states and satellites, who have similar backgrounds in nursing and community nursing provision, are now looking to their European counterparts to help develop their services along 'European lines'. As these groups of countries face similar challenges it seems logical to address their needs as a homogeneous group, but readers must be aware that there is considerable variation between the needs of, say, East Germany and Estonia. It is also a mistake to believe that learning is one way, there is much the west can learn from the east.

Nursing in the Soviet model of health care was very subservient to the medical profession. Nurses have been taught and managed mainly by doctors. Head nurses were frequently doctors and doctors gave nursing orders. At the conference it was clear that nurses from the 'New Europe' were envious of the professional status of European and American nurses. They viewed organizations like the UKCC and the National Boards as means to achieve many of their aspirations and gave dire warnings to the more cynical UK delegates who expressed their frustration at these bodies, that life with is much better with than without professional organizations.

This theme of power, or rather the lack of it, was clearly identified by Salvage. She pointed out that even in a country like the United Kingdom which has a strong nursing representation with nurse or ex nurse MPs and nurse government advisors, nurses still have to fight to ensure their voice is heard. Nurses from both old and new Europe would do well to take note of Salvage's (1993) comment that 'Lack of formal power at the top is to be reflected elsewhere, for example in the absence of a nursing contribution to decision making in the health care team' (p. 4).

Primary health care in the new Europe

Clearly primary health care in east European states has had a much lower status than hospital care, the main roles are to act as a filter, deal with the lower level interventions and refer on to specialists. In certain areas of the former Soviet republics due to geographical vastness the main bulk of primary health care is carried out by Feldschers. Feldschers are a grade of health care worker almost unique to the former Soviet Union and can be likened to being midway between a nurse and a doctor. In city areas Feldschers can be found working in hospitals as paramedics or physicians' assistants, carrying out many duties that nurses in the UK consider as part of their daily work, dressings, medication, intravenous therapy, etc. They also perform extended role procedures that are increasingly being incorporated into UK nurses' work. Feldschers may be likened to the primary health care nurse practitioner in the USA. They are often the only health care provision in areas not attractive to doctors because of low salaries and extreme conditions. Usually these primary health care Feldschers are local women who return to their home community following training, working as respected community members and wise women. Salvage (1993) reports her findings of their worth following a visit to Kazakhstan and Kyrgyzstan and comments that 'the Feldscher was the front line of PHC, working in health centres in small rural towns and villages with a team of midwives and nurses, backed up by a visit from the doctor every so often. The Feldschers assess, diagnose and evaluate; they have some prescribing powers; they offer health advice and ante natal-care' (p. 8).

Unfortunately there is talk of decreasing, rather than developing the Feldscher role. International aid support is being directed at the provision of trained doctors, mirroring western primary health care. It is ironic that the west sees nurse practitioners as innovative yet the east views them as old fashioned. As Salvage (1993) notes 'Once again the work of the nurse is invisible and undervalued' (p. 8). The nurse practitioner and other community nurses in this country might learn much from the way Feldschers have developed their role.

The role of the World Health Organization in European nursing

The World Health Organization has done much to create a vision of the role of the European nurse and given clear understanding of nursing contribution to improving peoples' health. The famous WHO meeting at Alma Ata in 1978 identified that the primary health care approach was the best way to achieve health for all by the year 2000 (WHO, 1978). It was particularly notable as it focused on targets and needs of populations, not narrow professionalism. Figure 19.1 summarizes the six main themes of the 38 targets to be achieved in the health of WHO member states populations by the year 2000.

Primary health care at Alma Ata was not seen as simply gatekeeping or as the first point of contact with the health care system. Primary health care was seen as a much wider concept than health care and included provision

---

38 TARGETS – 6 MAIN THEMES:

1   **Equity**
    Reducing health inequalities within and between countries

2   **Health promotion**
    and prevention of disease

3   **Community partcipation**

4   **Multisectoral cooperation**

5   **International cooperation**

6   **Primary health care**
    Should be the focus of health care system – 'meeting the basic health needs
    of each community through services provided as close as possible to where
    people live and work, readily accessible and acceptable to all'

Figure 19.1 Health for all by the year 2000. *Source:* WHO (1978)

of those basic human rights and structures that underpin health, for example
food, transport, education, housing, etc. 'Health for all nurses' should be
liaising with and be active in assessing community need and not limit their
activities to illness-related assessments and interventions. Nurses should for
example be involved in ensuring that the water supplies are safe in
developed as well as underdeveloped countries, particularly if their client
groups are susceptible.

The first WHO European conference on nursing took place in Vienna in
1988, following which WHO published the conference findings, which
highlighted the mission for achieving health for all (Fig. 19.2). The mission
statement clearly advocates two points: the nurse's role in helping clients to
achieve their potential (nursing is seen as much more than crisis
intervention); and interventions should be community based.

There is little that nurses can disagree with in the WHO Health For All
Nursing's Mission, as most uphold the principles highlighted within it. It is
worthwhile to reflect on philosophical changes that inspired its creation and
to consider progress towards achieving the goals outlined. Salvage (1993)
states that:

The key concept underlying the development of the Health For All Nurse
is the need to create a nursing role which is appropriate to the needs of
the people, rather than to the needs of the health care system.
Fundamentally it means a transformation of the nurse's traditional role
as a servant to a doctor and general dogs body, into that of a well-
educated professional whose unique and distinctive contribution to health
care is respected by all colleagues and is regarded as an equal partner in
the health care team. The focus of her practice is not being a medical

To help individuals, families and groups to determine and achieve their physical, mental and social potential, and to do so in the context of the environment in which they live and work.

The nurse's functions:

• Promotion and maintenance of health

• Prevention of ill-health

• Care during illness and rehabilitation

This requires the nurse to:

1. Provide and manage direct nursing care
2. Teach patients and clients
3. Teach other health workers
4. Participate fully in the health care team
5. Develop nursing practice based on critical thinking and research

Figure 19.2 Health for all: nursing mission. *Source*: WHO (1993)

assistant, but working alongside the patient or community – jointly with other professionals where necessary – to improve people's health. (p. 13)

In an age of rapid change UK nurses must ensure the characteristics new Europeans see as a desirable role model are protected and developed and vice versa.

The second paper on the theme of European nursing at the 1993 good practices conference was presented by Verheij, a Dutch social scientist, who has investigated organizational structures in community nurses throughout Europe. This study was commissioned with intentions of informing the Netherlands Government of good practices in community nursing which they may wish to adopt in their health care reforms. The paper provided an overview of common concerns and solutions throughout Europe offering a refreshing non-nursing perspective.

Verheij makes the point that community nursing is much the same wherever it takes place. Patient care needs are much the same. A UK district nurse would soon feel at home taking over a Wijkverpleegkundige (home nurse) morning round in the Netherlands. Although superficially the same, there are major differences in the way community nurses are funded, organized and trained throughout Europe. If we accept that the European care needs are similar it is interesting to compare and contrast solutions as it allows us to stand back and reflect upon our own service. A difficult thing to do when one is immersed in the system.

To prove that health needs are similar, one needs to compare statistics of the countries concerned. Verheij commented on the demographic changes taking place in the over 65s, seeing this as a driving force for health care reform in many countries including our own. Table 19.1 illustrates that all countries are being faced with this problem in varying degrees. Note that the UK has one of the lowest predicted levels of growth of the over 65s. Verheij (1993) comments that 'A growing demand is of course not a problem as such. It only becomes one if this demand cannot be met by sufficient supply. And this is increasingly the case in many countries' (p. 32).

Table 19.1 Percentage of population over 65 in nine countries

	1987	2000	2010	Year 2020	2030	2040	2050
Norway	16.2	15.2	15.1	18.2	20.7	22.8	21.9
UK	15.3	14.5	14.6	16.3	19.2	20.4	18.7
Germany	15.1	17.1	20.4	21.7	25.8	27.6	24.5
Belgium	14.3	14.7	15.9	17.7	20.8	21.9	20.8
France	13.8	15.3	16.3	19.5	21.8	22.7	22.3
Finland	13.1	14.4	16.8	21.7	23.8	23.1	22.7
Netherlands	12.5	13.5	15.1	18.9	23.0	24.8	22.6
USA	12.3	12.2	12.8	16.2	19.5	19.8	19.3
Canada	10.7	12.8	14.6	18.6	22.4	22.5	21.3

Source: Verheij (1993) p. 31

Solutions to the increasing demand for community care and cost containment

The problem faced by all countries in Europe, if not the world, is how to deal with increasing health care demand and contain costs. Verheij suggests four main solutions that have been applied to community nursing and uses these to form a framework to discuss the major solutions as applied in different countries (Fig. 19.3).

Funding	By limiting the cost of a unit of care, it may be possible to do more with less money
Cooperation	By means of more cooperation the work can be made more efficient
Division of tasks	By developing a more efficient way of dividing tasks among various types of personnel, more can be done with the same budget. The generalist–specialist dilemma and levels of expertise are highly related topics
Attractiveness of the profession	Making the work of home nurse more attractive and increasing the workforce

Figure 19.3   Verheij's solutions. *Source:* Verheij (1993)

Funding

Not surprisingly it appears that how nurses are funded makes a great difference to what nurses do. If payment for psychosocial and preventive activities is low or non-existent it appears to be a direct correlation in the nurse's activities. There is a truism in the saying 'he who pays the piper calls the tune'.

It is not only who pays for nursing care but methods of reimbursement for nursing activities that makes a difference. Verheij identifies two types of reimbursement for nursing activities, fee for service and fixed budget. Figure 19.4 shows which country uses which.

Fee for service	Fixed budget
Belgium	UK
Germany	Finland
USA	Norway
France (partly)	Netherlands
	Canada
	France (partly)

Figure 19.4   Verheij's types of reimbursement. *Source*: Verheij (1993)

Fee for service reimbursement

There are various types of fees for service reimbursements. In its simplest form there is a list of tasks and procedures with fixed costs, similar to Diagnostic Related Groups in the USA. In France this list is known as a 'Nomenclature'. If the care given is on the list, the cost of the treatment or nursing agency fees can be claimed back from the Government by the patient. Some nurses are employed by charity status organizations who claim fees directly so none or only supplementary costs are incurred by patients. Verheij notes that nomenclatures of several countries covers mainly technical tasks. The result is that psychosocial and preventive activities are performed less often in Belgium than in the Netherlands which has a fixed budget system similar to the UK.

Reimbursement can also be based on the number of home visits undertaken. In Germany there is a distinction between hygienic care 'Grundpflege' and technical care 'Behandlungspflege' which are reimbursed at different rates. The effect on the work activities of community nurses is obvious.

A third type of fee for service is based on the number of days of patient care; this forms part of the system in Belgium reducing the potential discrimination of the long-term dependent patient under the 'nomenclature' system.

Fixed budgets

The fixed budget system of payment is found in the UK, Finland, Norway and the Netherlands. Budgets are allocated to organizations responsible for providing nursing care dependent on size and needs of the community. France has a fixed budget as well as the nomenclature system for the HAD Hospital à Domicile (Hospital at Home), and SAD Soins à domicile pour personnes agèes (elderly care at home). Reimbursement for HAD patients is about three times as high as for SAD.

Verheij comments on the dangers of neglecting psychosocial and preventive activities under fixed fees for service system. Diagnostic related groups or nomenclature system certainly has potential to contain costs. All patients with, say, a leg ulcer dressing will have the same level of reimbursement, despite the amount of resources required to carry out the care. Administrative costs are therefore reduced as the requirement to cost each individual care is removed. Even though costs of delivering care varies between patients, costly and cheap patients should balance each other out. However, quality of care must be threatened under such a system that appears to reward minimalist intervention.

Co-payment

Co-payment is a system in which people pay a contribution to or pay for an associated part of their care. In the UK there has been talk of co-payment in the form of charging for hospital hotel services – meals and drinks. Most European countries, including the UK, expect co-payment for drugs and social services but home nursing is usually free of charge (see Fig. 19. 5).

No co-payment	Dependent on Insurance	Yes co-payment
UK	Belgium	Belgium
Finland	France	Netherlands
Germany		
Norway		

Figure 19.5   Co-payment for community nursing. *Source*: Verheij (1993)

Belgium and the Netherlands are the only countries that charge a co-payment for community nursing. In these two countries additional insurance to cover co-payment is purchased by most people. Alternatively a small membership fee entitles members of home nursing organizations to free care.

Trends in payments for community nursing services

Throughout Europe, attempts have been made through various means to contain costs – or to use the fashionable positive expression, maximize 'value for money'. Germany and France are considering linking payment to the level of patient dependency. Belgium introduced a scheme like this in 1991, however there is no evidence that this has resulted in reduced costs.

Germany has introduced measures to encourage informal care. Patients can receive 400 marks a month to organize their own care (be their own care manager). Informal carers who have been caring for a dependent for at least a year can receive a grant to organize care cover while they take a holiday. Unfortunately this initiative has not saved money. Most people who applied for this grant were not in receipt of formal care. This proves that there must have been high levels of invisible, informal caring taking place in the community.

Most countries are either considering or carrying out some form of competitive elements in health care. The market economy and competitive tendering is now widespread. In the Netherlands community care has been traditionally supplied by both the private sector and charitable Cross Associations supported by government grant. In future the Cross Associations will compete with private associations for contracts in the hope that this will contain costs. Effect on quality is however unknown.

Cooperation

Cooperation between care agencies is an obvious way of reducing costs and problems of role overlap and conflict. Increasing elderly populations require increased home help and nursing services. Most countries except the UK have recognized the value of not only promoting cooperation between agencies, but of amalgamating the services into one. Countries that have integrated the home help and nursing services such as Norway and Germany report no problems of role conflict (Verheij and Kerkstra, 1992). In the Netherlands and Finland there is much discussion on the division of tasks, as Verheij (1993) states 'The question is whether uncomplicated nurses activities should always be a nursing job, and whether help with activities of daily living should always be a task for home helpers' (p. 38).

Division of tasks

In all countries there are two levels of home care nurse, the level of training varies between three and five years for a first level nurse and between one and three years for a second level nurse. Criteria for a second level nurse in Verheij and Kerkstra's study (1992) is unclear and appears to include auxiliary, enrolled and staff nurse equivalents. In most countries there is special educational preparation for public health nursing (health visiting). Special educational preparation for home nursing (district nursing) is less common, consisting of mainly in service and short courses. However, inclusion of home nursing is now incorporated in basic pre-registration education in both Norway and the UK. In most countries first level nurses assess patients and technical care, while second level nurses attend to patients continuing care and hygiene needs. Interestingly, in Belgium there appears to be no task difference between first and second level nurses.

There is much discussion, particularly in the Netherlands, about who should do assessment visits in the future: first level nurses involved in patient care, a manager, or a special assessment team. Puchasers are demanding more standardized, objective and less individual assessments. They prefer separation of assessment and delivery of care. Nurses, however, object to the loss of autonomy. In several countries nurses are not allowed to take direct referrals. Referrals from general practitioners is only being allowed, particularly in countries where there is a strong private health care economy (Germany, France and Belgium), as it is a condition of insurance companies' reimbursement.

In all countries except the Netherlands, there is a clear distinction between child health and elderly care. This is however changing as Dutch nurses are specializing in either elderly or child care. The specialization spilt between preventive and curative care seems much less popular. Verheij found difficulty in the idea that a well elderly person in the UK could be visited by a health visitor and a sick one by a district nurse, a view that can be sympathized with given the philosophical difficulties in making a clear definition of health. Converse development is taking place in Finland where, after several years of specialization (child and elderly), there is a move towards a generalist nurse to reduce travelling costs and provide less fragmented care.

Making the job more attractive

Surprisingly, community nursing as a career choice is not as popular elsewhere as in the UK, where there are often more applicants than posts. In many countries community nursing is an unpopular choice because of dependency on doctor prescriptions, pressures of work and lack of career opportunity. In some countries hospital nurses are seen as higher status and are paid more than home nurses. Efforts are being made to increase the attractiveness of community nursing in many countries, particularly former Soviet states. Equal pay, education and a career structure, which are all taken for granted in the UK, are seen by Verheij (1993) as making the job more attractive.

Discussion

In the final part of this chapter the following will be discussed: the reasons why there is little European nurse employment mobility, the significance of Europe for UK nurses, and a brief overview of the European Union (EU).

Why are there not more UK nurses working in Europe?

Despite being members of the EEC since the 1970s employment mobility amongst European nurses remains low. Pritchard and Wallace (1994) reviewed research (notably Buchan et al., 1992) in relation to nurses wishing to take advantage of the EU, regulations which allow them to work in other EU countries. Interestingly, the research highlights that the low level of movement for employment is due to the lack of recognition of post-registration qualifications.

EU Directives 77/452/EEC and 77/453/EEC deal with mutual recognition of formal general nursing qualifications and laws and regulatory instruments associated with nursing. They do not, however, recognize post-registration specialist professional qualifications. There are also some differing expectations of prerequisites for community nursing. For example, a district nurse from the UK who chooses to work in the Netherlands will need to have experience of well baby care and, in Germany, will require home help experience. Clearly, the skills and training are not equitable within different countries. In addition to these obstacles there are potential language problems. Even fluent speakers may find dialects and technical jargon a barrier to safe practice. It is difficult, therefore, initially to gain employment at anything but a basic level. A further problem is that, generally speaking, nurses have little understanding of the workings of the EU and its importance to nursing.

Brief outline of the aims and legislation mechanisms of the European Union

The aim of the EU is to ensure four freedoms of movement between member states. These are freedom of movement of goods, services, labour and capital through the elimination of internal frontiers, creating an economic and social union (Pritchard and Wallace, 1994), the intention being to secure mutual economic and social benefit for member states. By joining together, Europe becomes the largest trading centre in the world. The way the EU seeks to control the member states is through EU law. Despite a popular belief to the contrary, there is concern to protect rights and interests of individual countries, but there is greater concern that the economic and social 'playing field' should be as 'level' as possible. If not one member state could, for example, gain advantage over the rest by manufacturing products more cheaply if health and safety directives are disregarded.

There are four main types of legislation:

- A *Regulation* is an EU law which overrides any national law and is binding on all member states.
- A *Directive* requires a member state to put in place legislation complying to EU guidelines.
- A *Decision* is binding only to named countries, companies or individuals.
- *Recommendations* are statements not laws, and they are not legally binding.

Nursing education and the EU

The EU has come in for some criticism in the past for imposing inflexible laws in the interest of harmonization between the various member states. A more helpful catch phrase that has crept into use recently throughout the EU, according to Keithly (1994), is 'recognition not harmonisation'. This has led to a shift away from directives which state the content of a nursing curriculum towards a recognition of outcomes. Examples of this new thinking is the directive (92/51/EEC) which recognizes higher education in nursing. The increased flexibility of this new approach allows for development of exciting shared modules or student exchange throughout Europe, a potential which Keithly (1994) notes is only slowly being exploited.

The formal link between nursing and the EU is the Permanent Committee of Nursing (PCN) which advises the EU on nursing's contribution to the health of Europe and general nursing issues. There is a nurse representative from each member state.

Nurse training is represented by the Advisory Committee on Training in Nursing (ACTN) which has a remit to ensure comparable high standards of training across the EU and amend nurse training in line with current developments.

Comparative nursing studies

It is surprising, given the interest, that there is not more international comparative nursing research like Verheij's. Comparisons between how different countries provide community nursing should provide examples of good practice. There are however problems of comparing 'like with like' which undermines the validity of the research, an incompatibility of concepts and data exist. In Verheij and Kerkstra's study (1992), for instance, it is apparent that in some countries 'home nurses' are more an amalgamation of social worker and care attendant. In other countries 'home nurses' are highly skilled carers whereas in others they have a mainly supervisory role to health care assistants. Van der Zee *et al.* (1994) claim to have solved the problem by using the same measurement tool in three countries, namely Belgium, Germany and the Netherlands. Their study was conducted in the region around Maastricht where the three countries border upon one another. Results are interesting but the ability to extend the technique to include the UK is unlikely, as presumably there are more similarities between areas with close geographical boundaries. Comparative studies provide a wealth of pragmatic information and introduce unique solutions to common problems (for example, Sigsby, 1994). They do not necessarily provide the answers, as an ideal solution may fail in a different environment, due to social and organizational differences.

Comparisons between nursing in Europe and the UK

There is much to be learned from studying nursing in Europe. Among the examples we may or may not wish to emulate there are some warnings. The effects of a lack of strong nursing leadership upon the status and professional development of nurses is clear. Nurse leadership in the UK, so coveted by east European nurses, is being reduced as a result of organizational and philosophical change. Nurses may for a time enjoy illusions of freedom that current changes are bringing but may find in future that the profession becomes subservient and may lose 'its voice'. Professional organizations and initiatives such as Clinical Supervision (Butterworth and Faugier, 1992) are examples of strategies which can be employed to maintain and improve the quality of services. Moves such as joint medical and nursing education should be examined carefully as interesting comparisons can be made with countries which do this already. This does not mean, however, that an approach should not be pursued on the grounds that it has not been successful elsewhere. It is to be expected that initiatives in different socio-economic climates will result in different results. For example, joint training for health care professionals has several positive potentials: improved communication, role understanding and reduction in role overlap. On the other hand it has the potential to erode the nursing contribution to health care if all health care professionals embrace the medical model and nurses are considered to be 'failed doctors'.

Another major difference between the UK and a large proportion of Europe is a strong emphasis on nursing specialization in the UK as opposed to a more generalist approach to community care in the rest of Europe. Keithly (1994) reports that an EU Advisory Committee on the Training of Nurses (ACTN) review of nurse training found that whilst the UK had many hundreds of courses available to nurses, no other European country could offer such choice. A tradition of strong nursing leadership with its associated ability to attract resources has led to the high standard and clinical diversity of UK nursing. It is possible that the very moves towards European harmonization may lead to erosion of the quality and quantity of nursing courses and practice. Debates on the specialist vs. generalist nurse is an example how Europe may affect UK practice. It will be interesting to see if the Post Registration Education and Practice (PREP) Community Nursing qualification is the first step towards a generalist qualification in the UK.

Driven by a need to address the problems caused by a shrinking economically active population supporting an increasingly large dependent population, every country is implementing cost containment measures in health care. Nijkamp *et al.* (1991) notes that shifting responsibility away from societal responsibility for health care to local government and individuals appears to be the only successful method of cost containment in health care. Initiatives such as *Health of the Nation* (DOH, 1991) and the NHS and Community Act (1990) are aimed at achieving this end. Debates on community care, skill mix and multiskilling are not restricted to the UK

At the time of writing community health care remains free at the point of delivery. Prescription charges are the only exception. The principle that the state pays only a percentage of the cost of health care is fairly common in Europe. The difference is met in the form of co-payments which are paid by the individual, by 'top up' insurance or, in the case of home care (Belgium and the Netherlands), by joining a local charitable organization which provides home care to its members, and those others who are either in financial difficulty or are willing to pay a fee. If this concept seems alien, it is worthwhile to reflect that prior to the advent of the welfare state, community nursing in the UK was organized on a charity or fee for service basis, and co-payments already exist for social care.

Conclusion

The Netherlands and the former USSR states have set an excellent example that the UK nurse might emulate. They have looked outside their country and investigated how community nursing is provided in other countries so that they can develop systems based on 'good examples'. Although community nursing in the UK is a well established excellent service which many wish to emulate, we must not forget that there is much we can learn from other countries. As Europe grows larger it is hoped that nurses from different countries will become closer, help one another and share ideas.

Looking at Europe allows us to widen our debate on new ways of working and serves as a comparative aid to analysing current practice. This is no longer a luxury or interesting pastime for academics; as Europe moves closer together, nurses should be involved in raising standards not compromising on the lowest common denominator. A final thought: many recent health care reforms in this country seem to have been imported from the USA. As we are European, is it not time we turned to Europe more?

Points to consider

1 Is separating the assessment of need from the delivery of care appropriate?

2 What are the advantages, disadvantages and constraints on community nurses implementing the principles outlined in the World Health's Health for All and Nursing's Mission, in the new NHS?

3 Is there a role for a Feldscher or nurse practitioner in community nursing? In what areas could such a practitioner make a contribution and what should be the boundaries of their practice?

4 Consider the likely affect of different methods of funding on community nursing care.

5 Compare the implications for community nurses and their clients of employment by GP, social service, or charitable organization.

References

Buchan, J., Seccombe, I. and Ball, J. 1992: The international mobility of nurses – a UK perspective. *IMS Report No 230*. University of Sussex.

Butterworth, T. and Faugier, J. (eds) 1992: *Clinical supervision*. Manchester: Chapman and Hall.

DOH 1991: *Health of the nation*. London: Department of Health

Keithly, T. 1994: European nursing: a new perspective. *Journal of Nurse Management*, **2**, 6, 293–7.

Nijkamp, P., Pacolet, J., Spinnewyn, H., Vollening, A., Wildcrom, C. and Winters, S. 1991: *Services for elderly in Europe – a cross national comparative study*. Belgium: Commission of the European Communities, Higher Institute of Labour Studies, Catholic University of Leuven.

Pritchard, A.P. and Wallace, M.J. 1994: Moving around Europe – an overview of European Union nursing legislation. *Accident and Emergency Nursing*, **2**, 4, 211–15.

Salvage, J. 1993: Nursing in Europe. In *Community nursing monograph number five*, 1–28. Manchester UK: University of Manchester, School of Nursing Studies.

Sigsby, L.M. 1994: A comparison of nursing – implications for elder care in Sweden and the United States. *Scandinavian Journal of Caring Sciences*, **8**, 3, 131–5.

Van der Zee, J., Kramer, K., Derksen, A., Kerkstra, A. and Stevens, F.C.J. 1994: *Journal of Advanced Nursing*, **20**, 791–801.

Verheij, R. 1993: An account of a research project. In *Community nursing monograph number five*. Manchester UK: University of Manchester, School of Nursing Studies, 29–45.

Verheij, R. and Kerkstra, A. 1992: *International comparative study of community nursing*. Aldershot: Avebury, Ashgate Publishing Limited.

WHO 1978: Declaration of Alma Ata. *Health For All* Series No.1. Geneva: World Health Organization.

WHO 1993: *Nursing in action: strengthening nursing and midwifery to support health for all*. Copenhagen: World Health Organization Regional Office for Europe.

77/45 2-3/EEC 1977: *Official Journal of the European Communities* 15 July, 20:L176

92/51/EEC 1992: *Official Journal of the European Communities* 18 June, 25:L109.

20 Towards the next millennium

Rita Bell

This chapter is intended to reflect the many complexities facing community health care nurses in the 1990s. They are facing challenging times but, clearly, they retain a prime position at the forefront of primary health care. Evidence, such as presented in earlier chapters, suggests that it is not feasible to maintain the status quo and indicates that change is essential in order to address the multifarious health needs in present day nursing in the community.

The following text attempts to analyse the context of community nursing and speculate upon the direction necessary to take community nursing forward into the next millennium, taking into account the emerging market culture in community health care and the changing health needs of present day society. It is proposed that community nurses can influence their professional role development to shape community nursing as they move towards the next century, as a means of actively responding to the health needs of the community and the demand for quality nursing care in the client's home surroundings.

The road may well be hazardous and not without dilemmas and some confusion, but historically, community nurses have demonstrated their ability to be flexible and responsive to change.

This chapter presents a model which is designed to offer a logical, cost-effective and rational approach to the changing workplace. The model capitalizes upon the many positive features inherent in professional practice in the community which have been accrued over the years as a result of developments in professional identity. Yet it supports the role of development in accommodating the competencies required to sustain service delivery in the community setting both now and in the future.

Introduction

Nurses in the primary health care setting are currently experiencing unprecedented change both from within their working environment and as members of a developing profession. According to Moores (1992), nursing, midwifery and health visiting is taking place in a world of constant change and development which implies that practice must be dynamic, relevant and responsive to relate to the changing needs of clients, patients and their families. This paper proposes that the last decade of the twentieth century has offered a remarkable opportunity for community nurses to develop as professionals, thus taking full account of the complexity of the working environment, including the climate of change and the numerous dilemmas currently facing community nurses. There appear to be significant forces influencing community nursing which are currently the subject of intense debate both within and outside the profession. These powerful influences signal the need for change, thus heralding the emergence of a new breed of community nurses in the next millennium.

Primary health care in the 1990s

CHANGES IN POST-REGISTRATION EDUCATION

In the 1990s, community nurse education will change in response to major developments in pre-registration education in the form of Project 2000 (UKCC, 1986; Cain *et al.*, 1995). Although this new programme was introduced in 1986, its impact has only just started to take effect in the community, particularly in terms of the recruitment of staff nurses with diploma level qualifications and a limited amount of community experience. Inevitably, this has had major implications for the future of specialist community nurses such as health visitors and district nurses who undergo professionally recognized post-registration education to work in the primary health care setting as specialist practitioners. The introduction of first level nurses directly into the community as a result of Project 2000 programmes will have a major influence upon skill mix initiatives in the community. This calls for role development as specialist practitioners particularly in relation to leadership qualities, clinical competencies and · managerial skills. However, this dilemma has recently been addressed to some extent by the United Kingdom Central Council for Nurses, Midwives and Health Visitors which recommends major changes in community nurse education as an active response to changes in health and client needs as well as changes in nurse education (UKCC, 1994). In other words, the profession recognizes the critical contribution specialist community nurses are capable of making to the health and well-being of the community in the 1990s and beyond. There is little doubt that a radical rethink of skills is necessary to address the health needs of the community in the closing years of the 20th century and subsequently lead community health care nurses positively into the next millennium (Trnobranski, 1994; Carey, 1994). Education will play a crucial part in these developments and appropriate study programmes are imperative to ensure safe, autonomous nursing practice in the community.

However, there appears at present to be some confusion over titles and roles of community nurses which is the subject of some controversy. Although the notion of community nursing is generally accepted there is emerging an additional specialty in the form of the nurse practitioner. There is growing interest surrounding the potential development of this role but there are some concerns over interpretation and understanding of the concept of the nurse practitioner in practice, particularly in relation to how this role is perceived alongside district nursing, health visiting and practice nursing. However, this debate implies that there are gaps in the current community nursing provision which require urgent attention. Are we in danger of introducing another role or grade in community nursing which could be misconstrued and create overlap and stress to clients, nursing staff and medical staff? What are the advantages and disadvantages of this new role in the community?

THE WORKING ENVIRONMENT: PRIMARY HEALTH CARE AND THE COMMUNITY NURSE

The impact of the NHS reforms and the subsequent 'shift to Primary Health Care' designed by the policy makers has greatly influenced the development of nursing roles outside the hospital setting (Department of Health, 1989a, 1989b, 1989c, 1991b, 1992). A climate of political change and reforms is having a profound effect upon the provision of community health care in the United Kingdom particularly in relation to the skills necessary to support quality community nursing (Trnobranski, 1994). According to the Department of Health Heathrow Debate in 1993, changes in health care provision will determine a dramatic change in the way nurses function with specific reference to facilitating skills in the community. The current climate of service delivery presents the community practitioner with a complex working environment, stretching their management ability and research skills if they are to influence the health status of the community population in these times of inequalities of health combined with market economy and consumer participation.

However, there are many positive and stimulating aspects to community nursing which offer opportunities for role development. McMurray (1990) notes that the health of the community is a multifaceted, dynamic and challenging concern which offers today's practitioners a unique opportunity to redefine their roles in accordance with the locality they serve. In addition, the introduction of the UKCC (1992) Scope for Professional Practice guidelines has offered professional credence for nurses to expand and develop their skills to meet the needs of clients and patients (Trnobranski, 1994). This is particularly relevant in primary health care where community practitioners have a diverse range of skills and a high level of competency to cope with the heavy demands of practice in non-institutional settings and delivery of care to clients in their own homes.

Historically, evidence suggests nursing in the community is different and these differences include the nature of the client/nurse relationship, the distinct emphasis on health and well-being and the lack of direct peer or managerial support (Baly et al., 1987; MacKenzie, 1989; McMurray, 1990; DNA, 1993; Cain et al., 1995). This poses a crucial question: how is the role of the community nurse defined?

Careful scrutiny of current practice suggests that a community nurse is an appropriately qualified professional nurse who coordinates care to individuals, families, groups and communities, assisting clients to make informed choices about health which are culturally appropriate, viable, cost effective and practical (Bryar, 1994). However, in spite of developments in community nurse education, change is long overdue. This is acknowledged by Poulton (1994) who draws attention to the conclusion of a study in the West Midlands in the mid 1980s which indicates that 'nurses could play a much larger and more autonomous part in the care of patients than they currently do' (p. 4).

Furthermore, efforts to introduce nurse prescribing in Britain can be seen as an attempt to change the law to enable nurses to make a more effective contribution to primary health care and actively develop their role to match the health needs of the 1990s (Bryar, 1994; Poulton, 1994).

In recent years, a number of government reports have drawn attention to the potential contribution of community nurses to the health and well-being of the population (DHSS, 1986; DOH, 1991b; NHSME, 1993a; NHSE, 1993b).

Undoubtedly, role development rests heavily upon the community practitioner having a working knowledge of the community, its residents, the organization, the distribution of health care services and the network of provision. This places a heavy responsibility on community nurses and requires a high level of motivation in these complex and often frustrating times and relies upon commitment and dedication by professionals choosing to work in this setting.

Nevertheless, Walton Spradley (1991) notes that community health care nursing offers today's practitioner unprecedented challenges recommending a change of stance by the practitioners. More specifically, it is argued that caring community agencies are at present faced with the challenge of how best to manage innovation and change and they must consider how best they can imaginatively expand their repertoire of skills in response to changes in health needs and social policy directives. It is proposed that in spite of the confetti of policy documents and evidence of report fatigue, these are exciting times for community nurses and they must be encouraged to take up this challenge and positively respond to the changing set of circumstances in primary health care.

NEED FOR CHANGE

Schofield (1992) notes that primary health care is more than a set of services delivered as part of the National Health Service provision, therefore, the complexity of the environment must be recognized by community nurses if they are to ensure quality care provision. Reflection upon community nursing in the 1990s highlights at least two specific issues which warrant scrutiny. First, O'Neill (1983) warned that without considered action, there is grave danger of a health crisis in the next millennium and proposes this is no idle threat. Secondly, according to Maraldo (1991), working in the community is influenced by a number of current trends which may impact on professional practice. These trends include consumerism, changing attitudes and values, competition and increased privatization. Indeed, in some instances, current trends may be perceived by some community nurses as major obstacles and threats to quality practice.

Health crisis in primary health care

O'Keefe *et al.* (1992) predict a pending health crisis in the coming decade which must be taken seriously by community nurses. This would require taking full account of key factors which have the potential to underpin the predicament including:

- shift in emphasis from biomedical/curative approaches to preventative approaches;
- 'epidemiological transition' from childhood illnesses to chronic and degenerative disorders;
- iceberg of sickness;
- environmental pollution;
- user dissatisfaction;
- widening gap between demand and supply;
- demographic 'time bomb'. (O'Keefe *et al.*, 1992. Chapter 1)

George and Miller (1994) go further and state that Britain's health care levels compare poorly with the international scene, particularly in relation to variations in health by class, race, region, aspects of quality and quantity of provision. This confirms the importance of community nurses accurately analysing their work profile and utilizing a reliable assessment as a basis for role intervention (Bryar, 1994; DOH, 1993a; DOH, 1993b; DOH, 1993c) According to community managers, this still appears to be deficient in some instances (NHSE, Northern and Yorkshire Region, 1994).

OBSTACLES AND THREATS

The final decade poses a number of potential areas of concern to community nurses. Challenges include issues of competition in the current market economy.

The acute sector of health care provision

In the present climate of competition, threats may be emerging form the acute sector in the form of 'outreach' services. According to Jackson and Lavender (1994), many treatments are undertaken in acute hospitals which need not be carried out there. Furthermore, many users of hospital services do not need access to such specialist resources on all occasions, for example diabetic care. Similarly, a range of procedures can be carried out in the home in some cases without high levels of medical and nursing input. Indeed, some may consider that in order to promote earlier and faster hospital throughput, community services should be managed by the acute sector and contracted to private home nursing agencies. However, what does this mean to the very large number of the population who never reach hospital and would this take account of the learning that has taken place as a result of the historical development of community nursing services?

O'Keefe et al. (1992) refer to the anxieties expressed by Hancock (1990) and state that the organization of primary health care should not be undermined by the re-orientation taking place in the acute sector. Again, these issues present community services with a demanding situation if they are to influence the pattern of events thus securing their place in the community services. This has particular meaning for community staff in this current climate of uncertainty, limited opportunities and job insecurity. Is this suggesting that community nursing should be provided using a range of models to meet the breadth of community health needs?

Relationships with the voluntary sector

Increased competition is also creating a potential rift between statutory and voluntary agencies which must not be overlooked. Although O'Keefe et al. (1992) suggest a competitive model which will increase the marginalization of voluntary services, it could be viewed as an opportunity for real growth. Community nurses have traditionally worked closely with voluntary agencies but, in this present climate, the notion of partnerships could be difficult when finance is at the top of the agenda. This raises questions such as who will win the business contracts in the market system? What does this mean for high dependency services if we are to take full account of the predicted demographic trends of the 1990s? How will this affect the roles and responsibilities of the community nurses of the future?

CHANGE PROCESS AND THE IMPACT OF NHS REFORMS

Robust evidence of the impact of the NHS reforms is limited at present but the implications for health care professionals are now emerging, particularly in relation to role expectations and workload. According to Bowman (1995), a superficial glance at current initiatives, including the NHS and Community Care Act of 1990 (DOH, 1990), indicates that incurring changes will place heavy demands on nurses. Inevitably, services must be developed which meet the actual needs of the community (Audit Commission, 1992). It is argued that the scale of these reforms will result in a dramatic change in perceptions both among the users and health professionals (Bowman, 1995). In particular, The Patient's Charter document (DOH, 1991a) will require nurses to change their attitudes and realize that the service is now client led and is not the dictatorial service it has been in the past. The Charter philosophy emphasizes user consultation and patients are empowered by the Charter to demand their needs are met. In the primary health care setting this has been further supported by the introduction of frameworks for Local Community Care Charters in 1994 which clearly place community nurses at the forefront of service delivery (DOH/DOE, 1994). The implications of Charter initiatives on community nurses must not be underestimated, particularly in relation to local standards and skill mix initiatives. Changing patterns of primary health care clearly indicate the need to review roles and reconsider boundaries in community nursing (Lynch and Perry, 1992; Malin, 1994; Titterton, 1994; Cain *et al.*, 1995; Reed and Gilleard, 1995) Undoubtedly, the mix of skills required to provide current day primary health care is changing, particularly in relation to direct access, the range of patients and clients and the diversity of needs and conditions (Richardson and Maynard, 1995). This has led to the belief that the community requires a new dimension in community practice to accommodate the clinical requirements of the population and support the general practitioners. Much has been written about the need to develop the nurse practitioner concept in the community. The debate about boundaries between doctors and nurses in many instances reflects the desire of doctors to hold on to tasks which could well be performed by others for fear of undermining the medical profession (Normand, 1993).This concern is made more relevant by the fact that many tasks traditionally carried out by doctors could be directed towards community nurses and the debate also extends to the use of care workers and nursery nurses in the primary health care setting.

The changing face of community nursing

What will community nursing look like at the beginning of the next century? In order to foretell the future, we must understand the present and also study the past (Dunlop, 1995). What does reflection upon community health care nursing and the primary health care workplace reveal?

What appears certain is that primary health care, both as a concept and in practice, is at the very heart of health care and health service development (NHSE, 1994). Community health care nurses will continue to form an essential part of the health care system albeit subject to a logical refashioning of skills and competency levels. It is clear that community nurses will be key workers in strategies for improving health and this is confirmed in the recent report of the Standing Nursing and Midwifery Advisory Committee (NAHAT, 1995; DOH, 1995). However, it is suggested that community health care nursing requires a radical rethink incorporating the role of nurse practitioner if it is to remain viable as it moves into the next millennium. Salvage (1991) considers the role of nurse practitioner as critical in meeting the World Health Organization slogan Health For All by the Year 2000. The Liverpool study in 1994 confirms the unique opportunity facing community nurses which signals the importance of change and development in this crucial professional field (Kirwan, 1994). This is acknowledged by the UKCC (1994) in their proposals for a 'new' specialist community nurse at post-registration level in spite of a reluctance to recognize the title nurse practitioner. This in itself is creating confusion both in the workplace and educational institutions. Surely, there is a need for agreement and rationalization in terms used to describe this post-registration community practitioner.

Fawcett-Henessy (1990) goes further and suggests that the development of the nurse practitioner role has arisen from inadequacies in the provision of medical care, particularly in relation to the lack of suitably qualified medical practitioners in accident and emergency departments, patient dissatisfaction with quality and difficulties of access. Nevertheless, it has to be stated that overall current evidence does not suggest that this is the sole reason for development in this field. This new breed of practitioner is not designed to act as a substitute for medicine but as a means of capitalizing upon the existing body of knowledge and skills to improve and develop practice in the primary health care setting in response to the health needs of the population. According to McMurray (1990), the most noticeable trend affecting practice has been the emphasis on the extension of role of the nurse, which raises the question of how should the term community nurse practitioner be defined?

There is no commonly accepted definition of the nurse practitioner's role, and the term is applied to a wide range of nursing practice both in hospital and primary health care (Bryar, 1994). According to the literature, the role of nurse practitioner is constantly evolving and implies different relationships between the general practitioner and the community nurse particularly in relation to diagnostic ability and direct access by the public. Stillwell (1992) states that a nurse practitioner in primary health care practises in an advanced, expanded role and makes professionally autonomous decisions for which she is wholly responsible but is linked with advanced level skills in diagnosing. However, according to DNA (1989), there has not been much work in this area and in some cases it is difficult to see the difference between nurse practitioner roles and aspects of district nursing and health visiting, albeit subject to development. Therefore, in view of these areas of controversy and professional recommendations to develop community nurse education, it would appear essential that the UKCC (1994) specialist community practitioner model and the evolving nurse practitioner role be developed in tandem to avoid confusion and misinterpretation. This chapter proposes that a combination of current models lends itself to a comprehensive role definition for community nurses as follows:

> A community specialist nurse practitioner is an autonomous, independent health care professional who clearly understands the uniqueness of practice in the community in contrast to the hospital setting. Therefore, a community specialist practitioner is committed to working within the UKCC (1992) Scope for Professional Practice as applied to the community and is capable of theory based practice underpinned by the principles of the new disciplines of community nursing outlined by the UKCC (1994) Community PREP document.

The ultimate attribute of this new breed of practitioner will be a raised level of problem solving to that of community nurse consultant.

Community health care nurses are in a prime position to lead the field in securing WHO Health for All by the Year 2000. The National Association of Health Authorities in 1995 makes reference to the potential of nurses, midwives and health visitors in the promotion of public health and reiterates the findings of the Standing Nursing and Midwifery Advisory Committee in relation to their position as key workers. This new breed of practitioners will be well placed to assist in achieving national and international targets for health promotion and will possess a number of essential attributes:

- professional confidence and self-awareness and the ability to gain public and professional trust;
- comprehensive knowledge base relevant to specialist community practice as defined by UKCC (1994);
- attitudes and values developed to ensure professional performance in the community;
- repertoire of skills including diagnosing/prescribing/counselling and health promotion.

Butterworth (1990) highlights the view of the Royal College of Nursing in this debate which recognizes that future nurses in primary health care will necessarily be capable of providing:

- direct access to nursing care offering client choice;
- accurate assessment of clients' problems using extended skills of diagnosis when appropriate;
- an autonomous nursing service accepting full responsibility for accepting and discharging patients and where necessary referring to other agencies.

Redefinition of role

Community nursing is a developing profession which requires a new approach towards the next millennium. According to Lanara (1993), 'the next century will require that nurses undertake increasing responsibilities and that they are competent to provide the most appropriate and 'excellent' services to individuals within a framework of holistic care in the most complex and diverse settings' (p. 85). The climate of political and professional variations is having a profound effect upon community nursing and in the 1990s is calling for a diversity of skills, including the development of clinical and management ability, to satisfy the range of community health needs (see Fig. 20.1).

Although, according to Bryden (1992), the future is difficult to predict, it is imperative that community nurses appreciate that there could be a crisis in health in the very near future. However, in view of the finite resources in the health service, they must be prepared to consider radical alternatives

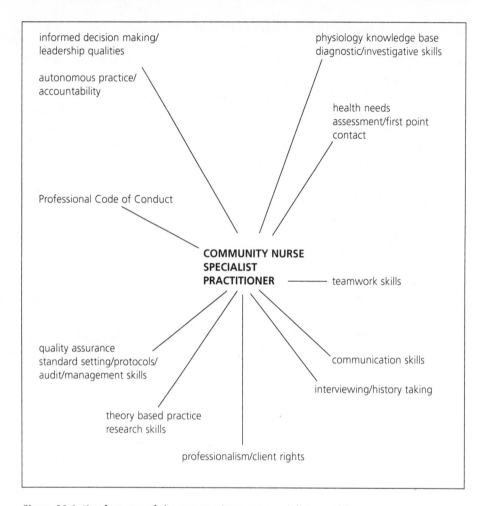

Figure 20.1 Key features of the community nurse specialist practitioner

to the way that they offer their services to accommodate effectively the needs of the population and yet secure value for money in this world of rationing and constraints.

What is clear is that this will require a comprehensive set of competencies and responsibilities and the recognition that nurses will function as both generalists and specialists in a variety of settings including primary health care. Consumerism, competition and market efficiency is becoming a way of life. Trnobranski (1994) presents a case for redefinition of the role of some community nurses to that of nurse practitioner, but this paper suggests that the way forward must be through the development and redefinition of the role of all branches of community nursing, thus maximizing the potential of all specialist community practitioners and taking full account of the diversity of needs in the primary health care setting.

Primary health care is about activities designed to address issues of equity, acceptability, cost effectiveness and consumer participation (WHO, 1988a). Community nurses are well placed to assist in achieving national and international targets for health promotion and there is a general acceptance that this new breed of practitioners will be educated to effect informed decision making, recognize the normal in health and refer as appropriate thus taking their place in the forefront of primary health care. Inevitably, this requires the right level of education to ensure these advanced levels of competencies. This must recognize the reality of community health care nursing and service providers need to accept their responsibilities in achieving role development and change.

What does the future hold for community nurses? Dilemmas versus role development

According to Maraldo (1991), the final decade of the century presents many dilemmas to community nurses, particularly in relation to the nature of the working environment, new professional directives and constant political change. Nevertheless, in spite of the complexities and serious predictions, primary health care is moving forward at a rapid pace. It is up to community health care nurses to make the most of the many challenges and opportunities presented in the primary health care setting. The profession has been given the opportunity to take itself forward with professional integrity, confidence and surety into the next century and it cannot afford to fail (Bowman, 1995).

Looking to the future, we are entering an exciting era of health care (Allen, 1991; Howkins, 1995). In primary health care, surely, this calls for community nurses to take control of their role development and rethink the range of skills required to satisfy the health needs of the 'real world' in the 1990s. Community health care nurses require many clinical competencies quite distinct from the acute setting in order to satisfy the multifarious health needs of the population (Kenyon et al., 1991). The 'real world' is constantly changing and each locality or neighbourhood may be different.

What it the true nature of the workplace in primary health care?

Undoubtedly, health care now and into the next millennium will include a new range of clinical competencies which should be determined by local need if the shift to primary health care is to be realized and the general public are to be given the choice of health care services and venue. This will require a flexible mode of working and a variety of models which may include the merging of roles on occasions but does this mean as a profession we should be introducing yet another breed of community nurses called nurse practitioners? Or should community nurses take control of their own destiny and develop skills which truly match the community health needs, thus providing a community nursing service which really is accessible, acceptable, cost effective and includes the consumer viewpoint in programmes of care? What does this mean in relation to the concept of nurse practitioner developments in the community?

How will this fit with the proposed changes in community nurse education? There is no doubt that looking to the future requires a 'forward thinking vision'. According to the DNA (1993):

> We need to look upon community nursing as complementary to general practice and assess the existing skill mix within the practice and patient needs in order to provide the most appropriate service. (p. 7)

Do community health care nurses have the motivation, power base and active support to move forward into the 21st century?

Primary health care is a challenging working environment and the way forward must be determined by community nurses themselves.

This chapter supports the view that community nurses must grasp the nettle and tackle role development if they are to accommodate the health needs surrounding the next millennium and take their rightful place at the forefront in primary health care delivery.

They owe it to themselves and the profession, but more importantly, the public they serve.

References

Audit Commission 1992: *Community care: managing the cascade of change.* London: HMSO.

Allen, L. 1991: Hospital at Home – the manager's view. In DNA (1991) *Hospital at Home: a selection of conference papers.* Edinburgh: District Nursing Association.

Baly, M.E., Rowbottom, B. and Clark, J.M. 1987: *District nursing* (2nd edn). London: Heinemann.

Bowman, M.B. 1995: *The professional nurse: coping with change, now and in the future.* London: Chapman and Hall.

Bryar, R. 1994: An examination of the need for new nursing roles in primary health care. *Journal of Advanced Nursing,* **8**, 1.

Bryden, P. 1992: The future of primary health care. In Straky, K. *Continuity and crisis in the NHS.* London: Open University.

Butterworth, A. 1990: Patients' needs or professionalisation. *Nursing Standard,* **21**, 14, February, 36–7.

Cain, P., Howkins, E. and Hyde, V. 1995: *Community nursing: dimensions and dilemmas.* London: Edward Arnold.

Carey, L. 1994: *Nurse practitioners – their role in general practice.* Conference paper. London, August 1994.

Department of Health 1989a: *Working for patients* (White Paper) (Cam). London: HMSO.

Department of Health 1989b: *Promoting better health.* London: HMSO.

Department of Health 1989c: *Caring for people: community care in the next decade.* London: HMSO.

Department of Health 1990: *NHS and Community Care Act*. London: HMSO.

Department of Health 1991a: *Patient's charter*. London: HMSO.

Department of Health 1991b: *An introduction to the Children's Act*. London: HMSO.

Department of Health 1992: *The health of the nation: strategy for health in England*. London: HMSO.

Department of Health 1993a: *The health of the nation: one year on – a report on the progress of health of the nation*. London: HMSO.

Department of Health 1993b: *Working together for better health*. London: DOH.

Department of Health 1993c: *The Heathrow debate: the challenges of nursing and midwifery in the 21st century*. London: HMSO.

Department of Health 1995: *Making it happen – public health: the contribution, role and development of nurses, midwives and health visitors*. London: DOH.

Department of Health/Department of the Environment 1994: *Framework for local community care charters in England* LAC (94) 24, HSG (94) 47, 17/94.

DHSS 1986: *Neighbourhood nursing – a focus for care*. Report of the Community Nursing Review. DHSS: London.

DNA 1989: *Key issues in district nursing*: Paper 1 District Nursing Association.

DNA 1993: *Consumer choice: fact or fiction*. District Nursing Association, Edinburgh.

Dunlop, J.M. 1995: Public health in the third millennium. *Public Health*, **109**, 165–7.

Fawcett-Henessy, A. 1990: *The role of the nurse practitioner*. Kings Fund/WHO seminar paper in South East Thames Regional Health Authority (1994) Nurse Practitioner Projects: 1992–1994. SETRHA.

George, V. and Miller, S. 1994: *Social policy towards 2000: squaring the welfare circle*. London: Routledge.

Hancock, C. 1990: Cited in O'Keefe, E. *et al.* (1992): *Community health: issues in management*. Business Education Limited, Chapter 7, p. 223.

Head, 1988: *Nurse practitioners: new pioneers*. Nursing Times, June 29, **84**, 26, 26–8.

Howkins, E. 1995: The political imperatives in community nursing. In Cain, P. Howkins, E. and Hyde, V. (1995) *Community nursing: dimensions and dilemmas*. London: Edward Arnold.

Jackson, P. and Lavender, M. 1994: *The public services yearbook*. London: Chapman and Hall.

Kenyon, V. *et al.* 1991: Clinical competencies in community health nursing. In Walton Spradley, B. *Readings in community health care nursing* (4th edn). Philadelphia: Lippincott Co.

Kirwan, M. 1994: *Nurse practitioner pilot project: Marlborough surgery*, UK Conference paper. Nurse Practitioners : Practising for the Future. Cafe Royal, London, August 1994.

Lanara, V.A. 1993: The nurse of the future: role and function. *Journal of Nursing Management* 83–7.

Lynch, B. and Perry, R. 1992: *Experiences in community care*. London: Longman.

Mackenzie, A. 1989: *Key issues in district nursing*. London: District Nursing Association (UK).

Malin, N. (ed.) 1994: *Implementing community care*. London: Open University Press.

McMurray, A. 1990: *Community health care nursing: primary health care in action*. London: Churchill Livingstone.

Maraldo, P.J. 1991: The nineties: A decade in search of meaning. In Walton Spradlley, B. 1991: *Readings in community health nursing* (4th edn). Philadelphia: Lippincott Co.

Moores, Y. 1992: *The extended role of the nurse/scope for professional practice*. P/CEO(92)4. London: Department of Health.

NAHAT 1995: *Making it happen*. National Association of Health Authorities and Trusts Briefing paper No. 81, May 1995.

NHSE 1993a: *New world, new opportunities: nursing in primary health care*. London: HMSO.

NHSE 1993b: *Vision for the Future*. London: HMSO.

NHSE 1994a: *Community PREP conference report*. Northern and Yorkshire Regional Health Authority University of Leeds.

NHSE 1994b: *Developing NHS purchasing and GP fundholding. Towards primary care-led NHS*. London: Department of Health.

Normand, C.E.M. 1993: Changing patterns of care: the challenges for health care professionals. In Malek, M. (1993) *Managerial issues in the reformed NHS*. Chichester: Wiley.

O'Keefe, E. *et al*. 1992: *Community health: issues in management*. Sunderland Tyne and Wear: Business Education Ltd.

O'Neill, P. 1983: *Health crisis: year 2000*. London: Heinemann.

Otterwill, R. and Wall, A. 1991: *The growth and development of community health services*. Business Education Publishers Ltd.

Poulton, B.C. 1994: *A needs based approach to developing and evaluating the nurse practitioner role*. RCN Conference paper. August 1994.

Reed, R. and Gilleard, C. 1995: Elderly patients' satisfaction with a community nursing service. In Wilson, G. (ed.), *Community care: asking the users*. London: Chapman and Hall.

Richardson, G. and Maynard, A. 1995: *Fewer doctors? more nurses? A review of the knowledge base of doctor–nurse substitution*. University of York.

Salvage, J. (ed.) 1991: *Nurse practitioners, working for change in primary health care*. London: Kings Fund Centre London.

Schofield, D. 1992: Implications of Government White Papers on the future of primary health care. In Spurgeon, P. *The changing face of the NHS in the 1990s*. London: Longman.

SETRHA 1994: *Nurse practitioner projects 1992–1994*. London: South East Thames Regional Health Authority Directorate.

Stillwell, B. 1992: In Bryer, R. (1994) An examination of the need for new nursing roles in primary health care: the role of the nurse practitioner. *Journal of Interprofessional Care*, **8**, 1.

Titterton, M. (ed.) 1994: *Caring for people in the community: the new welfare*. London: Kingsley Publishers.

Trnobranski, P.H. 1994: Nurse practitioner: redefining the role of community nurse? *Journal of Advanced Nursing*, **19**, 134–9.

UKCC 1986: *Project 2000: a new preparation for practice*. London: UKCC.

UKCC 1992: *The scope for professional practice*. London: UKCC.

UKCC 1994: *The future of professional practice – the Council's standards for education and practice following registration*. London: UKCC.

Walton Spradley, B. 1991: *Readings in community health care nursing* (4th edn). Philadelphia: Lippincott.

WHO 1988a: *From Alma Ata to the year 2000: reflection at the mid-point*. Geneva: WHO.

WHO 1988b: *European Conference on Nursing* (Summary Report). Vienna 1988. Copenhagen: WHO.

WHO/ICN 1989: *Nursing in primary health care: ten years after Alma Ata and perspectives for the future*. Geneva: WHO.

Index